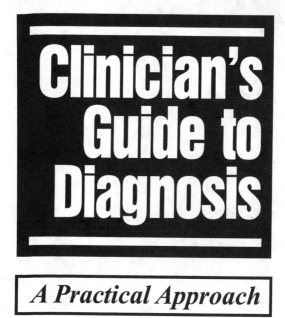

Clinician's Guide to Diagnosis

A Practical Approach

lexi-comp

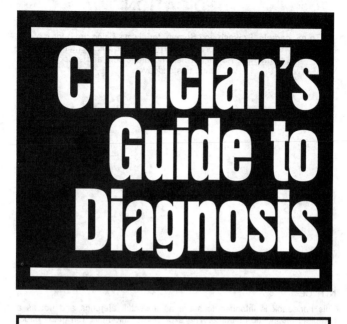

Clinician's Guide to Diagnosis

A Practical Approach

Samir Desai, MD
Assistant Professor of Medicine
Department of Medicine
Baylor College of Medicine
Houston, Texas

Staff Physician
Veterans Affairs Medical Center
Houston, Texas

LEXI-COMP INC
Hudson (Cleveland)

DEDICATION

To my parents, Prakash and Suman, for always being there for me;
to my brother, Parag, for reminding me what's important in life;
and to my wife, Rajani, for her encouragement and support
during this endeavor.

NOTICE

This handbook is intended to serve as a useful reference and not as a
complete diagnostic resource. The explosion of information in many direc-
tions, in multiple scientific disciplines, with advances in diagnosing techniques, and continuing evolution of knowledge requires constant scholarship.
The authors, editors, reviewers, contributors, and publishers cannot be
responsible for the continued currency of the information or for any errors or
omissions in this book or for any consequences arising therefrom. Because of
the dynamic nature of diagnostic medicine as a discipline, readers are
advised that decisions regarding diagnosis and treatment must be based on
the independent judgment of the clinician. The editors are not responsible for
any inaccuracy of quotation or for any false or misleading implication that may
arise due to the text.

Lexi-Comp Inc
1100 Terex Road
Hudson, Ohio 44236
(330) 650-6506

ISBN 1-930598-51-3

CLINICIAN'S GUIDE TO DIAGNOSIS

TABLE OF CONTENTS

FOREWORD

Samir Desai's text entitled *Clinician's Guide to Diagnosis: A Practical Approach* provides a fresh approach to the ill patient because it is symptom-based not disease-based. The vast majority of texts assume the clinician already has arrived at a diagnosis and then provides information about that disease. However, if the diagnosis is unclear, the practitioner might have to read through many different disease entities to see which disease his/her patient's presentation most closely matches. Even after going through this process, there is no guarantee that the clinician will have considered every pertinent illness and, as such, may have overlooked the very one afflicting the patient. This text takes a ground up approach, starting with the patient's symptoms and then working through the diagnosis. A text which simply presented long lists of conditions which could cause a symptom such as jaundice would be of little use. This is where Desai's text excels. It takes the initial presenting symptom and proceeds in a logical fashion using physiology as the basis for developing the symptom complex into a known disease entity, which, after all is the very basis of Internal Medicine.

The *Clinician's Guide to Diagnosis: A Practical Approach* will be a helpful compendium not only for students and residents, but also for the senior clinician. I intend to consult it the next time I'm given an impossible CPC to solve.

Blase A. Carabello, MD
Chief, Medical Service
Veterans Affairs Medical Center
Houston, Texas

The W.A. "Tex" and Deborah Moncrief, Jr Professor of Medicine
Vice Chairman
Department of Medicine
Baylor College of Medicine

ABOUT THE AUTHOR

Samir Desai, MD, obtained his medical degree from the Wayne State University School of Medicine, Detroit, Michigan. After completing his residency in Internal Medicine at Northwestern University in Chicago, Illinois, he had the privilege of serving as chief medical resident. While chief medical resident, he was actively involved in medical education as a Clinical Instructor of Medicine.

Following his chief medical residency, Dr Desai joined the faculty at the Baylor College of Medicine. As an Assistant Professor of Medicine, he remains active in medical education, working closely with medical students, interns, and residents at the VA Medical Center in Houston, Texas - one of the major teaching hospitals at the Baylor College of Medicine. He is also one of the principal authors of the *Clinician's Guide to Laboratory Medicine: A Practical Approach* which along with the *Clinician's Guide to Diagnosis: A Practical Approach* is part of the Lexi-Comp "Clinician's Guide" series.

PREFACE

It is with great pleasure that I introduce you to the *Clinician's Guide to Diagnosis: A Practical Approach.* This new book is part of the Lexi-Comp "Clinician's Guide" series which also includes the *Clinician's Guide to Laboratory Medicine: A Practical Approach.* This series of books is dedicated to providing clinicians with practical approaches to commonly encountered problems.

The impetus for this book came from my own experiences as a medical student and house officer. As a young clinician, it was a challenge for me to develop the logical thought processes that seemed to come so naturally for my attending physicians. I marveled at the ease with which these seasoned clinicians approached patients with various symptoms, sifting effortlessly from symptom to diagnosis. I recall wondering if and when I would feel comfortable in my ability to link a patient's symptom with a disease.

With the passage of time, I have come to realize that these accomplished clinicians benefited from experience. Experience and time provide all clinicians with the ability to develop their own approaches to clinical problems. Now as an attending physician who has the great opportunity to teach medical students and house officers, I see these young clinicians facing the same struggles that I encountered during my training.

Out of these struggles was borne the "Clinician's Guide" series. The initial book in this series, the *Clinician's Guide to Laboratory Medicine,* provided a step-by-step approach to the evaluation of abnormal laboratory tests. In this new book, the *Clinician's Guide to Diagnosis,* we take a step back, so to speak, from the *Clinician's Guide to Laboratory Medicine* to consider the symptoms that clinicians commonly encounter. The *Clinician's Guide to Diagnosis* offers a step-by-step approach that guides the clinician from symptom to diagnosis through a series of logical steps. These approaches have been designed to mimic the logical thought processes of experienced clinicians.

A book such as this one assumes that the evaluation of a symptom can proceed through a series of steps. The accomplished clinician realizes, however, that the practice of medicine is not easily reduced to a series of steps. Every patient is unique. As such, the approach to a patient's clinical problem should always be individualized.

It is certainly not my intent to convey to the reader that the approaches offered here are the only ones available in the evaluation of symptoms. I recognize that there may be disagreement among clinicians with regards to these approaches. If the purpose of the book, which is to provide acceptable approaches to the symptoms most commonly encountered, is kept in mind, it will accomplish its goal of bridging the chasm between the theory and practice of medicine, particularly for medical students and house officers.

In addition to medical students and house officers, it is my feeling that other clinicians such as nurse practitioners, physician assistants, and established physicians will also find this book useful. It is my hope that these groups will find that this source provides practical approaches that are not readily available in standard textbooks, guidance to help make informed clinical diagnoses, and readily accessible information at the point of care.

Please feel free to email me with questions or comments at cgd-feedback@lexi.com.

— Samir Desai, MD

ACKNOWLEDGMENTS

The creation of the *Clinician's Guide to Diagnosis: A Practical Approach* was an ambitious project that required the effort, time, and energy of many individuals working together to ensure that the goals of this book would be fulfilled. It certainly would not have been possible without the vision of Robert D. Kerscher, president of Lexi-Comp, Inc. Several years ago, he shared in my belief that the *Clinician's Guide to Laboratory Medicine* would be a significant addition to the libraries of healthcare professionals. The *Clinician's Guide to Diagnosis*, the second book in the Lexi-Comp "Clinician's Guide" series, is no less a product of his own vision.

Of equal importance were the efforts of Lynn Coppinger. In fact, I can truly say that her unrelenting enthusiasm played a large role in driving the project from its early stages to completion. I am grateful to her for spurring me on during the latter stages of this book's preparation. I continue to be amazed with her superb work and attention to detail. This work has come to fruition largely because of her dedication, commitment, and professional expertise. Matthew Kerscher, product manager, also deserves considerable credit. It is his insight, experience, and fresh ideas that have played a major role in the growth of the "Clinician's Guide" series. Of course, Lynn and Matt, are just two members of the first-class team at Lexi-Comp that played key roles in the development of this book. Special thanks are also extended to Tracey Reinecke for her assistance with the cover design, Jeanne Wilson for her work on the web page product, Ginger Stein, for her proofreading skills, and Dave Marcus for his expertise in indexing.

I would also like to thank the medical students and residents at the Baylor College of Medicine. It is their unbridled curiosity and enthusiasm that provided me with the inspiration for this book. I am especially grateful to Drs Timothy Connolly and Mary Ann Gaska for their review of certain chapters.

I am blessed to have the opportunity to work with an outstanding faculty at the Baylor College of Medicine. Members of the Baylor Internal Medicine department that deserve special thanks include Drs Jeffrey Bates, Sandy Lithgow, Paul Haidet, and Douglass Mann. I am also grateful to Louis Wu and Carmelita Kussad for their efforts in the development of this book.

Not all clinicians are fortunate enough to have a chairman like Dr Blase Carabello. He has given me every opportunity to work closely with medical students and house officers in both the inpatient and outpatient setting at the VA Medical Center in Houston, one of the major teaching hospitals at the Baylor College of Medicine. He has offered me constant encouragement in my endeavors, allowing me to grow professionally. He is precisely the seasoned and accomplished clinician that young clinicians aspire to become.

— Samir Desai, MD

HOW TO USE THIS HANDBOOK

Each chapter of the *Clinician's Guide to Diagnosis*, offers a practical approach to the evaluation of a particular symptom. All of the approaches are written in a step-by-step format, designed to provide rapid answers to the questions that commonly arise at the point of care.

Each step begins with a question. The reader is encouraged to answer the question based upon the information gathered from the patient's clinical presentation. An example from the chapter entitled "Hematuria" is given below.

Step 1 - What is Hematuria?

Hematuria is defined as the presence of blood in the urine. It may either be gross or microscopic. When it is gross, it understandably causes considerable anxiety in both patients and clinician's alike. In particular, there is concern that the hematuria may be caused by a serious condition (eg, malignancy). It is important to realize, however, that the causes of gross and microscopic hematuria are the same. Therefore, a thorough evaluation is necessary regardless of whether the patient presents with gross or microscopic hematuria.

If the patient complains of gross hematuria, ***Proceed to Step 2***.

If the patient has microscopic hematuria, ***Proceed to Step 3***.

As shown in the example above, the body of the step contains the information that is necessary to answer the question as it relates to the patient at hand. At the end of each step is a decision point. The next step in the evaluation will differ depending upon which decision point is chosen. In the example given above, the reader who has a patient with gross hematuria will travel to step 2. The reader who has a patient with microscopic hematuria, however, will skip step 2 (thus bypassing information that is relevant to patients with gross hematuria) and travel to step 3.

The steps to these chapters are designed to guide the reader from symptom to diagnosis. By proceeding through the series of steps, the long list of causes of a particular symptom will be quickly narrowed until the correct diagnosis is ultimately established. This book contains over 35 algorithms. The algorithms serve to help the reader quickly organize a strategy for approaching the particular symptom. Each algorithm closely parallels the information in its respective chapter. The algorithms are located at the end of each chapter. Also at the end of each chapter is a list of references that can be referred to for further information.

There may be times when the reader wishes to access information without proceeding through a series of steps. In these cases, the reader is encouraged to visit the extensive Topic Index where the symptom or disease of interest can be quickly located. In other words, it is not necessary for the reader to always start at step 1 when searching for information.

AMENORRHEA

STEP 1: *What is Amenorrhea?*

Amenorrhea can be divided into primary and secondary types. Primary amenorrhea refers to the situation where menses has not occurred by the age of 16. Secondary amenorrhea is said to exist when a previously menstruating woman has not had menstrual periods for more than 6 months. The reader is referred to other texts for the evaluation of primary amenorrhea. What follows is one approach to the patient with secondary amenorrhea.

Proceed to Step 2

STEP 2: *Are There Any Clues in the Patient's History That Point to the Etiology of the Amenorrhea?*

Clues in the patient's history that point to the etiology of the amenorrhea are listed in the following table.

Historical Clue	Condition Suggested
Acne Greasy or oily skin Hirsutism Obesity	Polycystic ovarian syndrome
History of chemotherapy	Ovarian failure
History of radiation therapy	Ovarian failure
History of diabetes mellitus, Addison's disease, or thyroid disease	Ovarian failure (autoimmune etiology)
Galactorrhea	Hyperprolactinemia
Weight loss	Functional amenorrhea
Excessive exercise	Functional amenorrhea
Psychological stress	Functional amenorrhea
Symptoms of early pregnancy	Pregnancy
Cessation of menstruation followed by hot flashes, vaginal dryness, or mood swings	Menopause
Rapid progression of hirsutism	Adrenal or ovarian androgen-secreting tumor
Bodybuilder	Exogenous androgen use
Medication history	Amenorrhea secondary to medication use (eg, danazol, deproprovera, LHRH agonists, oral contraceptives)
Severe dieting	Functional amenorrhea
Fatigue Nervousness Palpitations Sweating Weight loss	Hyperthyroidism

(Continued)

(continued)

Historical Clue	Condition Suggested
Constipation Hoarseness Loss of hair Memory impairment Sensation of cold Weakness Weight gain	Hypothyroidism
Headache Neurological symptoms Visual field defect	CNS lesion (hypothalamic or pituitary)
History of pelvic inflammatory disease or endometriosis	Asherman's syndrome
History of cautery for cervical intraepithelial neoplasia or obstructive cervical malignancy	Cervical stenosis
Debilitating illness	Functional amenorrhea

Proceed to Step 3

STEP 3: Are There Any Clues in the Physical Examination That Point to the Etiology of the Amenorrhea?

Clues in the patient's physical examination that point to the etiology of the amenorrhea are listed in the following table.

Physical Examination Finding	Condition Suggested
Tachycardia	Hyperthyroidism
Bradycardia	Hypothyroidism Physical or nutritional stress
Coarse skin Coarseness of hair Dry skin Edema of the eyelids Weight gain	Hypothyroidism
Exophthalmos Hyper-reflexia Lid lag or retraction Soft, moist skin Tremor	Hyperthyroidism
Galactorrhea	Hyperprolactinemia
Bradycardia Cold extremities Dry skin with lanugo hair Hypotension Hypothermia Minimum of body fat Orange discoloration of skin (hypercarotenemia)	Anorexia nervosa

(Continued)

Physical Examination Finding	Condition Suggested
Painless enlargement of parotid glands Ulcers or calluses on skin of dorsum of fingers or hands	Bulimia
Signs of virilization: Clitoromegaly Frontal balding Increased muscle bulk Severe hirsutism	Adrenal or ovarian androgen-secreting tumor
Centripetal obesity Hirsutism Hypertension Proximal muscle weakness Striae	Cushing's syndrome

If the history and physical examination provide clues to the etiology of the amenorrhea, the clinician should evaluate accordingly.

If the etiology of the amenorrhea is not clear after a thorough history and physical examination, **Proceed to Step 4.**

STEP 4: *Is the Patient Pregnant?*

The most common cause of secondary amenorrhea is pregnancy. Pregnancy is usually suspected on the basis of the history and physical examination. Since the hCG that is secreted by the placenta enters the maternal circulation and is ultimately excreted in the urine, pregnancy can be diagnosed before symptoms and signs suggest it. It is now feasible to detect pregnancy 8-10 days after ovulation with determination of β-hCG in the urine.

Despite what the patient may say, every patient with secondary amenorrhea should have a pregnancy test. If the test is negative, then further evaluation is warranted.

If the pregnancy test is positive, **Stop Here.**

If the pregnancy test is negative, **Proceed to Step 5.**

STEP 5: *What are the Results of the Thyroid Function Tests?*

Secondary amenorrhea may be an early manifestation of hypothyroidism. In fact, many patients with hypothyroidism may have no other signs or symptoms suggestive of hypothyroidism. Thyroid function tests will also exclude hyperthyroidism as the cause of amenorrhea.

If the results of the thyroid function tests indicate hypothyroidism, **Stop Here**.

If the results of the thyroid function tests are not consistent with hypothyroidism, **Proceed to Step 6.**

STEP 6: *What is the* Serum Prolactin Level*?*

Once pregnancy has been excluded, a serum prolactin level should be obtained, particularly in the patient complaining of galactorrhea. The absence of galactorrhea should not dissuade the clinician from obtaining a serum prolactin level, since a fair number of patients with hyperprolactinemia do not have a history of galactorrhea.

Hyperprolactinemia is a common cause of secondary amenorrhea. Excessive secretion of prolactin may be the result of many different conditions. Before undertaking an extensive evaluation of hyperprolactinemia, it is wise to repeat the prolactin level, as nonspecific stimuli may cause an elevation. These include stress, sleep, and food intake.

If the patient has elevated prolactin levels, further evaluation is necessary to determine the etiology of the hyperprolactinemia.

If the patient does not have elevated prolactin levels, *Proceed to Step 7*.

STEP 7: *What is the Patient's Estrogen Status?*

Determining estrogen status can begin with assessment of the vaginal mucosa and cervical mucus. The following characteristics of the vaginal mucosa suggest adequate estrogen levels:

- Moist
- Rugated

The following characteristics of the cervical mucus suggest adequate estrogen levels:

- Mucus can be stretched
- Mucus ferns after drying

While these characteristics are helpful in providing information about estrogen status, more commonly, a progesterone challenge test is performed. In this test, either 10 mg of medroxyprogesterone acetate is taken orally once or twice a day or 100 mg of progesterone in oil is administered intramuscularly. In a woman with adequate estrogen levels and a normal outflow tract, withdrawal menstrual bleeding should be appreciated within 1 week of discontinuing the progesterone. The progesterone challenge test is superior to measurements of plasma estradiol, because estrogen levels fluctuate, and measuring estrogen levels is expensive.

If withdrawal bleeding occurs, then the patient has chronic anovulation with estrogen present. *Proceed to Step 8*.

If withdrawal bleeding does not occur, *Proceed to Step 11*.

STEP 8: *What is the Differential Diagnosis in the Amenorrheic Patient Who Responds to the Progesterone Challenge With Uterine Bleeding?*

Withdrawal bleeding that occurs in response to the progesterone challenge test indicates adequate estrogen production. In these patients, the most common cause of amenorrhea is polycystic ovarian syndrome (Stein-

Leventhal syndrome). In this syndrome, there is a mild to moderate excess in androgen levels. This results in the following clinical manifestations:

Stein-Leventhal Syndrome Clinical Manifestations	
Acne	Mild virilization (severe cases only)
Hirsutism	Obesity
Infertility	Oily skin
Irregular (absent) menses	

The diagnosis is supported by elevated LH levels with normal or low FSH levels. An LH:FSH ratio >2-3 argues for the diagnosis of polycystic ovarian syndrome.

Other causes of anovulation in the presence of estrogen include:

- Cushing's syndrome
- Late-onset congenital adrenal hyperplasia (21-hydroxylase or 11-β-hydroxylase deficiency)
- Ovarian tumors
- Adrenal tumors

Proceed to Step 9

STEP 9: *Which Patients Should Have Further Evaluation?*

Not all patients with chronic anovulation with estrogen present require testing to differentiate between polycystic ovary syndrome (PCOS) and the other causes listed above. However, there are certain features that should prompt further evaluation. These include the sudden onset of hirsutism, virilization (clitoral enlargement, temporal hair loss, deepening of the voice), and signs and symptoms of Cushing's syndrome.

If the above features are not present, the diagnosis is polycystic ovarian syndrome. *Stop Here.*

If any of the above features are present, *Proceed to Step 10*.

STEP 10: *What Tests Should be Performed to Differentiate Between the Causes of Chronic Anovulation With Estrogen Present?*

These disorders may be differentiated from polycystic ovarian syndrome by measurement of serum testosterone and dehydroepiandrosterone sulfate (DHEA-S). Testosterone levels >2 ng/mL should prompt a search for an ovarian tumor.

DHEA-S levels >7 µg/mL should prompt a search for an adrenal source. In these patients, a CT scan should be performed to exclude the presence of an adrenal tumor. A normal CT scan should be followed by measurement of a basal 17-hydroxyprogesterone level. A level >9 nmol/L supports the diagnosis of late-onset adrenal hyperplasia.

In patients suspected of having Cushing's syndrome, evaluation should begin with a 24-hour urine collection for cortisol.

If the testosterone, DHEA-S, and 24-hour urine free cortisol levels are all normal, polycystic ovarian syndrome is the likely diagnosis.

End of Section.

STEP 11: *What is the FSH Level?*

In the amenorrheic patient with a failure to bleed after a progesterone challenge test, a plasma FSH level should be obtained.

If the FSH level is low or normal, **Proceed to Step 12**.

If the FSH level is >40 IU/L in a female <40 years of age, the diagnosis is premature ovarian failure. If the patient is <30 years of age, a karyotype should be ordered to exclude the presence of a Y chromosome.

Besides ovarian failure secondary to chromosomal abnormalities, other causes of ovarian failure include:

- Autoimmune disease
- Chemotherapy
- Radiation therapy
- 17-α-hydroxylase deficiency
- 17-, 20-lyase deficiency
- Resistant ovary syndrome
- Galactosemia

The most common cause of premature ovarian failure is autoimmune disease. While this may occur as an isolated condition, in some cases, autoimmune ovarian failure is accompanied by other endocrine disorders such as hypothyroidism, hypoparathyroidism, and adrenal insufficiency. Therefore, it is reasonable to assess the function of other endocrine organs with appropriate testing. The other causes listed above are rare and are usually suspected based on characteristic signs and symptoms.

End of Section.

STEP 12: *What is the Differential Diagnosis in the Amenorrheic Patient Who Fails to Bleed After Progesterone Challenge and Who Has a Low or Normal FSH?*

A low or normal FSH in the amenorrheic patient, who fails to bleed after the progesterone challenge test, is either due to a hypothalamic-pituitary disorder or anatomic defect of the outflow tract.

The diagnosis of an anatomic defect of the outflow tract is usually apparent from the history and physical examination. Scarring or stenosis of the cervix may occur following surgery, cryosurgery, electrocautery, or laser therapy. Destruction of the endometrium that ensues results in Asherman's syndrome.

If the history and physical examination does not establish the diagnosis of an outflow tract defect, then further testing can be done. To delineate between a hypothalamic-pituitary disorder and a defect of the outflow tract, cyclic estrogen and progesterone can be given. Specifically, 1.25 mg of orally conjugated estrogens are administered for 4 weeks, along with 10 mg of medroxyprogesterone acetate during the last 10 days.

If withdrawal bleeding does not occur in the patient with an intact uterus, the diagnosis is likely an anatomic defect of the outflow tract. Confirmation of the diagnosis requires either hysteroscopy or hysterosalpingography. **Stop Here.**

If withdrawal bleeding occurs, **Proceed to Step 13**.

STEP 13: *What are the Results of the MRI of the Sella?*

When withdrawal bleeding occurs in the amenorrheic patient with a low or normal FSH, a hypothalamic-pituitary disorder is present. These disorders can be divided into structural and functional causes. Structural causes are essentially the same as those that cause hypopituitarism. These include:

Hypothalamic - Pituitary Failure Structural Causes	
Malignancy	Infiltration
Pituitary adenoma	Hemochromatosis
Hypothalamic tumors	Amyloidosis
Craniopharyngioma	Vascular event
Germinoma	Sheehan's syndrome
Meningioma	(postpartum pituitary necrosis)
Glioma	Carotid aneurysm
Metastatic cancer	
Inflammatory disease	
Granulomatous disease	
Tuberculosis	
Sarcoidosis	
Syphilis	
Lymphocytic hypophysitis	
Histiocytosis X / eosinophilic granuloma	

Functional etiologies of amenorrhea include:

Hypothalamic – Pituitary Failure Nonstructural Causes	
Anorexia nervosa / bulimia	Drug-related
Chronic debilitating illness	Exercise
AIDS	Malnutrition
Malabsorption	Stress
Malignancy	Weight loss
Uremia	

The clinician should obtain an MRI scan to differentiate between structural and functional etiologies.

End of Section.

REFERENCES

Aloi JA, "Evaluation of Amenorrhea," *Compr Ther*, 1995, 21(10):575-8.

Baird DT, "Amenorrhoea," *Lancet*, 1997, 350(9073):275-9.

Crosignani PG and Vegetti W, "A Practical Guide to the Diagnosis and Management of Amenorrhoea," *Drugs*, 1996, 52(5):671-81.

Kiningham RB, Apgar BS, and Schwenk TL, "Evaluation of Amenorrhea," *Am Fam Phys*, 1996, 53(4):1185-94 (review).

McIver B, Romanski SA, and Nippoldt TB, "Evaluation and Management of Amenorrhea," *Mayo Clin Proc*, 1997, 72(12):1161-9.

SECONDARY AMENORRHEA

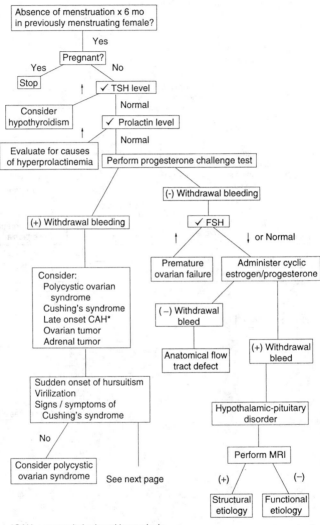

*CAH = congenital adrenal hyperplasia

SECONDARY AMENORRHEA
(continued)

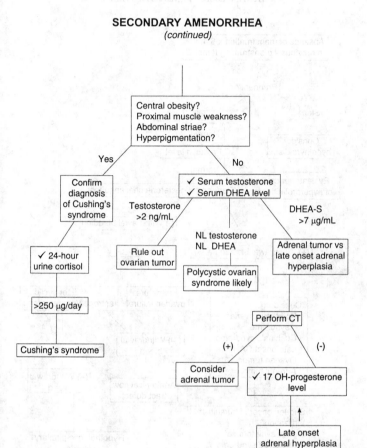

Central obesity?
Proximal muscle weakness?
Abdominal striae?
Hyperpigmentation?

Yes — Confirm diagnosis of Cushing's syndrome

No — ✓ Serum testosterone / ✓ Serum DHEA level

Confirm diagnosis of Cushing's syndrome → ✓ 24-hour urine cortisol → >250 µg/day → Cushing's syndrome

Testosterone >2 ng/mL → Rule out ovarian tumor

NL testosterone NL DHEA → Polycystic ovarian syndrome likely

DHEA-S >7 µg/mL → Adrenal tumor vs late onset adrenal hyperplasia → Perform CT

(+) → Consider adrenal tumor

(-) → ✓ 17 OH-progesterone level ← Late onset adrenal hyperplasia

BACK PAIN, LOW (ACUTE)

STEP 1: *How Common is Acute Low Back Pain?*

Acute low back pain is among the top ten reasons patients seek medical care. In the United States, the frequency of back pain is between 60% and 90% over a lifetime. In any given year, 20% to 50% of the working population experience back pain. Although most causes of acute low back pain are benign, the clinician must recognize features in the patient's clinical presentation that are suggestive of more serious disease.

Proceed to Step 2

STEP 2: *What are the Causes of Acute Low Back Pain?*

The causes of acute low back pain are listed in the following box.

Causes of Low Back Pain*	
Mechanical low back or leg pain (97%)†	
Lumbar strain, sprain (70%)	Spondylolisthesis (2%)
Degenerative processes of disks	Congenital disease (<1%)
and facets, usually	Severe kyphosis
age-related (10%)	Severe scoliosis
Herniated disc (4%)	Transitional vertebrae
Spinal stenosis (3%)	Spondylolysis
Osteoporotic compression fracture (2%)	
Nonmechanical spinal conditions (1%)	
Infection (0.7%)	Neoplasia
Epidural abscess	Lymphoma and leukemia
Osteomyelitis	Metastatic carcinoma
Paraspinous abscess	Multiple myeloma
Septic diskitis	Primary vertebral tumors
Shingles	Retroperitoneal tumors
Inflammatory arthritis (0.3%)	Spinal cord tumors
Ankylosing spondylitis	Paget's disease of the bone
Inflammatory bowel disease	
Psoriatic spondylitis	
Reiter's syndrome	
Visceral disease or referred (2%)	

*Figures in parentheses indicate the estimated percentages of patients with these conditions among all adult patients with low back pain in primary care. Percentages may vary substantially according to demographic characteristics or referral patterns in a practice.

†The term "mechanical" is used here to designate an anatomical or functional abnormality without an underlying malignant, infectious, or inflammatory disease.

Adapted from Deyo RA and Weinstein JN, "Low Back Pain," *N Engl J Med*, 2001, 344(5):363-70 (review).

Proceed to Step 3

STEP 3: *Does the Patient Truly Have Acute Low Back Pain?*

It is important to differentiate acute from chronic low back pain. The Agency for Health Care Policy and Research (AHCPR) defines acute low back pain as pain that has been present for less than 3 months. Pain that exceeds 3 months in duration is considered to be chronic.

The clinician should also determine the location of the back pain. Low back pain is an imprecise term, meaning different things to different people. It is important to ask the patient where the pain is located. Most authorities agree that low back pain is present when the pain is most prominent in the lumbosacral region. Pain that is localized to the back but above the T12 vertebra should not be considered to be low back pain.

If the patient does not have acute low back pain, *Stop Here.*

If the patient has acute low back pain, *Proceed to Step 4.*

STEP 4: *Does the Patient Have a Referred Source of Acute Low Back Pain?*

Referred back pain is an uncommon cause of acute low back pain, accounting for 2% of all cases. The causes of referred low back pain are listed in the following box.

Causes of Referred Low Back Pain	
Gastrointestinal illnesses	Gynecologic conditions
Appendicitis (retrocecal or pelvic)	Ectopic pregnancy
Biliary colic/cholecystitis	Endometriosis
Colon cancer	Pelvic cancer
Diverticulitis	Pelvic infection
Pancreatic cancer	Uterine myoma
Pancreatitis	Vascular
Penetrating peptic ulcer disease	Abdominal aortic aneurysm
Rectal cancer	Aortic dissection
Genitourinary	Miscellaneous
Prostate cancer	Retroperitoneal abscess
Prostatitis	Retroperitoneal hematoma
Pyelonephritis	Retroperitoneal tumor
Ureteral colic	

Since many of the previously mentioned causes of referred back pain are serious conditions, the clinician must be aware of features in the patient's clinical presentation that warrant consideration of these causes. Referred low back pain is a type of nonmechanical pain that differs from the mechanical type in that the latter usually has the following clinical features:

- Back pain usually begins after a mechanical event such as bending, falling, or lifting
- Movements of the back usually worsen the pain
- Bed rest often relieves the pain

The absence of these clinical features should prompt the clinician to consider nonmechanical or referred causes of acute low back pain. It is important for the clinician to realize, however, that the above features do not definitively differentiate between these two forms of acute low back pain. For example, the patient with referred acute low back pain may describe some worsening of the pain with changes in body position (ie, pain of pancreatitis may worsen with recumbency). This may be erroneously perceived as a mechanical type of pain because it changes with position or movement.

Also, pain that is of mechanical origin may not have the characteristic features described above. Therefore, the absence of these features does not exclude the mechanical causes of acute low back pain. Nevertheless, the features listed above still have considerable utility in differentiating mechanical from nonmechanical acute low back pain.

In most cases of referred low back pain, other clinical manifestations are present. Symptoms that should prompt the clinician to consider referred low back pain include dyspepsia, abdominal pain, change in bowel habits, hematuria, and flank pain. Physical examination of the abdomen (including rectal examination) and pelvic region often yields findings suggestive of a condition associated with referred low back pain.

If the patient has referred acute low back pain, **Stop Here**.

If the patient does not have referred acute low back pain, **Proceed to Step 5**.

STEP 5: *Are There Any Clues in the Patient's History That Point to the Etiology of the Acute Low Back Pain?*

Clues in the patient's history that point to the etiology of the acute low back pain are listed in the following table.

Historical Clue	Condition Suggested
History of malignancy*	Metastatic cancer Carcinomatous meningitis Epidural metastases Metastatic plexus lesions Paravertebral tumor masses Vertebral metastases
Weight loss	Malignancy Tuberculosis of the spine
Fever	Acute transverse myelitis Bacterial endocarditis Causes of referred acute low back pain Connective tissue disease (ie, ankylosing spondylitis) Epidural abscess Subdural empyema Vertebral osteomyelitis
History of osteoporosis	Vertebral compression fracture
Corticosteroid treatment	Vertebral compression fracture
Back pain radiating below knee	Nerve root compression or irritation
Intravenous drug abuse	Bacterial endocarditis Epidural abscess Vertebral osteomyelitis

(Continued)

(continued)

Historical Clue	Condition Suggested
Age <20	Higher incidence of congenital, developmental, and bony abnormalities (eg, spondylolysis, spondylolisthesis)
Older age (>50)	Likelihood of serious disease increases with age
Anticoagulant therapy	Epidural hematoma
	Retroperitoneal hematoma
Radiation of pain to the following: Calf Heel Posterior part of the thigh Sole of the foot 4th and 5th toes	S1 nerve root compression or irritation
Radiation of pain to the following: Dorsum of the foot First or second toes Groin Hip Lateral calf Posterolateral thigh	L5 nerve root compression or irritation
Radiation of the pain to the anterior part of the thigh and knee	Lesion affecting the L4 nerve root (compression or irritation)
Back pain follows trauma	Collapse or wedging of an osteoporotic vertebra
	Herniated intervertebral disc
	Low back strain
	Vertebral fracture
Back pain began after age 40	Argues strongly against ankylosing spondylitis
Pain worse with coughing, sneezing, straining at stool (Valsalva maneuvers)	Suggests nerve root compression
Diarrhea	Spondylitis associated with inflammatory bowel disease
Skin rash	Spondylitis associated with psoriasis
History of conjunctivitis	Spondylitis associated with Reiter's syndrome
History of uveitis	Ankylosing spondylitis
Pain radiates from abdomen to the back	Consider referred causes of acute low back pain
Pain worse with movement of the spine	Mechanical cause of acute low back pain
Pain unaffected by movement of the spine	Referred cause of acute low back pain
Pain during menstruation	Endometriosis
Worse in the morning Significant morning stiffness Worse with inactivity Relieved or improved with activity	Ankylosing spondylitis Other causes of inflammatory arthritis

*Malignancies that frequently involve the spine include metastatic cancer of the breast, prostate, lung, kidney, colon, and thyroid gland. Multiple myeloma, Hodgkin's lymphoma, and non-Hodgkin's lymphoma warrant consideration as well.

Proceed to Step 6

STEP 6: *Are There Any Clues in the Patient's Physical Examination That Point to the Etiology of the Acute Low Back Pain?*

Clues in the patient's physical examination that point to the etiology of the acute low back pain are listed in the following table.

Physical Examination Finding	Condition Suggested
Difficulty walking on heels	Weakness in L5 innervated muscles
Difficulty walking on toes	Weakness in S1 innervated muscles
Positive straight leg raise test	Nerve root compression or irritation (sensitive but not very specific for nerve root compression or irritation)
Fever	Acute transverse myelitis
	Bacterial endocarditis
	Causes of referred acute low back pain
	Connective tissue disease (ie, ankylosing spondylitis)
	Epidural abscess
	Subdural empyema
	Vertebral osteomyelitis
Positive crossed straight leg raise test	Insensitive but highly specific for nerve root compression or irritation
Chest expansion of less than 2.5 cm	Ankylosing spondylitis (specific but not very sensitive)
Rectal examination*	Indicated for assessment of rectal tone, prostate (for mass), rectum (for mass)
Absence of knee reflex	L4 nerve root compression or irritation
Absence of Achilles or ankle reflex	S1 nerve root compression or irritation
Decreased strength of ankle and great toe dorsiflexion	L5 nerve root compression or irritation
Decreased plantar flexion strength	S1 nerve root compression or irritation

*A rectal examination is not indicated in all patients with back pain. It should be performed, however, in patients who have severe back pain, neurologic complaints, neurologic deficits, or other red flags (see Step 7). A diminished or absent rectal tone should prompt the clinician to consider spinal cord or cauda equina compression.

Proceed to Step 7

STEP 7: *Are There Any Alarm Features (Red Flags) in the Patient's Clinical Presentation?*

Of utmost importance in the evaluation of the patient presenting with acute low back pain is the identification of alarm features (also known as red flags) in the patient's clinical presentation that increase the likelihood of serious disease. These are the patients with acute low back pain that require further evaluation. Alarm features in the patient presenting with acute low back pain are listed in the following box.

Alarm Features (Red Flags) in the Patient with Acute Low Back Pain
History
Age >50 years or <20 years
Bowel / bladder incontinence*
Fever
History of chronic infection
Major trauma in a young patient
Minor or major trauma in the elderly patient
Pain awakening patient from sleep
Pain worse at night
Pain worse at rest
Past medical history of cancer
Risk factors for spinal infection
Immunosuppression
Intravenous drug use
Recent bacterial infection
Unexplained weight loss
Unrelenting pain despite appropriate treatment or even supernormal analgesics
Urinary retention
Physical Examination
Abdominal mass
Focal neurologic deficits
Major motor weakness
Perianal/perineal sensory loss
Unexpected laxity of the anal sphincter
Pelvic mass
Rectal mass
Unexplained fever
Unexplained weight loss

*On occasion, a patient may present with bowel and/or bladder incontinence but no other findings suggestive of spinal cord compression or cauda equina syndrome. In these cases, it may be difficult to determine if the incontinence is due to serious spinal pathology or some other condition. An elevated postvoid residual (>100 mL) in such a patient should prompt serious consideration of spinal cord compression or cauda equina syndrome.

If the patient has alarm features, **Proceed to Step 8**.

If the patient does not have alarm features, **Proceed to Step 11**.

STEP 8: *Does the Patient Have Radicular Pain?*

In Step 7, alarm features or red flags suggestive of serious spinal pathology were discussed. One of these features is the presence of focal neurological signs or symptoms. Many patients with radicular low back pain have accompanying neurologic signs or symptoms. However, not all of these patients should be considered to have alarm features since most will have symptom resolution with conservative therapy over a period of several months. This step will help separate radicular low back pain into the following two groups:

- Those likely to have symptom resolution with conservative therapy
- Those who require further investigation and evaluation because of the possibility of serious spinal pathology

Radicular low back pain is a manifestation of any process causing lumbosacral nerve root compression or irritation. It should be suspected whenever back pain is accompanied by leg (pain radiating below the knee) and/or foot pain. Most often, patients describe the pain as shooting, sharp, burning, tingling, or numbness.

The most widely used physical examination maneuver to support the presence of radicular low back pain is the straight leg raise test. During this maneuver, the leg is passively raised (flexion at hip with knee fully extended) while the opposite leg lays flat. The test is considered positive if the characteristic pain is elicited when the leg is raised to between 30° and 60° of elevation. Each leg should be tested. Nerve root compression is likely when the straight leg raise test is positive. It is even more likely when the crossed straight leg raise test is positive.

If the patient does not have radicular low back pain, **Proceed to Step 9**.

In patients with radicular low back pain, motor, reflex, and sensory changes corresponding to the involved nerve root are often appreciated. The presence of these focal neurologic deficits, as mentioned above, should not necessarily be considered alarming. The majority of these cases are due to herniated disks. Most patients with herniated disks will have symptom (including neurologic) resolution with conservative therapy over a period of a few months. The challenge lies in identifying patients with herniated disks that should not be treated with conservative therapy and the minority of patients who have radicular low back pain not due to herniated disks (ie, tumor, infection, fracture).

The presence of any of the following features in the patient's clinical presentation should prompt the clinician to consider further evaluation and investigation:

- Alarm features (red flags) listed in the box in Step 7
- Severe or significant neurologic deficit
- Progressive neurologic deficit

In the presence of one or more of these features, conservative therapy is not recommended. The absence of all of these features suggests that the radicular low back pain is not due to serious spinal pathology.

If the patient with radicular low back pain has alarm features, severe or significant neurologic deficit, or progressive neurologic deficit, **Proceed to Step 9**.

If the patient with radicular low back pain does not have alarm features, severe or significant neurologic deficit, or progressive neurologic deficit, **Proceed to Step 12**.

STEP 9: *What Laboratory Testing Should be Performed in the Patient With Acute Low Back Pain Who Has Alarm Features?*

The presence of one or more of the alarm features listed in the box in Step 7 should prompt the clinician to consider a potentially serious spinal condition such as malignancy, fracture, infection, spinal cord compression, or cauda equina syndrome. The following tests may be indicated in the evaluation of these patients:

- CBC

  The white blood cell count may be elevated in patients with infection (ie, vertebral osteomyelitis, spinal epidural abscess). A normal white blood cell count, however, should not exclude these possibilities. The white blood cell count is usually normal in patients with malignancy.

- Erythrocyte sedimentation rate (ESR)

  Although the ESR is a nonspecific test, many experts recommend the test to screen for serious disease in patients with acute low back pain who have alarm features. The ESR is elevated in many patients with infection. The ESR may also be elevated in some patients with malignancy (ie, multiple myeloma) or spondyloarthropathy (ie, ankylosing spondylitis). It is important to realize that a normal ESR does not exclude the presence of serious disease.

- Plain radiographs of the lumbar spine

  Plain radiographs of the lumbar spine are indicated in patients with acute low back pain having alarm features. This is especially true in patients with signs and symptoms suggestive of tumor, infection, fracture, or neurologic dysfunction. In most cases, anteroposterior (AP) and lateral views suffice. The role of these radiographs are to aid the clinician in the detection of serious spinal pathology such as infection, malignancy, fracture, or spondyloarthropathy. In general, plain radiographs of the lumbar spine should be the initial radiologic test in the evaluation of acute low back pain with alarm features. However, the presence of significant neurologic deficits warrants performance of MRI as the initial imaging modality of choice. Plain radiographic findings in patients with serious spinal disease are listed in the following table.

Condition	Plain Radiographic Findings
Vertebral osteomyelitis*	Disk space narrowing
	Erosions of vertebral body end-plates
	Fusion of vertebrae
	New bone formation
	± paravertebral soft tissue mass
	Reactive sclerosis
Epidural abscess†	Findings consistent with associated vertebral osteomyelitis
	Paraspinal mass
Epidural spinal cord compression (malignancy)	Destruction of vertebral body cortical edges
	Mixed lesions
	Osteoblastic lesions
	Osteolytic lesions
	Paraspinal soft tissue mass
	Pedicle destruction (winking owl sign)
	Vertebral body compression fractures
Osteoporosis/vertebral compression fracture	Anterior wedging of vertebral bodies in thoracic spine
	Diffuse osteopenia#
	Prominence of vertebral trabeculae
	Vertebral body compression fractures

*Radiographic findings may not be detectable for up to eight weeks following the onset of infection. 90% of patients will have radiographic abnormalities by four weeks.

†Unremarkable plain radiographs of the spine are not uncommon in patients with epidural abscess.

‡At least 30% of the bony matrix must be destroyed or replaced by tumor before radiographic abnormalities consistent with malignancy can be demonstrated.

#Bone density must decrease by at least 30% before osteopenia is apparent.

Proceed to Step 10

> **STEP 10:** *What are the Conditions That the Clinician Should Consider When the Patient With Acute Low Back Pain Has Alarm Features?*

The conditions that the clinician should consider in the evaluation of acute low back pain with alarm features are discussed in further detail in the remainder of this step.

Vertebral Osteomyelitis

The incidence of vertebral osteomyelitis is increasing. Although it is a rare cause of back pain in patients <50 years of age, it can occur and deserves consideration, especially in intravenous drug users. Risk factors for the development of vertebral osteomyelitis are listed in the following box.

Risk Factors for the Development of Vertebral Osteomyelitis	
Corticosteroid therapy	Intravenous drug use
Diabetes mellitus	Older age
Dialysis	Spine or disk surgery
Immunocompromise	Trauma
Infection	Urinary tract instrumentation
Antecedent bacteremia due to other causes	
Contiguous spread of paraspinal infection	
Genitourinary tract infections	
Infective endocarditis	

Back pain is the most common symptom of vertebral osteomyelitis. Classically, the pain increases with movement and abates with rest. Symptoms are usually present for weeks to months (as long as two years) prior to presentation. Up to 10% of patients, however, report an illness duration of less than one week. Systemic symptoms such as fever and night sweats may be present in up to 50%. Fever may be absent, however, in many patients, especially those of older age.

Laboratory tests are of limited value in establishing the diagnosis. Leukocytosis is not present in all cases of vertebral osteomyelitis. The ESR, however, is elevated in over 90% of patients. Studies have shown that the average ESR ranges from 80-90 mm/hour. Blood cultures may reveal the etiologic agent.

Plain radiographs of the spine are abnormal in most patients with vertebral osteomyelitis. However, the abnormal findings are often nonspecific. Bone scanning has a sensitivity over 90% but the specificity only approaches 80%. The results of the bone scan often do not allow the clinician to differentiate vertebral osteomyelitis from other causes of back pain such as malignancy or trauma. One advantage of the bone scan over plain radiography is that the bone scan is often positive within 24 hours of the onset of the infection.

MRI is superior to both plain radiographs and bone scans of the spine in the diagnosis of vertebral osteomyelitis. It has a sensitivity and specificity of 96%

and 93%, respectively. When positive blood cultures are lacking, bone biopsy should be considered to identify the etiologic pathogen. Bone biopsy can be unrevealing in patients with vertebral osteomyelitis, especially when antibiotic therapy has been started prior to biopsy. Sampling error is another reason for a negative bone biopsy.

When bone biopsy cultures are positive, studies have shown that *S. aureus* is the bacterial organism most commonly isolated. Coagulase negative staphylococci and gram-negative organisms (usually of urinary tract origin) are less commonly found.

Epidural Abscess

Epidural abscess may be caused by bacteria, fungi, or mycobacteria. Bacterial infection is most commonly encountered. Like vertebral osteomyelitis, epidural abscess has a male predilection. Risk factors for epidural abscess are listed in the following box.

Risk Factors for Epidural Abscess
Alcoholism
Cirrhosis
Diabetes mellitus
Infection
Contiguous spread (eg, vertebral osteomyelitis)
Documented sepsis
Endocarditis
Intra-abdominal infection
Intravenous drug abuse
Pulmonary infection
Skin and soft tissue infection
Urinary tract infection
Vascular catheter
Post-procedure
Remote surgery of spine
Trauma
Nonpenetrating
Penetrating

The number of days that pass from symptom onset to hospital presentation varies. Although patients may present with symptoms that have been present for months, the median duration of illness prior to patients seeking medical care is about 10 days. Back pain, which is present in 75% of patients at the time of admission, is the most commonly encountered symptom in patients with epidural abscess. A history of back trauma is not uncommon. Eighty percent of patients have fever.

The most feared complications of epidural abscess are neurologic. Patients may progress from back pain to weakness. Paralysis may then ensue. Because the neurologic deficits of epidural abscess are often irreversible, it is important that the clinician establish the diagnosis at the earliest stage possible. Four clinical stages of epidural abscess have been described, as shown in the following box.

Clinical Stages of Epidural Abscess
• Stage 1
Fever and focal back pain or spinal pain at the level of the affected spine
• Stage 2
Nerve root compression with nerve root pain
• Stage 3
Spinal cord compression with accompanying deficits in motor and sensory nerves and bowel and bladder sphincter function
• Stage 4
Paralysis

The results of one study, which examined the signs and symptoms of epidural abscess present at the time of hospital admission, are shown in the following table.

Symptoms / Signs	Number of Patients (%)
Backache	72
Radicular pain	47
Weakness	35
Sensory deficit	23
Bladder dysfunction	28
Paralysis	21
Neck stiffness	21
Bowel dysfunction	9

Adapted from Darouiche RO, Hamill RJ, Greenberg SB, et al, "Bacterial Spinal Epidural Abscess. Review of 43 Cases and Literature Survey," *Medicine*, 1992, 71(6):369-85 (review).

A pathogen is identified in about 90% of cases when material from the epidural abscess is cultured, especially if the cultures are obtained prior to the institution of antibiotic therapy. Blood cultures may also be positive. The etiologic organisms often identified in patients with epidural abscess are listed in the following table.

Organism	Number of Isolates
Staphylococcus aureus	28
Coagulase negative staphylococcus	4
Escherichia coli	3
Pseudomonas aeruginosa	2
Streptococcus agalactiae	2
Streptococcus pneumoniae	1
Nongroupable viridans streptococci	1
Enterobacter cloacae	1
Proteus mirabilis	1
Bacteroides urealyticus	1
None identified	1
TOTAL	45

Adapted from Darouiche RO, Hamill RJ, Greenberg SB, et al, "Bacterial Spinal Epidural Abscess. Review of 43 Cases and Literature Survey," *Medicine*, 1992, 71(6):369-85 (review).

Epidural Spinal Cord Compression

Compression of the thecal sac by a malignancy in the epidural space satisfies the definition of malignant epidural spinal cord compression. By no means is malignancy the only cause of epidural spinal cord compression. For example, an epidural abscess or hematoma may present similarly. In the remainder of this step, however, the term "epidural spinal cord compression" will refer to that caused by malignancy. Of major concern in these patients is irreversible loss of neurologic function due to involvement of either the spinal cord or cauda equina (cauda equina syndrome is discussed later in this step). Epidural spinal cord compression affects approximately 5% of all patients with cancer.

Epidural spinal cord compression may be caused by many different malignancies. The most common causes are listed in the following box.

Most Common Malignant Causes of Epidural Spinal Cord Compression	
Breast cancer	Non-Hodgkin's lymphoma
Lung cancer	Prostate cancer
Multiple myeloma	Renal cell cancer

Although the malignant cause of epidural spinal cord compression is known in most cases, in up to 20% of cases, the manifestations of epidural spinal cord compression may be the initial presentation of an underlying malignancy.

The initial symptom noted in the majority of patients is back pain (95% of patients). It usually antedates the other symptoms of epidural spinal cord compression by one or two months. Although the pain is often nonspecific (patients may also complain of radicular pain), pain that worsens with recumbency and percussion tenderness are two features that should prompt the clinician to consider malignant epidural spinal cord compression. Patients with vertebral metastases are certainly prone to the development of compression fractures. This complication should be suspected when the pain acutely worsens.

At the time of presentation, approximately 75% have weakness. In most of these cases, physical examination reveals symmetric weakness. Early in the course of the condition, the weakness may be mild, affecting the iliopsoas or hamstring muscle groups. Slight hyper-reflexia of the patellar or Achilles deep tendon reflexes may also be noted. With further progression, an upper motor neuron type of muscle weakness may develop, characterized by spasticity, hyper-reflexia, and Babinski's sign.

Ascending numbness and paresthesias may also be noted. Autonomic dysfunction such as urinary retention may occur as well. Bowel and/or bladder incontinence are less common. These autonomic symptoms are usually late findings.

The signs and symptoms of malignant epidural spinal cord compression are listed in the following table.

Sign or Symptom	First Symptom (%)	Symptom at Diagnosis (%)
Pain	96	96
Weakness	2	76
Autonomic dysfunction	0	57
Sensory disturbance	0	51
Ataxia	2	3
Flexor spasm	0	2

Adapted from Byrne TN, "Spinal Cord Compression From Epidural Metastases," *N Engl J Med*, 1992, 327(9):614-9 (review); also from Gilbert RW, Kim JH, and Posner JB, "Epidural Spinal Cord Compression From Metastatic Tumor: Diagnosis and Treatment," *Ann Neurol*, 1978, 3(1):40-51.

Establishing the diagnosis of malignant epidural spinal cord compression requires radiologic imaging. It is important to understand that radiologic evaluation is indicated even if the neurologic examination is normal. Plain radiographs of the spine often reveal abnormalities. However, the false-negativity rate of radiography in the diagnosis of epidural spinal cord compression may be as high as 17%. Although there are many reasons for this false-negativity rate, chief among these reasons is the fact that 30% to 50% of bone must be destroyed before plain radiographs of the spine can demonstrate findings consistent with malignancy.

MRI has replaced CT myelography as the radiologic imaging modality of choice in patients with epidural spinal cord compression. It is useful in differentiating malignancy from other causes of epidural spinal cord compression such as disc herniation, suppurative bacterial infections, hemorrhage, and tuberculosis. When an MRI is performed, imaging of the entire spine should be performed since 10% of patients with metastatic disease of the spine will have asymptomatic epidural metastases elsewhere. CT myelography may be indicated in patients who are claustrophobic or in those who cannot lay on their back.

Cauda Equina Syndrome

Recall that the spinal cord terminates at the L1 level. Below this level, a process within the spinal canal can involve the nerve roots, resulting in the cauda equina syndrome. This syndrome is characterized by asymmetric lower extremity weakness and hyporeflexia. Multiple nerve roots may be compromised, resulting in saddle anesthesia (decreased sensation over upper posterior thighs, perineum, and buttocks), bowel/bladder incontinence, urinary/fecal retention, or decreased rectal tone. Malignancy, central disk herniation, epidural abscess, and epidural hemorrhage are some of the more common causes of the cauda equina syndrome. When findings consistent with the cauda equina syndrome are present, prompt MRI of the spine is indicated.

Vertebral Fractures

Although a severe flexion-compression force is needed to cause a vertebral fracture in normal bone, in bones that are osteoporotic, even minimal trauma may result in a vertebral compression fracture. Common precipitants include bending, coughing, or falling.

The pain of a vertebral compression fracture is characteristically acute and severe. Patients are fairly reliable at localizing the pain to the site of the fracture. Although the pain may be localized, in other cases, radiation of the pain into the abdomen or flanks may be noted. It is quite uncommon for the pain to radiate into the lower extremities. The pain is often worsened by bending, coughing, straining, or prolonged sitting. The spinous process that is involved can usually be detected by physical examination, which will reveal percussion tenderness. The natural history of the pain is persistence of pain for one to two months followed by a gradual resolution.

Plain radiographs of the spine usually reveal a wedge fracture of a vertebral body (anterior wedging). Collapse or involvement that is primarily posterior should prompt consideration of an underlying malignancy and a pathologic fracture.

Both men and women are at increased risk for osteoporosis with advancing age. In women, postmenopause is also a major risk factor. There are many conditions that are associated with osteoporosis, as shown in the following box.

Causes of Osteoporosis	
Connective tissue disease	Gastrointestinal conditions
Ehlers-Danlos syndrome	Malabsorption
Marfan syndrome	Obstructive jaundice (chronic)
Osteogenesis imperfecta	Primary biliary cirrhosis
Rheumatoid arthritis	Hematologic disorders
Endocrine disorders	Hemolytic anemia
Acromegaly	Leukemia
Anorexia nervosa	Lymphoma
Hypercortisolism	Multiple myeloma
Hyperparathyroidism	Immobilization
Hyperprolactinemia	Medications
Hyperthyroidism	Alcohol
Hypogonadism	Anticonvulsants
Hypothalamic amenorrhea	Chemotherapy
Premature ovarian failure	Cyclosporine
	Glucocorticoids
	Gonadotropin-releasing
	hormone agonists
	Heparin
	Thyroxine

End of Section.

STEP 11: *Does the Patient Have Radicular Low Back Pain?*

Radicular low back pain is a manifestation of any process causing lumbosacral nerve root compression or irritation. It should be suspected whenever back pain is accompanied by leg pain (pain radiating below the knee) and/or foot pain. Most often, patients describe the pain as shooting, sharp, burning, tingling, or numbness.

The most widely used physical examination maneuver to support the presence of radicular low back pain is the straight leg raise test. During this maneuver, the leg is passively raised (flexion at hip with knee fully extended) while the opposite leg lays flat.

The test is considered positive if the characteristic pain is elicited when the leg is raised to between 30° and 60° of elevation. Each leg should be tested. Nerve root compression is likely when the straight leg raise test is positive. It is even more likely when the crossed straight leg raise test is positive.

If the patient has radicular low back pain, *Proceed to Step 12.*

If the patient does not have radicular low back pain, *Proceed to Step 14.*

STEP 12: *Does the Patient Truly Have Radicular Back Pain?*

The clinician, however, should be aware of some pitfalls in the interpretation of the straight leg raise test. Some patients may experience discomfort or pain with straight leg raising that is not radicular. A common example is when the discomfort begins beyond 60° of elevation. This type of response is often observed because of hamstring tightness. The elicitation of pain with leg elevation of less than 30° is also not consistent with radicular pain since this degree of elevation has not been found to significantly stretch the nerve roots.

If the straight leg raise test is equivocal, there are other maneuvers that may be performed. All of these maneuvers stretch the nerve roots. These maneuvers are described in the following box.

Physical Examination Maneuvers to Detect Radicular Low Back Pain
Straight leg raise
Straight leg raise with dorsiflexion of the foot*
Straight leg raise with flexion of the neck*
Flip sign†

*The addition of these maneuvers to the standard straight leg raise can cause further stretch of the nerve roots.

†With the patient in the sitting position, the clinician passively extends the knee while noting the patient's postural response to this movement. When no postural adjustment accompanies passive extension of the knee, the flip sign is absent. When full passive extension of the knee causes the patient to fall back, the patient is considered to have a positive flip sign.

The clinician should realize, however, that not all leg pain is due to nerve root irritation. In fact, most patients presenting with acute low back pain and leg pain do not have nerve root irritation. 70% of patients with back pain report some radiation of pain into the legs. In most of these cases, the pain is dull and poorly localized. The pain may extend into the buttocks or thighs but rarely does it extend below the knee. These are features that allow the clinician to separate true radicular pain from other causes of low back pain that are often accompanied by nonspecific radiation to the leg.

If the patient has radicular pain, *Proceed to Step 13.*

If the patient does not have radicular pain, *Proceed to Step 14.*

STEP 13: *Which Nerve Root is Involved?*

Once the presence of radicular pain has been established, the clinician can use the following information to determine the nerve root involved:

- Pattern of radicular pain
- Sensorimotor involvement
- Reflex changes

Taken together, these findings often allow the clinician to determine the nerve root involved, as shown in the following table.

Level of Disc Herniation	Nerve Root Compressed	Pain	Numbness	Weakness	Reflexes (Decreased or Absent)
L3-4	L4	Sacroiliac joint, hip, posterolateral thigh, anterior aspect of leg	L4 dermatome	Extension of knee (quadriceps)	Knee jerk
L4-5	L5	Sacroiliac joint, hip	L5 dermatome (includes great toe)	Dorsiflexion of great toe	None
L5-S1	S1	Lateral aspect of leg and foot	S1 dermatome (includes lateral toes)	Unusual (plantar flexion of foot)	Ankle jerk

Adapted from Vanden Briuk KD and Edmonson AS, "The Spine," *Campbell's Operative Orthopedics*, 6th ed, Edmonson AS and Crenshaw AH (eds), St Louis, MO: CV Mosby Co, 1980; also from *Principles of Ambulatory Medicine*, 5th ed, Barker RL, Burton JR, and Zieve PD (eds), Baltimore, MD: Williams and Wilkins, 1999, 922.

Most cases of radicular low back pain are due to intervertebral disc herniation. Ninety-five percent of disc lesions affect L5 and S1 nerve roots. Only 5% of disc lesions affect L2, L3, or L4 nerve roots. The clinician should realize that not all patients with radicular pain will have motor, sensory, and reflex signs consistent with nerve root irritation or compression. These signs may be absent when nerve compression is not sufficient to affect nerve function.

Eighty percent of these patients respond to conservative management. Conservative therapy includes the following:

- Limiting physical activity (bed rest with patient in semi-Fowler's position)
- NSAID use
- Muscle relaxants
- Narcotic analgesics if pain is severe

If the above measures fail to result in an improvement in the back pain, the clinician may consider epidural corticosteroid injections. Radicular pain that persists despite conservative management may warrant surgery. In general, an imaging procedure, preferably an MRI of the spine, should be performed if radicular pain continues despite one to two months of conservative therapy. The majority of these patients are free of pain within two months.

End of Section.

STEP 14: *What are the Results of Conservative Treatment?*

Patients who do not have radicular low back pain should be considered to have a simple backache. Simple backache has also been termed acute lumbosacral strain, back strain, back sprain, and mechanical back pain. Clinical features consistent with simple backache are listed in the following box.

Clinical Features Consistent with Simple Backache
History
Dull or aching
Gradual in onset (over hours) but can occur suddenly after, for example, heavy lifting
Improved with rest
Located in low back
Mild to moderate pain
± radiation to thighs or buttocks
Worse with movement
Physical Examination
Mild to moderate tenderness over involved area
No other abnormalities noted
No percussion tenderness over spine or specific vertebral body
± paravertebral spasm

Establishing a specific diagnosis is not important in these patients because the treatment of these patients is the same, irrespective of the etiology. Most of these patients will improve with conservative therapy. Conservative therapy includes the passage of time, analgesic medications (preferably anti-inflammatory medications), muscle relaxants, and rapid return to normal activities.

The majority of these patients will improve within 10 days. Some, however, require up to six weeks for amelioration of symptoms. Eight-five percent of these patients will recover completely. Because back pain will resolve in most of these patients, there is no need to obtain plain radiographs of the lumbar spine. Plain radiographs of the lumbar spine should be considered, however, if the pain persists for more than six weeks.

The clinician should instruct the patient to return for further evaluation should any of the alarm features listed in the box in Step 7 occur.

End of Section.

REFERENCES

"Acute Low Back Problems in Adults: Assessment and Treatment. Agency for Health Care Policy and Research," *Clin Pract Guide Quick Ref Guide Clin*, 1994, 14(iii-iv):1-25.

Principles of Ambulatory Medicine, 5th ed, Barker RL, Burton JR, and Zieve PD (eds), Baltimore, MD: Williams and Wilkins, 1999, 922.

Borenstein DG, "A Clinician's Approach to Acute Low Back Pain," *Am J Med*, 1997, 102(1A):16S-22S.

Braddom RL, "Perils and Pointers in the Evaluation and Management of Back Pain," *Semin Neurol*, 1998, 18(2):197-210.

Bratton RL, "Assessment and Management of Acute Low Back Pain," *Am Fam Phys*, 1999, 60(8):2299-308.

Byrne TN, "Spinal Cord Compression From Epidural Metastases," *N Engl J Med*, 1992, 327(9):614-9 (review).

Connelly C, "Patients With Low Back Pain: How to Identify the Few Who Need Extra Attention," *Postgrad Med*, 1996, 100(6):143-6, 149-50, 155-6.

Darouiche RO, Hamill RJ, Greenberg SB, et al, "Bacterial Spinal Epidural Abscess. Review of 43 Cases and Literature Survey," *Medicine*, 1992, 71(6):369-85 (review).

Della-Giustina DA, "Emergency Department Evaluation and Treatment of Back Pain," *Emerg Med Clin North Am*, 1999, 17(4):877-93.

Della-Giustina DA and Kilcline BA, "Acute Low Back Pain: A Comprehensive Review," *Compr Ther*, 2000, 26(3):153-9 (review).

Deyo RA and Weinstein JN, "Low Back Pain," *N Engl J Med*, 2001, 344(5):363-70 (review).

Gilbert RW, Kim JH, and Posner JB, "Epidural Spinal Cord Compression From Metastatic Tumor: Diagnosis and Treatment," *Ann Neurol*, 1978, 3(1):40-51.

Mazanec DJ, "Evaluating Back Pain in Older Patients," *Cleve Clin J Med*, 1999, 66(2):89-91, 95-9.

McGregor AH and Hughes SP, "Initial Assessment of Back Pain: An Overview," *Hosp Med*, 1998, 59(6):492-5.

Patel AT and Ogle AA, "Diagnosis and Management of Acute Low Back Pain," *Am Fam Phys*, 2000, 61(6):1779-86, 1789-90.

Rose-Innes AP and Engstrom JW, "Low Back Pain: An Algorithmic Approach to Diagnosis and Management," *Geriatrics*, 1998, 53(10):26-8, 33-6, 39-40.

Rosomoff HL and Rosomoff RS, "Low Back Pain. Evaluation and Management in the Primary Care Setting," *Med Clin North Am*, 1999, 83(3):643-62.

Staiger TO, Paauw DS, Deyo RA, et al, "Imaging Studies for Acute Low Back Pain. When and When Not To Order Them," *Postgrad Med*, 1999, 105(4):161-2, 165-6, 171-2.

Tehranzadeh J, Andrews C, and Wong E, "Lumbar Spine Imaging. Normal Variants, Imaging Pitfalls, and Artifacts," *Radiol Clin North Am*, 2000, 38(6):1207-53.

Vanden Briuk KD and Edmonson AS, "The Spine," *Campbell's Operative Orthopedics*, 6th ed, Edmonson AS and Crenshaw AH (eds), St Louis, MO: CV Mosby Co, 1980.

Yelland M, "The Investigation of Low Back Pain in General Practice. The Use of Plain Films," *Aust Fam Physician*, 1998, 27(7):620-3.

LOW BACK PAIN (ACUTE)

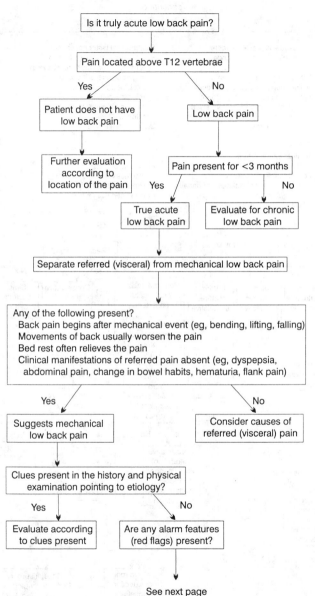

Is it truly acute low back pain?

↓

Pain located above T12 vertebrae

Yes → Patient does not have low back pain

No → Low back pain

Patient does not have low back pain
↓
Further evaluation according to location of the pain

Low back pain
↓
Pain present for <3 months

Yes → True acute low back pain

No → Evaluate for chronic low back pain

↓

Separate referred (visceral) from mechanical low back pain

↓

Any of the following present?
  Back pain begins after mechanical event (eg, bending, lifting, falling)
  Movements of back usually worsen the pain
  Bed rest often relieves the pain
  Clinical manifestations of referred pain absent (eg, dyspepsia, abdominal pain, change in bowel habits, hematuria, flank pain)

Yes → Suggests mechanical low back pain

No → Consider causes of referred (visceral) pain

↓

Clues present in the history and physical examination pointing to etiology?

Yes → Evaluate according to clues present

No → Are any alarm features (red flags) present?

↓

See next page

LOW BACK PAIN (ACUTE)
(continued)

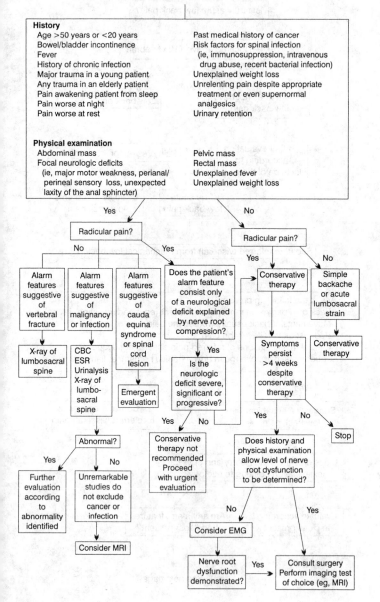

History
Age >50 years or <20 years
Bowel/bladder incontinence
Fever
History of chronic infection
Major trauma in a young patient
Any trauma in an elderly patient
Pain awakening patient from sleep
Pain worse at night
Pain worse at rest

Past medical history of cancer
Risk factors for spinal infection
(ie, immunosuppression, intravenous
drug abuse, recent bacterial infection)
Unexplained weight loss
Unrelenting pain despite appropriate
treatment or even supernormal
analgesics
Urinary retention

Physical examination
Abdominal mass
Focal neurologic deficits
(ie, major motor weakness, perianal/
perineal sensory loss, unexpected
laxity of the anal sphincter)

Pelvic mass
Rectal mass
Unexplained fever
Unexplained weight loss

Yes | No

Radicular pain?

Radicular pain?

No | Yes | Yes | No

Alarm features suggestive of vertebral fracture → X-ray of lumbosacral spine

Alarm features suggestive of malignancy or infection → CBC ESR Urinalysis X-ray of lumbo-sacral spine → Abnormal? → Yes: Further evaluation according to abnormality identified / No: Unremarkable studies do not exclude cancer or infection → Consider MRI

Alarm features suggestive of cauda equina syndrome or spinal cord lesion → Emergent evaluation

Does the patient's alarm feature consist only of a neurological deficit explained by nerve root compression? → Yes → Is the neurologic deficit severe, significant or progressive? → Yes: Conservative therapy not recommended Proceed with urgent evaluation / No

Conservative therapy → Symptoms persist >4 weeks despite conservative therapy → Yes / No → Stop

Simple backache or acute lumbosacral strain → Conservative therapy

Does history and physical examination allow level of nerve root dysfunction to be determined? → No: Consider EMG → Nerve root dysfunction demonstrated? → Yes → Consult surgery Perform imaging test of choice (eg, MRI) / Yes: Consult surgery Perform imaging test of choice (eg, MRI)

BREAST MASS / LUMP

STEP 1: *How Common is Breast Cancer?*

Breast cancer is the second most common malignancy in women (after skin cancer). Over a lifetime, one in eight women will develop breast cancer. Early detection of breast cancer leads to an improved outcome. As such, the clinician and the patient should focus on maintaining breast health by performing the following:

- Monthly breast self-examinations

- Clinical breast examination

    A clinical breast examination should be performed yearly in all women >40 years of age; women between the ages of 20-40 should have a clinical breast examination every three years

- Screening mammography (age appropriate)

Although mammography is important in the screening and diagnosis of breast cancer, most patients with breast cancer initially present with a breast mass or lump appreciated either during self-examination or during a breast exam at their physician's office. In fact, 70% of breast cancer cases present with the discovery of a lump or mass, most of which are detected by the woman herself. As the public becomes more educated about breast cancer, the number of women presenting to clinicians with the complaint of breast mass or lump may increase. As such, it behooves the clinician to become familiar with the evaluation of the patient presenting with breast mass or lump. Irrespective of how the lump or mass was detected, the challenge lies in differentiating a benign from malignant lesion.

Proceed to Step 2

STEP 2: *What Aspects of the History are Important in the Evaluation of the Patient Presenting With a Breast Mass?*

The risk of developing breast cancer increases with age as shown in the following table.

Age	Risk (%)
Risk to age 50	2.5
Risk to age 70	8
Risk to age 110	12

The likelihood of a breast mass being malignant in the younger woman (<25) is close to zero. In contrast, nearly 75% of breast masses evaluated in the older woman (>70) are found to be malignant.

As the public becomes more educated about breast cancer, women are becoming more cognizant about the factors that impact upon their individual risk of developing breast cancer. These factors are considered in the following table.

Factors	Relative Risk
Family history of breast cancer	
First-degree relative	1.8
Premenopausal first-degree relative	3.0
Postmenopausal first-degree relative	1.5
Premenopausal first-degree relative (bilateral breast cancer)	9.0
Postmenopausal first-degree relative (bilateral breast cancer)	4.0-5.4
Menstrual history (age in years)	
Menarche before age 12	1.7-3.4
Menarche after age 17	0.3
Menopause before age 45	0.5-0.7
Menopause from age 45-54	1.0
Menopause after age 55	1.5
Menopause after age 55 with more than 40 menstrual years	2.5-5.0
Oophorectomy before age 35	0.4
Anovulatory menstrual cycles	2.0-4.0
Pregnancy history	
Term pregnancy before age 20	0.4
First-term pregnancy at age 20-34	1.0
First-term pregnancy after age 35	1.5-4.0
Nulliparous patient	1.3-4.0
Noninvasive breast disease	
Atypical lobular hyperplasia	4.0
Lobular carcinoma *in situ*	5.2
Other neoplasms	
Contralateral breast cancer	2.0-10.0
Cancer of the major salivary gland	4.0
Cancer of the uterus	2.0
Radiation	Varies depending on the dosage

Adapted from *Breast Disease*, Marchant DJ (ed), Philadelphia, PA: WB Saunders Co, 1997, 119.

Although assessing risk factors for breast cancer is important, the information gleaned from the history and risk factor assessment does not allow the clinician to rule breast cancer in or out. As such, further evaluation is always necessary in the patient presenting with a breast mass, irrespective of the risk. The major considerations in the differential diagnosis of a breast mass include breast cancer, fibrocystic changes, cyst, fibroadenoma, and fat necrosis. The approach that follows will help distinguish benign from malignant breast disease.

Proceed to Step 3

STEP 3: *Does the Patient Truly Have a Breast Lump or Mass?*

Prior to embarking on an evaluation, the clinician should ensure that a breast mass or lump is truly present. In some cases, the mass or lump that is perceived by the patient is really a normal variant of breast tissue.

In premenopausal women, the glandular tissue of the breast is normally nodular. This nodularity is especially prominent in the upper outer quadrants of the breast. Not uncommonly, this nodularity may be mistaken for a dominant breast lump or mass. When nodularity is benign, it often waxes and wanes during the menstrual cycle. Nodularity is usually more pronounced during the luteal or latter half of the menstrual cycle. As a result, the most ideal time for clinical breast examination in premenopausal women is 5-10 days after the onset of menses.

A dominant breast mass usually persists throughout the menstrual cycle. The presence of a dominant breast mass is also supported when palpation of the same region of the contralateral breast is unremarkable.

If a breast mass or lump is not present during the follicular phase of the menstrual cycle in the premenopausal woman, *Stop Here.*

If a breast mass or lump persists throughout the menstrual cycle in a premenopausal women <35 years of age, *Proceed to Step 4.*

If a breast mass or lump persists throughout the menstrual cycle in a premenopausal woman >35 years of age, *Proceed to Step 9.*

If a breast mass is appreciated in the postmenopausal woman, *Proceed to Step 9.*

STEP 4: *Is the Mass Solid or Cystic?*

In the premenopausal woman <35 years of age, a breast mass that persists throughout the menstrual cycle requires further evaluation. Although a benign etiology is more common in this age group, it is important to realize that 40,000 women <50 years of age are diagnosed with breast cancer every year in the United States. While the clinical breast examination allows the clinician to confirm the presence of a breast mass, it is inaccurate in differentiating a benign from malignant etiology.

Once a breast mass is confirmed by clinical breast examination, the clinician should try to ascertain whether the mass is solid or cystic. Because the physical examination is not reliable in making this distinction, the clinician should perform either an ultrasound study or fine-needle aspiration of the mass.

If an ultrasound study of the mass is performed, *Proceed to Step 5.*

If fine-needle aspiration of the mass is performed, *Proceed to Step 9.*

STEP 5: *What are the Results of the Ultrasound?*

Ultrasonography can be used to distinguish a cystic from solid lesion. In this setting, entire radiologic screening of the breast is not necessary. Rather the clinician should direct the ultrasound study towards the palpable mass. It is important to realize, however, that not all palpable masses are detected by ultrasound, particularly if the mass is solid and small. A palpable mass that is not visualized by ultrasound should be presumed to be solid.

If ultrasonography reveals the breast mass to be solid, **Proceed to Step 12.**

When a cystic lesion is demonstrated on ultrasound, the clinician should determine if the cyst is simple or complex. Criteria for the diagnosis of a simple cyst are listed in the following box.

Ultrasonographic Criteria for the Diagnosis of a Simple Cyst
Absence of internal echoes
Bright posterior walls
Round or oval contour
Smooth walled
Through transmission (posterior acoustic enhancement)
Well circumscribed margins

All criteria listed above must be met to establish the diagnosis of a simple cyst. Even when the radiologic features of the cyst are consistent with a simple cyst, many recommend that the cyst should be aspirated to confirm that it is benign. In addition, aspiration will allow the clinician to completely evaluate the breast during a breast examination. Aspiration may also be performed for symptomatic relief when the cyst manifests with pain. When the radiologic findings are consistent with a complex cyst, excision of the cyst rather than aspiration should be considered. In these cases, there is concern that the complex cyst may represent intracystic carcinoma.

If the ultrasound findings are consistent with a simple cyst, **Proceed to Step 6**.

If the ultrasound findings are suggestive of a complex cyst, the patient should be referred for consideration of cyst excision. **Stop Here**.

STEP 6: What are the Results of the Fine-Needle Aspiration (FNA)?

Many authorities recommend fine-needle aspiration of a simple cyst demonstrated on ultrasound for the following reasons:

- To confirm the benign nature of the cyst
- To allow optimal and complete examination of the breast free of interfering masses
- To provide symptomatic relief when the cyst is causing pain
- To provide expeditious diagnosis

The color of the fluid obtained from cyst aspiration varies depending upon the age of the cyst. Lighter fluid tends to be aspirated in cysts of more recent onset while older cysts usually contain darker fluid. Aspiration of bloody fluid requires further evaluation. When the aspirate is bloody, intracystic carcinoma is a concern. In these cases, it is important not to evacuate all of the fluid from the cyst. Rather the procedure should be stopped when bloody fluid is aspirated. That which is obtained should be sent for cytologic examination. Both mammography and excisional biopsy should be performed.

If nonbloody fluid is obtained, **Proceed to Step 7.**

If bloody fluid is obtained, the patient should be referred for mammography and excisional biopsy. **Stop Here.**

STEP 7: *Is There a Residual Mass?*

The aspiration of nonbloody fluid does not definitively establish that the cystic lesion is benign. After aspiration, the clinician should assess for the presence of a residual mass. When a palpable mass persists after withdrawal of cystic fluid, intracystic carcinoma remains a concern. The presence of a residual mass should prompt the clinician to perform mammography and excisional biopsy.

If there is no residual mass after aspiration, **Proceed to Step 8.**

If there is a residual mass after aspiration, the patient should be referred for mammography and excisional biopsy. **Stop Here.**

STEP 8: *Has the Cyst Recurred at Follow-Up?*

Recurrence of the cyst at one to two month follow-up is another indication for further evaluation. In these cases, the cyst should be reaspirated. The patient should then be reassessed in one to two months for recurrence. Recurrence should prompt consideration of intracystic carcinoma. Recurrence after the second aspiration requires the clinician to perform mammography and excisional biopsy.

If there is no cyst recurrence at follow-up, **Stop Here.**

If the cyst recurs even after the second aspiration, the patient should be referred for mammography and excisional biopsy.

End of Section.

STEP 9: *What are the Results of the Fine-Needle Aspiration (FNA)?*

Fine-needle aspiration of a palpable mass may be performed to differentiate a cyst from solid mass. FNA establishes the diagnosis of a simple cyst when the criteria in the following box are met.

Criteria for the Diagnosis of a Simple Cyst by FNA
Aspiration of straw-colored fluid (nonbloody)
Lesion disappears completely after aspiration
Lesion does not reappear on follow-up physical examination

Criteria for the diagnosis of a solid mass by FNA are listed in the following box.

Criteria for the Diagnosis of a Solid Mass by FNA
No fluid aspirated
If there is any aspirate, it will be solid
Mass will persist following aspiration

If nonbloody fluid is obtained, **Proceed to Step 7.**

If bloody fluid is obtained, **Proceed to Step 10.**

If criteria for the diagnosis of a solid mass by FNA are met in a woman <35 years of age, **Proceed to Step 11.**

If criteria for the diagnosis of a solid mass by FNA are met in a woman >35 years of age, **Proceed to Step 13.**

STEP 10: *What is the Major Concern in Patients Who Have Bloody Fluid Aspirated During FNA of a Palpable Breast Mass?*

Aspiration of bloody fluid requires further evaluation. When the aspirate is bloody, intracystic carcinoma is a concern. In these cases, fluid should be sent for cytologic examination. Both mammography and excisional biopsy should be performed.

End of Section.

STEP 11: *Should Mammography or Ultrasound be Performed?*

Many experts recommend ultrasound over mammography in the evaluation of a solid breast mass in a woman <35 years of age. This is because mammography is of limited utility in women <35 years of age. The increased density of breast tissue in younger women does not allow a proper evaluation of the breast mass by mammography. Mammography has a higher false-positive and false-negative rate in younger women.

For these reasons, then, some experts recommend ultrasound as the initial breast imaging modality in the younger woman with a palpable breast mass. In this setting, the ultrasound should not be performed to screen the entire breast. Instead it should be directed towards the palpable mass. If the ultrasound reveals findings suspicious for cancer, the clinician should refer the patient for mammography and excisional biopsy.

The decision to proceed with either ultrasound or mammography in the evaluation of a breast mass in the younger woman should be made after a discussion with a breast imaging radiologist. It is important to realize that a negative radiologic imaging test, irrespective of the type, does not rule out breast cancer.

Proceed to Step 12

STEP 12: *What are the Results of the Biopsy?*

Biopsy evaluation is indicated in every solid breast mass. Biopsy techniques available to the clinician include the following:

- Fine-needle aspiration biopsy (FNAB)
- Core needle biopsy
- Open biopsy

Some of the factors involved in determining which biopsy technique to perform include the following:

- Size of the lesion
- Location of the lesion
- Size of the breast
- Availability of experienced cytopathologist if FNAB is planned

The combination of fine-needle aspiration biopsy, clinical breast examination, and breast ultrasound is known as the modified triple test. When all three arms of the modified triple test are consistent with a benign etiology, it is reasonable to observe the patient. If a suspicious finding is noted on any of the three tests, mammography and excision is recommended.

End of Section.

STEP 13: *What are the Results of Mammography?*

A diagnostic mammogram should be performed in all women >35 years of age who are presenting with a breast mass. It is important to realize that the purpose of the mammogram is not to rule out breast cancer within the identified mass. Instead, mammography is required to identify other occult lesions in the ipsilateral or contralateral breast. If fine-needle aspiration is planned, it is preferable to obtain the mammogram prior to aspiration to avoid false-positive findings related to bleeding within the breast tissue. If fine-needle aspiration is performed before mammography, most radiologists recommend waiting at least 2-4 weeks before obtaining a mammographic study. It is important to realize that a negative mammogram does not exclude the presence of breast cancer.

Proceed to Step 14

STEP 14: *What are the Results of the Biopsy?*

Biopsy of the solid breast mass should be performed irrespective of the mammographic findings. Biopsy techniques available to establish the diagnosis include the following:

- Fine-needle aspiration biopsy (FNAB)
- Core needle biopsy
- Open biopsy

Which test to perform is dependent upon local expertise. If FNAB is planned, the results of the FNAB may be combined with the findings noted on clinical breast examination and mammography. This is referred to as the classic triple test. The classic triple test is highly accurate when each test gives the same result. In one study, breast cancer was present in only 0.7% of cases when all three tests indicated a benign lesion. Over 99% of women who have findings suspicious for breast cancer on all three tests will be found to have breast cancer.

If any of the above tests yield suspicious results, the patient should be referred for further evaluation.

If the results of the above tests are consistent with a benign lesion, the patient should be reassessed at 3-6 months to ensure that the mass is stable or regressing.

REFERENCES

Breast Disease, Marchant DJ (ed), Philadelphia, PA: WB Saunders Co, 1997, 119.

Conry C, "Evaluation of a Breast Complaint: Is It Cancer?" *Am Fam Phys*, 1994, 49(2):445-50, 453-4.

Donegan WL, "Evaluation of a Palpable Breast Mass," *N Engl J Med*, 1992, 327(13):937-42.

Evans WP, "Breast Masses. Appropriate Evaluation," *Radiol Clin North Am*, 1995, 33(6):1085-108.

Giard RW and Hermans J, "The Value of Aspiration Cytologic Examination of the Breast. A Statistical Review of the Medical Literature," *Cancer*, 1992, 69(8):2104-10.

Layfield LJ, Glasgow BJ, and Cramer H, "Fine-Needle Aspiration in the Management of Breast Masses," *Pathol Annu*, 1989, 24(Pt 2):23-62.

Morrow M, "The Evaluation of Common Breast Problems," *Am Fam Phys*, 2000, 61(8):2371-8, 2385.

BREAST MASS / LUMP

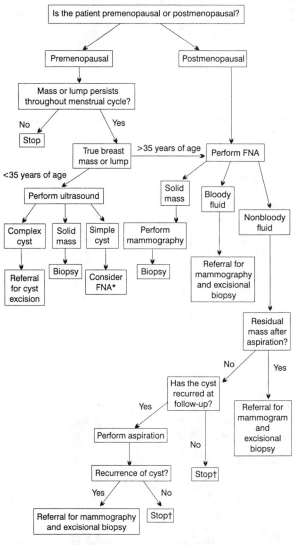

*Many authorities recommend FNA of a simple cyst demonstrated on ultrasound to confirm the benign nature of the cyst, to allow optimal and complete examination of the breast free of interfering masses, and to provide symptomatic relief when the cyst is causing pain.

†All women >35 years of age who present with a breast mass should have a mammogram.

BREAST PAIN

STEP 1: *How Common is Breast Pain?*

The most common breast symptom that prompts women to seek medical care is breast pain or mastalgia. In a study performed in 1985, approximately 65% of women reported having mastalgia. Only 50% of these women, however, sought medical attention for the breast pain. As public awareness of breast cancer increases, more women are likely to present to the primary care physician with this complaint.

Proceed to Step 2

STEP 2: *Does the Patient Truly Have Breast Pain?*

Not uncommonly, women complain of breast pain that does not originate from the breast. There are many conditions that may manifest with referred pain to the breast, some of which may be life-threatening. The clinician should perform a thorough history and physical examination in an effort to exclude conditions presenting with referred pain to the breast. Many of these conditions are listed in the following box.

Causes of Anterior Chest Pain That May Be Perceived by a Woman as Breast Pain	
Cervical radiculopathy	Hiatal hernia
Cervical rib	Myalgia
Cholelithiasis	Neuralgia
Coronary artery disease	Pleurisy
Costochondritis	Psychological pain
Herpes zoster	Tietze's syndrome

If the patient has referred pain to the breast, *Stop Here*.

If the patient truly has breast pain, *Proceed to Step 3*.

STEP 3: *Is the Breast Pain a Manifestation of Breast Cancer?*

Breast pain raises concern about the possibility of breast cancer. In one study, 15% of women with operable breast cancer reported having breast pain. However, only 7% of these patients presented with breast pain alone. Although studies have shown that breast pain alone is a rare presentation of breast cancer, it can occur. As such, a systematic approach is necessary to ensure that the clinician does not miss the rare patient who presents with breast pain alone as their initial manifestation of breast cancer.

Proceed to Step 4

STEP 4: *What are the Results of the Clinical Breast Examination?*

In patients presenting with breast pain, a thorough examination of the breast should be performed. Elicitation of any of the following findings raises concern that the breast pain is a manifestation of breast cancer:

- Breast mass
- Nipple discharge
- *Peau d'orange* (indentation of skin over a mass that often looks like an orange peel)
- Inverted nipple (new onset)
- Scaling, crusting, or ulceration of skin surrounding nipple (suggestive of Paget's disease)
- Asymmetry
- Change in breast contour
- Skin retraction
- Local area of redness
- Supraclavicular or axillary lymphadenopathy

It is important to realize that a normal clinical breast examination does not exclude breast cancer in women who present with breast pain.

If the history and physical examination are abnormal, then the work-up should proceed according to the abnormality noted. *Stop Here.*

If the history and physical examination are normal, *Proceed to Step 5*.

STEP 5: *What is the Age of the Patient?*

When the clinical breast examination is normal, further evaluation depends on the age of the patient.

If the patient is ≥35 years of age, *Proceed to Step 6*.

If the patient is <35 years of age, *Proceed to Step 7*.

STEP 6: *What are the Results of the Mammogram?*

All patients who are ≥35 years of age should have a mammogram. The only exception to this rule is in the woman who has had a mammogram within the year prior to her presentation with breast pain. The role of mammography in the older woman with breast pain is to evaluate the breast for findings suspicious of breast cancer. A normal mammogram should prompt the clinician to reassure the patient that the breast pain is not a manifestation of breast cancer.

If the mammogram is abnormal, further evaluation is warranted. The reader should consult an appropriate resource regarding further management.

If the mammogram is normal, *Proceed to Step 8*.

STEP 7: *Should Mammography Be Performed in the Younger Woman (<35 years of age)?*

When the clinical breast examination is normal, an imaging study is not required in the younger woman (<35 years of age) presenting with breast pain. The clinician should inform the patient that the pain is not due to malignancy.

Proceed to Step 8

STEP 8: *How is Mastalgia Classified?*

Once breast cancer has been excluded in a patient presenting with breast pain, the clinician should consider the benign causes of mastalgia. Benign mastalgia may be subdivided into one of the following types:

- Cyclical mastalgia
- Noncyclical mastalgia
- Chest wall pain

The frequency of these types of mastalgia is provided in the following table.

Type of Mastalgia	Frequency (%)
Cyclical mastalgia	67
Noncyclical mastalgia	26
Chest wall pain	7

These types of mastalgia will be discussed below.

Cyclical Mastalgia

The symptoms of cyclical mastalgia typically begin in the third decade of life. Although most patients describe the pain as dull, burning, or aching, some report a sharp or shooting pain. Women who have cyclical mastalgia complain of bilateral breast pain that is usually difficult to localize. Not uncommonly, the pain is noted to radiate to the axilla or arm. The pain usually begins five or more days before menses, often subsiding after the menstrual period. In some patients, however, the pain may persist throughout the menstrual cycle with an exacerbation occurring before menses. As women approach menopause, there is often an exacerbation of the pain. With menopause, many women report the resolution of the symptoms. Cyclical mastalgia resolves spontaneously in only 22% of women prior to menopause.

Noncyclical Mastalgia

When breast pain is unrelated to menses or occurs in the postmenopausal woman, noncyclical mastalgia is said to be present. In contrast to cyclical mastalgia which tends to begin in younger women, noncyclical mastalgia has a predilection for women between the ages of 40-50 years. Unlike cyclical mastalgia, the pain is usually localized and unilateral. Noncyclical mastalgia is less common than cyclical mastalgia.

Chest Wall Pain

Chest wall pain may include a variety of conditions including costochondritis, lateral extramammary pain syndrome, and cervical radiculopathy. Chest wall pain, irrespective of the type, is not considered to be true mastalgia. However, the pain often emanates from the area of the breast that overlies the chest wall pathology.

Tietze's syndrome is one consideration in patients with chest wall pain. This syndrome has often been used interchangeably with costochondritis. Both conditions are usually associated with unilateral pain located in the medial quadrant of the breast. Radiation of the pain to the shoulder is not uncommon. Coughing, sneezing, and inspiration may aggravate the pain. While both Tietze's syndrome and costochondritis are characterized by tenderness of one or more costal cartilages, the presence of localized swelling supports the diagnosis of Tietze's syndrome.

REFERENCES

Conry C, "Evaluation of a Breast Complaint: Is It Cancer?" *Am Fam Phys*, 1994, 49(2):445-50, 453-4.

Dixon JM, "Managing Breast Pain," *Practitioner*, 1999, 243(1599):484-6, 488-9, 491.

Mansel RE, "ABC of Breast Diseases. Breast Pain," *BMJ*, 1994, 309(6958):866-8.

Morrow M, "The Evaluation of Common Breast Problems," *Am Fam Phys*, 2000, 61(8):2371-8, 2385.

Steinbrunn BS, Zera RT, and Rodriguez JL, "Mastalgia. Tailoring Treatment to Type of Breast Pain," *Postgrad Med*, 1997, 102(5):183-4, 187-9, 193-4.

BREAST PAIN

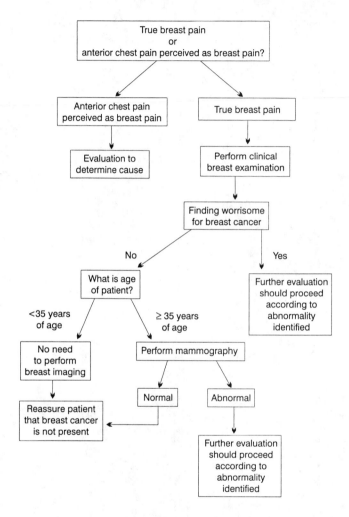

CHEST PAIN (ACUTE)

STEP 1: *How Common is Chest Pain?*

Chest pain accounts for approximately 5 million visits to the emergency room per year. This represents 5% of all emergency room visits. Although the majority of these cases are due to benign conditions, it can be quite challenging to differentiate these conditions from the serious causes of chest pain.

Proceed to Step 2

STEP 2: *What are the Causes of Chest Pain?*

The causes of chest pain are listed in the following box.

Causes of Chest Pain	
Cardiac	Neurologic
Aortic dissection	Brachial plexus syndrome
Aortic stenosis	Herpes zoster
Hypertrophic cardiomyopathy	Intercostal neuritis
Mitral valve prolapse	Radicular syndrome
Myocardial infarction	Thoracic disc disease
Pericarditis	Psychiatric
Pulmonary hypertension	Anxiety
Stable angina	Cardiac neurosis
Unstable angina	Depression
Gastrointestinal	Hyperventilation
Biliary colic	Malingering
Cholecystitis	Panic attacks
Esophageal rupture	Pulmonary
Esophageal spasm	Intrathoracic malignancy
Gastroesophageal reflux disease	Pleurisy
Pancreatitis	Pneumonia
Peptic ulcer disease	Pneumothorax
Musculoskeletal	Pulmonary embolism
Costochondritis	Tracheitis/tracheobronchitis
Muscle strain	Miscellaneous
Sternal or rib fractures	Mediastinal emphysema
Thoracic outlet syndrome	Mediastinal tumors
Tietze's syndrome	Mediastinitis
Trauma	

Proceed to Step 3

STEP 3: *Is the Chest Pain Caused by a Serious Condition?*

The approach to the patient presenting with chest pain should begin with consideration of the serious causes (ie, those that are potentially life-threatening). The serious causes of chest pain include the following:

- Aortic dissection
- Esophageal rupture
- Pneumothorax
- Pulmonary embolism
- Unstable angina/acute myocardial infarction

Every patient with recent or ongoing chest pain should be considered to have a life-threatening cause of chest pain until proven otherwise. If the patient is presenting to the emergency room, the following should be performed or obtained:

- Rapid assessment of airway, breathing, and circulation
- Continuous cardiac monitoring
- Intravenous access
- Administration of supplemental oxygen
- Vital signs
- 12-lead EKG
- Baseline cardiac markers if ischemia is suspected
- Administration of 160-325 mg of aspirin to be chewed and swallowed if ischemia is suspected (and no contraindications present)
- Administration of sublingual nitroglycerin if ischemia is suspected (and contraindications such as systolic blood pressure <90 mm Hg, severe tachycardia, and severe bradycardia are not present)

Once these issues have been addressed and the clinician is confident that no immediate life threats are present, a more extensive evaluation may then be pursued. It is worth reiterating that all patients should be considered to have a potentially life-threatening cause until proven otherwise. The only exception to this rule might be in the patient who unequivocally has a benign cause of chest pain such as chest wall pain.

This approach deals exclusively with the serious causes of chest pain. Should the patient not have any of the serious causes of chest pain, the clinician should search for one of the other causes listed in the box in Step 2. If the patient has pleuritic chest pain (pain that is induced or worsened by inspiration), proceed to the chapter on Chest Pain (Pleuritic) *on page 77.*

Proceed to Step 4

STEP 4: *Are There Any Clues in the History That Point to a Serious Cause of the Chest Pain?*

In this step, the key elements in the history that should prompt consideration of the serious causes of chest pain are considered.

Unstable Angina

Patients with unstable angina usually present in one of two ways:

- New onset chest pain

- Change in the pattern of the patient's stable angina

  Prior to discussing unstable angina in more detail, it is important to understand what stable angina is. The chest pain of stable angina is typically precipitated by exertion, heavy meals, or emotional upset. The pain is of gradual onset, climbing to a plateau before subsiding. Adjectives used to describe the pain include "heaviness", "crushing", or "tightness". Classically, the pain is retrosternal but radiation to both sides of the chest is not uncommon. The pain may also radiate to the arms, neck, jaw, or interscapular region. Occasionally, the pain may only be located in one of these areas. Most episodes of stable angina resolve within 20 minutes. Palliative factors include rest and sublingual nitroglycerin.

Unstable angina differs from stable angina in that the former may have one or more of the following characteristics:

- Increase in frequency of chest pain
- Increase in severity of chest pain
- Increase in duration of chest pain
- Chest pain at rest
- Chest pain is provoked by a lower level of physical activity
- Chest pain awakens the patient at night

Although stable angina responds readily to rest and the administration of sublingual nitroglycerin, the pain of unstable angina is less likely to do so. Most episodes of unstable angina last <30 minutes in duration. On occasion, the pain may be more prolonged or particularly severe, making it difficult for the clinician to differentiate unstable angina from myocardial infarction.

Acute Myocardial Infarction

Acute myocardial infarction is characterized by pain of variable intensity. While most patients describe severe pain, others report a mild discomfort. The duration of the pain usually exceeds 30 minutes. Adjectives used to describe the pain include "crushing", "feels like an elephant standing on my chest", "heaviness", or "squeezing". The clinician should realize, however, that adjectives which are not classic for the pain of acute myocardial infarction do not exclude the diagnosis. In fact, 22% of patients describe their pain as being "stabbing" or "sharp".

Classically, the pain is retrosternal but an epigastric location is not unusual. In these latter cases, it may be confused with gastrointestinal causes, leading to an erroneous diagnosis of "indigestion". Not uncommonly, there is radiation of the pain, most often to the sides of the chest. Many patients describe radiation of the pain down the arm. Although either arm may be involved, more commonly, patients describe radiation down the ulnar aspect of the left arm. Often accompanying this radiation is a tingling sensation in the hand or fingers. The pain may also radiate to the jaw, neck, shoulders, or interscapular region. Occasionally, the pain is only present in one of these locations.

Patients with a history of angina usually report that the pain is similar in location. However, the pain of acute myocardial infarction differs from that of stable angina in that the former is usually more severe and of longer duration. Furthermore, it responds less readily to rest and nitroglycerin.

Associated symptoms include nausea, vomiting, diaphoresis, weakness, palpitations, and shortness of breath. The clinician should realize that chest pain is not invariably present in patients with acute myocardial infarction. Up to 33% of patients have no symptoms whatsoever (silent myocardial infarction). Others have what are considered ischemic or anginal equivalents. These symptoms are considered in the following box.

Symptoms Considered Anginal or Ischemic Equivalents	
Alteration in mental status	Light-headedness
Diaphoresis	Nausea/vomiting
Discomfort in shoulder, arm, or jaw	Shortness of breath
Epigastric discomfort	Weakness (generalized)

Aortic Dissection

The incidence of aortic dissection is increasing as the population ages. Over 2000 new cases per year are reported in the United States. Aortic dissection should be a consideration in all patients with acute chest pain. Left untreated, it carries a significant mortality, as shown in the following table.

Time From Onset	Mortality Rate (%)
First 24 hours	21
Within 2 weeks	60
Within 3 months	>90

Not uncommonly, the diagnosis is not made before death. In fact, it is not suspected prior to death in as many as 33% of the cases. Although aortic dissection may occur in the absence of risk factors, in most cases, one or more risk factors are apparent. Risk factors for aortic dissection are listed in the following box.

Risk Factors for Aortic Dissection	
Age >50 years	Male gender
Coarctation of aorta	Noonan's syndrome
Cocaine use	Pregnancy
Congenital bicuspid or unicuspid	Syphilitic aortitis
aortic valve	Turner's syndrome
Connective tissue disease	Trauma
Ehler-Danlos syndrome	Iatrogenic
Marfan syndrome	Aortic incision
Osteogenesis imperfecta	Aortic valve replacement
Relapsing polychondritis	Cannulation
Systemic lupus erythematosus	Catheterization
Granulomatous arteritis	Cross clamping
HTN (70% to 90%)	Nonpenetrating abdominal or chest

Contrary to popular belief, most cases of aortic dissection do not occur after strenuous physical exertion. Chest pain is the most commonly encountered symptom, occurring in up to 90% of patients. The pain of aortic dissection is classically sudden in onset. The severity of the pain is often maximal from the onset. This is in contrast to the pain of acute myocardial infarction which often builds to a gradual plateau. Adjectives commonly used to describe the pain include "tearing", "cutting", "ripping", or "stabbing". Some patients are very uncomfortable, often writhing in agony or pacing relentlessly in an effort to find a position that offers them symptomatic relief.

The location of the pain seems to correlate with the location of the dissection. When patients complain of anterior chest pain only or pain that is most severe in the anterior chest, studies reveal involvement of the ascending aorta in over 90% of cases. When patients complain of interscapular pain only or pain that is most severe in the interscapular region, the descending aorta was found to be involved in over 90% of cases. Strongly predictive of ascending aorta involvement is any pain perceived in the throat, neck, jaw, or face. In contrast, pain in the back, abdomen, or lower extremities is highly suggestive of descending aorta involvement.

Quite characteristic of aortic dissection is migratory pain. In fact, 70% of patients with aortic dissection describe pain that migrates. The migration of the pain usually follows the path of the dissection.

Pulmonary Embolism

Over 600,000 cases of pulmonary embolism occur every year in the United States. Because the symptoms and signs of pulmonary embolism are nonspecific, in many of these cases, the diagnosis is missed, only to be made at the time of autopsy.

Most often, pulmonary embolism develops when thrombi travel from the deep venous system to the pulmonary arterial tree, causing obstruction of blood flow. Approximately 70% of patients have a clot that can be demonstrated in the lower extremities by venography. Although most cases are due to thrombi originating in the deep venous system of the lower extremities, approximately 10% are thought to arise elsewhere. The majority of these originate in the upper extremity veins, especially in patients with indwelling central venous catheters.

In many cases, risk factors for venous thromboembolism are present. These risk factors are considered in the following box.

Risk Factors for Deep Venous Thrombosis and Pulmonary Embolism	
Acute myocardial infarction	Lupus anticoagulant
Antithrombin III deficiency	Malignancy
Behcet's disease	Obesity
Congestive heart failure	Oral contraceptive use
Dysfibrinogenemia	Polycythemia vera
Essential thrombocytosis	Postoperative
Estrogen replacement (high dose)	Postpartum
Hemolytic anemia	Pregnancy
Heparin-induced thrombocytopenia	Protein C deficiency
History of deep venous thrombosis	Protein S deficiency
History of pulmonary embolism	Resistance to activated protein C
Homocysteinuria	Trauma
Immobilization	Venography
Indwelling central venous catheters	Venous pacemakers

The classic triad of dyspnea, chest pain, and hemoptysis is seen in <20% of patients. No features of the chest pain are diagnostic for pulmonary embolism. While some patients present with pleuritic chest pain, others may manifest with a retrosternal heaviness that mimics what is considered classic for acute myocardial infarction.

Symptoms encountered in patients proven to have pulmonary embolism by angiography are listed in the following table.

Symptom	Percent
Dyspnea	93
Chest pain, pleuritic	74
Apprehension	59
Cough	53
Hemoptysis	30
Sweating	27
Chest pain, nonpleuritic	14
Syncope	13

Adapted from "The Urokinase Pulmonary Embolism Trial: A National Cooperative Study," *Circulation*, 1973, 47(2 Suppl):II1-108; also from "Urokinase-Streptokinase Embolism Trial: Phase 2 Results. A Cooperative Study," *JAMA*, 1974, 229(12):1606-13.

Because the signs and symptoms of pulmonary embolism are nonspecific, further evaluation is certainly indicated, especially in the setting of risk factors for venous thromboembolism. The clinician should realize, however, that not all patients have an apparent predisposition at the time of diagnosis.

Pneumothorax

Pneumothorax is defined as the presence of free air between the visceral and parietal pleura. The causes of pneumothorax can be categorized into spontaneous and iatrogenic types, as shown in the following box.

Causes of Pneumothorax	
Spontaneous	
Primary	
Secondary	
Asthma	Interstitial lung disease
Chronic obstructive	Lymphangioleiomyomatosis
pulmonary disease	Marfan syndrome
Cystic fibrosis	Pleural malignancy
Histiocytosis X	Sarcoidosis
Infection	Trauma
Bacterial	Tuberous sclerosis
Pneumocystis carinii pneumonia	
Tuberculosis	
Iatrogenic	
Chest compression	Positive pressure ventilation
Intercostal nerve block	Subclavian cannulation
Needle aspiration (lung biopsy)	Transbronchial biopsy

The typical patient who develops a primary spontaneous pneumothorax is a young male smoker between the ages of 20-40 years. Although not all patients are symptomatic, most describe the sudden onset of unilateral chest pain and shortness of breath. The symptoms of secondary spontaneous pneumothorax are essentially the same. In contrast to primary spontaneous pneumothorax, these patients can precipitously decline because the pneumothorax occurs in the setting of an existing pulmonary disease. This underlying pulmonary disease limits these patients' pulmonary reserve.

When mediastinal shift and compression of the contralateral lung occurs because of the progressive accumulation of air under pressure, a tension pneumothorax is said to be present. The symptoms of tension pneumothorax are similar to that encountered in uncomplicated spontaneous pneumothorax but may be exaggerated.

Esophageal Rupture

The causes of esophageal rupture or perforation are listed in the following box.

Causes of Esophageal Perforation		
Boerhaave's syndrome*	Infection	Malignancy
Trauma†	Herpes simplex virus	Esophageal
Blunt	Cytomegalovirus	Lymphoma
Penetrating	Tuberculosis	Metastatic
Foreign body‡	Caustic injury#	
Radiation therapy	Iatrogenic§	

*Boerhaave's syndrome refers to spontaneous esophageal perforation.

†Trauma is responsible for up to 15% of cases. Penetrating injuries are much more common than blunt injuries.

‡Foreign body ingestion is the cause of esophageal perforation in about 15% of cases. Endoscopic removal of a foreign body may also be complicated by esophageal rupture.

#The risk of perforation is highest 3-5 days after the ingestion of the caustic substance. Instrumentation of the esophagus is associated with a higher risk of perforation in these patients.

§Instrumentation of the esophagus is the most common cause of perforation, accounting for nearly 50% of cases. Upper endoscopy, esophageal dilation, nasogastric tube, Sengstaken-Blakemore tube, endotracheal tubes, esophageal stents, and endoscopic ultrasound are just some of the techniques or procedures that have been complicated by perforation. Surgical injury from operations of the esophagus or contiguous structures is another iatrogenic cause.

In Boerhaave's syndrome, esophageal rupture classically follows vomiting. The typical patient is a middle-aged male with a history of recent excessive use of alcohol. Any factor that increases intraesophageal pressure can predispose to esophageal perforation. These factors include weight lifting, excessive coughing, hyperemesis gravidarum, seizures, and laughing. Between 80% and 100% of patients complain of pain. The location of the pain varies but, most commonly, patients describe severe chest or abdominal pain. Accompanying symptoms include nausea, vomiting, hematemesis, diaphoresis, dyspnea, odynophagia, and dysphagia. Any patient who reports pain after esophageal instrumentation should be considered to have esophageal perforation until proven otherwise.

Proceed to Step 5

STEP 5: *Are There Any Clues in the Physical Examination That Point to a Serious Cause of the Chest Pain?*

In this step, the key findings in the physical examination that should prompt consideration of the serious causes of chest pain are considered.

Unstable Angina

Physical examination findings of unstable angina are listed in the following box.

Physical Examination Findings of Unstable Angina	
Paradoxic splitting of S2	Dyskinetic apical impulse
S3	Transient systolic murmur of
S4	mitral regurgitation

These findings are not invariably present in patients with unstable angina. In fact, the examination may be unremarkable, especially when the patient is seen after the chest pain has resolved. In addition, these findings are nonspecific, commonly being appreciated in patients with stable angina or acute myocardial infarction. The presence of hypertension, diminished pulses, vascular bruits, xanthomas, or xanthelesmas makes an ischemic etiology more likely.

Acute Myocardial Infarction

Patients with acute myocardial infarction may appear restless, anxious, or distressed. Other physical examination findings that may be appreciated in patients with myocardial infarction are listed in the following table.

Physical Examination Finding	Clinical Significance
Hypertension	High sympathetic tone (especially in anterior myocardial infarction)
Hypotension	High vagal tone (especially in inferior myocardial infarction)
	Also consider pump failure
Tachycardia	High sympathetic tone (especially in anterior myocardial infarction)
	Also consider atrial or ventricular arrhythmias
Bradycardia	High vagal tone (especially in inferior myocardial infarction)
	Also consider heart block
Small volume pulses	Low cardiac output
Soft S1	Decreased left ventricular contractility
S3 Rales	Left ventricular systolic dysfunction
S4	Decreased left ventricular compliance
Elevated jugular venous pressure	Right ventricular infarction
Systolic murmur	Mitral regurgitation
	Ventricular septal rupture

Aortic Dissection

Physical examination findings that should prompt consideration of aortic dissection are listed in the following table.

Physical Examination Finding	Significance of Physical Examination Finding
Hypertension	Noted in up to 90% of distal aortic dissection Less commonly seen in proximal aortic dissection
Hypotension*	More commonly seen in proximal aortic dissection If present, consider the following: Cardiac tamponade Intrapleural rupture Intraperitoneal rupture
Pulse deficits†	Strongly suggestive of aortic dissection, especially proximal dissection
Murmur of aortic regurgitation‡	Suggestive of proximal aortic dissection
Focal neurologic findings consistent with CVA#	Suggestive of left common carotid or innominate artery involvement
Paraparesis or paraplegia	Suggestive of spinal artery involvement
Pericardial friction rub	Leakage of blood into the pericardial space

*Blood pressure measurement may be inaccurate with aortic dissection that involves the brachiocephalic vessels. This may result in falsely low blood pressure readings.

†50% of proximal aortic dissection are associated with pulse deficits. In contrast, pulse deficits are noted in only 15% of patients with distal dissection.

‡Aortic regurgitation is noted in up to 66% of patients with proximal aortic dissection.

#CVA is more commonly encountered in proximal aortic dissection, occurring in up to 6% of cases.

Pulmonary Embolism

Signs present in those proven to have pulmonary embolism by angiography are listed in the following table.

Sign	Percent
Tachypnea >16/minute	92
Rales	58
Accentuated second heart sound	53
Tachycardia >100/minute	44
Fever >37.8°C	43
Diaphoresis	36
S3 or S4 gallop	34
Thrombophlebitis	32
Lower extremity edema	24
Cardiac murmur	23
Cyanosis	19

Adapted from "The Urokinase Pulmonary Embolism Trial: A National Cooperative Study," *Circulation*, 1973, 47(2 Suppl):II1-108; also from "Urokinase-Streptokinase Embolism Trial: Phase 2 Results. A Cooperative Study," *JAMA*, 1974, 229(12):1606-13.

Pneumothorax

Physical examination findings consistent with primary spontaneous pneumothorax include hyper-resonance to percussion and decreased breath sounds. The signs of secondary spontaneous pneumothorax are the same. In some of these patients, however, the underlying lung disease (eg, COPD) may mask some of the physical examination findings of pneumothorax (eg, breath sounds may be reduced in both pneumothorax and COPD).

Patients with tension pneumothorax usually appear quite ill and may be noted to be in severe cardiovascular and respiratory distress. These patients are often agitated, restless, and cyanotic. Vital signs may reveal tachycardia, tachypnea, and hypotension. The hallmarks of tension pneumothorax include jugular venous distention, absent breath sounds on the ipsilateral side, and hyper-resonance to percussion. It is important to realize that hypotension is not invariably present, especially in those who are presenting early in the disease course.

Esophageal Rupture

Most patients with esophageal rupture appear acutely ill. Fever, tachycardia, tachypnea, and cyanosis are quite common. Subcutaneous emphysema may be noted. It is not uncommon for patients to present in shock.

Proceed to Step 6

> **STEP 6:** *Are There Any Findings on the EKG That Point to a Serious Cause of the Chest Pain?*

In this step, EKG abnormalities that should prompt consideration of the serious causes of chest pain are discussed.

Unstable Angina

Many patients with unstable angina have EKG changes, the most common of which are ST segment depression and T wave inversion. Although ST segment elevation does occur in patients with unstable angina, its presence should prompt consideration of acute myocardial infarction. There is an 80% prevalence of acute myocardial infarction in patients with at least 1 mm of new ST segment elevation.

The most characteristic finding is ST segment depression with or without T wave inversion. In the absence of ST segment depression, T wave inversion is less specific. However, it too may represent ischemia, particularly if the T wave inversion is deep and symmetrical. The prevalence of acute myocardial infarction is 20% among patients with new ST segment depression or T wave inversion.

The clinical significance of minor T wave inversion (<1 mm) or flattening is of limited value. Studies have shown that these findings are no more common in patients with unstable angina than in the emergency room population overall.

It is important to realize that a normal EKG does not exclude the diagnosis of unstable angina. The absence of findings consistent with ischemia does, however, place the patient at a lower risk for subsequent cardiac events. Patients with ST segment depression are at higher risk than those with T wave inversion alone. When EKG abnormalities are present in the patient with unstable angina, relief of the patient's pain is usually associated with either partial or complete resolution of the EKG abnormalities. Persistence of the EKG abnormalities beyond twelve hours is more suggestive of a non-Q wave myocardial infarction.

The clinician should realize that the EKG abnormalities found in unstable angina may be seen with non-Q wave myocardial infarction. In usual clinical practice, the differentiation between these two entities can only be made with the serial measurement of cardiac markers of injury.

Acute Myocardial Infarction

Approximately 75% of patients with acute myocardial infarction will have either ST segment elevation or depression noted on the initial EKG. This percentage will increase with subsequent EKGs done with the passage of time. About 25% of patients will have no initial EKG changes consistent with ischemia. The majority of these individuals (80%) will develop non-Q wave myocardial infarction.

Although the EKG is sensitive in the detection of changes consistent with ischemia, the findings are of low specificity. Although the presence of ST segment elevation is very suggestive of transmural ischemia/infarction, it is not specific for the diagnosis. In fact, ST segment elevation can be seen in patients with left ventricular aneurysm and pericarditis. Greater than 1 mm ST segment elevation in two or more contiguous leads should prompt consideration of primary PTCA or intravenous thrombolytic therapy, particularly in patients who have presented <12 hours from symptom onset (as long as ST segment elevation is not thought to be due to pericarditis or left ventricular aneurysm).

In the absence of mechanical intervention or reperfusion therapy, the ST segment elevation that is characteristic of transmural infarction usually returns to normal within 20 hours. This is also the type of infarction characterized by the appearance of Q waves. In these cases, Q waves are usually not noted until at least 10 hours pass from symptom onset. Once they have appeared, Q waves usually persist for the patient's lifetime. On occasion, Q waves may regress or even disappear completely many years after the infarction.

ST segment depression is suggestive of subendocardial ischemia but it may also be appreciated in patients with bundle branch block, left ventricular hypertrophy, and digoxin effect. ST segment depression may also occur in patients with unstable angina. Serial measurement of cardiac markers will help differentiate unstable angina from non-Q wave myocardial infarction in patients with ST segment depression.

To a certain extent, the findings noted on the EKG can predict the location of the infarct as well as the coronary artery involved, as shown in the following table.

Location of Infarction	EKG Leads	Coronary Artery
Extensive anterior	V1 - 6, I, aVL	Left main or proximal LAD
Anteroseptal	V1-3	LAD
Anterolateral	V4-6, I, aVL	LAD or left circumflex
High lateral	I, aVL	Obtuse marginal branch of left circumflex or diagonal of LAD
Inferior	II, III, aVF	Posterior descending artery (80%) or left circumflex (20%)
Right ventricular	Right precordial leads (ie, V4R)	Right coronary artery

Adapted from Chizner M, *Classic Teachings in Cardiology*, Cedar Grove, NJ: Laennec Publishing, 1996, 859.

Aortic Dissection

In 33% of patients with aortic dissection, the EKG may be normal. Another 33% of patients will have findings consistent with left ventricular hypertrophy.

In up to 2% of cases, dissection involving the ostium of a coronary artery may result in an acute myocardial infarction. When acute myocardial infarction does occur in the setting of aortic dissection, not uncommonly, the manifestations of the myocardial infarction overshadow that of the aortic dissection. This can lead to a catastrophic outcome if thrombolytic therapy is administered. For this reason, aortic dissection must be considered in every patient with myocardial infarction prior to the administration of thrombolytic therapy, particularly if the patient has suffered an inferior myocardial infarction (ischemic changes in the inferior leads are more common because dissection has a predilection to involve the right coronary artery).

Pulmonary Embolism

EKG abnormalities are present in 87% of patients with pulmonary embolism. The EKG abnormalities may be suggestive but are never diagnostic of pulmonary embolism. Tachycardia and nonspecific EKG findings are the most common abnormalities noted. Other findings that may be appreciated are listed in the following table.

EKG Abnormalities Noted in Pulmonary Embolism	
Tachycardia	P. pulmonale
Nonspecific ST-T wave abnormalities	SIQIIITIII pattern*
Right axis deviation	Atrial fibrillation
Right bundle branch block	Normal

*Refers to deep S wave in lead I and Q wave and T wave inversion in lead III.

Pneumothorax

On occasion, patients with pneumothorax, particularly the spontaneous type, may present with EKG abnormalities mimicking that seen in patients with anterior myocardial infarctions. In these cases, the R waves may be absent in the precordial leads.

Proceed to Step 7

STEP 7: *Are There Any Findings on the Chest Radiograph That Point to a Serious Cause of the Chest Pain?*

In this step, chest radiographic findings that should prompt consideration of the serious causes of chest pain are discussed.

Unstable Angina / Acute Myocardial Infarction

Many patients with unstable angina or uncomplicated acute myocardial infarction have unremarkable chest radiographs. In most cases, the heart shadow is of normal size. An enlarged heart shadow should prompt the clinician to consider the following possibilities:

- Severe coronary artery disease with prior myocardial infarction
- Coexisting valvular heart disease
- Concomitant nonischemic cardiomyopathy
- Hypertensive heart disease

Pulmonary vascular congestion may also be noted. In patients suspected of having unstable angina or acute myocardial infarction, the chest radiograph is also useful in excluding some of the other causes of chest pain. The chest radiograph may reveal abnormalities suggestive of aortic dissection, pneumothorax, pulmonary embolism, and other conditions.

Aortic Dissection

The chest radiograph will reveal abnormalities in approximately 85% of patients with aortic dissection. It is especially useful to compare the chest film with previous radiographs. Chest radiographic findings that suggest the presence of aortic dissection are listed in the following box.

Chest Radiographic Findings Suggestive of Aortic Dissection	
Aortic knob abnormalities	Esophageal deviation
Discrepancy in diameter of ascending and descending aorta compared to previous films	Increased aortic diameter
	Irregular aortic contour
	Left pleural effusion
Displacement of calcified intima	Mediastinal widening (80% to 90%)
Double density	Tracheal deviation

Even though the chest radiograph is abnormal in most patients with aortic dissection, rarely are the findings diagnostic for this condition. In addition, a normal chest radiograph should not prompt the clinician to discard this diagnosis. In fact, one study showed that the chest radiograph was unremarkable (normal or nonspecific findings) in up to 18% of patients with aortic dissection.

Pulmonary Embolism

Chest radiographic abnormalities are commonly encountered in patients with pulmonary embolism. Unfortunately, the findings are nonspecific. These findings are listed in the following box.

Chest Radiographic Findings Suggestive of Pulmonary Embolism	
Atelectasis	Normal†
Elevated hemidiaphragm*	Pleural effusion
Focal infiltrates	

*Nearly 50% of all patients will have an elevated hemidiaphragm at the time of presentation.

†At the time of presentation, normal chest radiographs are noted in approximately 30% of patients.

There are several radiographic findings that, although rare, are considered classic for pulmonary embolism. Westermark's sign refers to focal pulmonary oligemia. Hampton's hump, a finding suggestive of pulmonary infarction, is said to be present when a triangular, pleural-based density (with apex pointing to the hilum) is appreciated next to the diaphragm.

Pneumothorax

In patients with primary spontaneous pneumothorax, the chest radiograph usually confirms the diagnosis. On occasion, the chest radiograph may be unrevealing in the patient suspected of having pneumothorax. In these cases, the clinician may wish to obtain a chest radiograph in complete expiration. This film will make the pneumothorax more apparent.

Secondary spontaneous pneumothorax can also be confirmed by chest radiography. In patients with tension pneumothorax, the acuity of the presentation does not usually allow the clinician to confirm the diagnosis by obtaining a chest film. In these cases, the clinician often has to treat the patient presumptively because a delay in treatment may adversely affect the patient's outcome. If obtained, the chest radiograph will reveal complete lung collapse along with mediastinal shift.

Esophageal Rupture

The key to the diagnosis of esophageal rupture is consideration of the diagnosis. If suspected, the clinician should obtain the following radiographs urgently:

- Posteroanterior chest
- Lateral chest
- Upright abdominal

Chest radiographic findings suggestive of esophageal perforation are listed in the following box.

Chest Radiographic Findings Suggestive of Esophageal Rupture	
Hydropneumothorax	Pneumomediastinum
Hydrothorax	Pneumoperitoneum
Normal*	Subcutaneous/mediastinal emphysema
Pleural effusions	Subdiaphragmatic air

*Normal chest radiographs have been reported early in the course of esophageal perforation.

If the patient has a pneumothorax, **Stop Here.**

If the patient's clinical presentation is suggestive of unstable angina or acute myocardial infarction, **Proceed to Step 8.**

If the patient's clinical presentation is suggestive of aortic dissection, **Proceed to Step 9.**

If the patient's clinical presentation is suggestive of pulmonary embolism, **Proceed to Step 10.**

If the patient's clinical presentation is suggestive of esophageal perforation, **Proceed to Step 11.**

STEP 8: *Does the Patient Have Unstable Angina or Acute Myocardial Infarction?*

Measurement of the cardiac markers is essential in differentiating between unstable angina and acute myocardial infarction. Cardiac markers available to the clinician include the following:

- Creatine kinase (MB isozyme or CK-MB)
- Troponin
- Myoglobin

These cardiac markers are discussed in further detail in the remainder of this step.

Creatine Kinase

In most cases of acute myocardial infarction, increased CK-MB levels are noted 4-8 hours after symptom onset. Increased levels are seen in almost all patients by twelve hours after symptom onset. After peaking at about 24 hours, CK-MB levels return to normal by 72 hours.

Although CK-MB levels are fairly specific for the heart, it is present, albeit in small quantities, in noncardiac tissue. Therefore, false positive elevations may occur in noncardiac conditions. Furthermore, myocardial cell death not due to ischemic injury can also result in elevations of the CK-MB.

Troponin

The cardiac troponins (T or I) have been found to be more specific than CK-MB for heart injury. After myocardial injury, troponin levels rise at about the same time CK-MB levels rise. In contrast to CK-MB levels which return to normal within 3-4 days after symptom onset, troponin levels often remain elevated for up to two weeks. This longer duration of elevation allows the clinician to make the diagnosis of myocardial infarction when patients present several days after symptom onset.

Myoglobin

Since both cardiac and skeletal muscle contain large amounts of myoglobin, the use of myoglobin in the diagnosis of acute myocardial infarction lacks specificity. However, it is a sensitive marker of myocardial infarction. The absence of myoglobin elevation six hours after symptom onset strongly argues against the presence of an acute myocardial infarction.

Key information regarding these cardiac markers is summarized in the following table.

	Myoglobin	Troponin I	Troponin T	CK-MB
First Detected (Hours)	1-2	2-4	2-4	3-4
100% Sensitivity (Hours)	4-8	8-12	8-12	8-12
Peak (Hours)	4-8	10-24	10-24	10-24
Duration (Days)	0.5-1	5-10	5-14	2-4

Adapted from Adams JE, Abendschein DR, and Jaffe AS, "Biochemical Markers of Myocardial Injury: Is MB Creatine Kinase the Choice for the 1990s?" *Circulation*, 1993, 88(2):750-63 (review).

As mentioned earlier, the separation of non-Q wave myocardial infarction from unstable angina requires measurement of the cardiac markers of injury. Elevations of the cardiac markers in the patient presenting with a history and EKG findings compatible with acute myocardial infarction establishes the diagnosis of acute myocardial infarction. The clinician should realize, however, that 33% of patients with unstable angina will have elevated troponin levels but normal CK-MB levels.

End of Section.

STEP 9: *Does the Patient Have Aortic Dissection?*

For years aortography was considered the gold standard in the diagnosis of aortic dissection. With the advent of newer imaging techniques, it is now known that the sensitivity of aortography is not as high as was initially thought. Other techniques that have supplanted aortography include CT scanning, MRI, and transesophageal echocardiography. The sensitivity and specificity of these studies are listed in the following table.

Diagnostic Imaging Technique	Sensitivity (%)	Specificity (%)
Aortography	80-90	90-100
CT scanning	79-93	86-100
MRI	Nearly 100	Nearly 100
Transesophageal echocardiography (TEE)	92-100	82-95

Each of the above diagnostic techniques has advantages and disadvantages in establishing the diagnosis of aortic dissection, as shown in the following table.

Advantage	Aortography	CT	MRI	TEE
Readily available	Fairly	Quite	Fairly	Very
Rapid	Fairly	Quite	Fairly	Very
Performed at patient's bedside	No	No	No	Yes
Iodinated I.V. contrast	Yes	Yes	No	No
Cost	High	Reasonable	Moderate	Reasonable

Adapted from *Cardiology*, Crawford MH and DiMarco JP (eds), St Louis, MO: Mosby, 2001, 1.12.6.

In clinical practice, most hospitals perform CT or TEE in patients suspected of having aortic dissection. Although MRI has excellent sensitivity and specificity in the diagnosis, concerns regarding patient safety and the inability to perform the test in patients with pacemakers and metallic valves has limited it use. Aortography is now seldom performed but should be considered if the diagnosis remains uncertain despite performance of the noninvasive tests. Because none of the tests have 100% sensitivity and specificity, the clinician should consider repeat imaging or the performance of a complementary test if the initial imaging test chosen is not consistent with aortic dissection, especially if clinical suspicion for aortic dissection is high.

End of Section.

STEP 10: *Does the Patient Have Pulmonary Embolism?*

Laboratory test abnormalities that have been appreciated in patients with pulmonary embolism are listed in the following box.

Laboratory Test Abnormalities Noted in Pulmonary Embolism	
Leukocytosis*	Arterial hypoxemia#
Elevated liver function tests	Arterial hypocapnia#
Polycythemia†	Positive plasma D-dimer§
Thrombocytopenia/thrombocytosis‡	

*The white blood cell count may be elevated to as high as 20 x 10^9 cells/L. A normal white blood cell count, however, is not uncommon.

†Pulmonary embolism does not lead to an increase in the hemoglobin/hematocrit. Polycythemia is, however, a well recognized risk factor for venous thromboembolism.

‡Most patients with pulmonary embolism have normal platelet counts. Thrombocytosis is a risk factor for pulmonary embolism (ie, essential thrombocytosis). Thrombocytopenia should raise concern for the possibility of heparin-induced thrombosis.

#In the past, arterial blood gas analysis revealing arterial hypoxemia and hypocapnia were considered hallmarks of pulmonary embolism. The PIOPED study showed that many patients with pulmonary embolism have normal PaO_2 and $PaCO_2$ levels. The alveolar-arterial oxygen difference also has limited utility in the diagnosis of pulmonary embolism.

§A positive D-dimer test is present in most patients with pulmonary embolism. However, the test is not specific, with positive test results being appreciated in many different conditions including acute myocardial infarction, pneumonia, and other systemic diseases. Therefore, a positive result provides very little diagnostic information in the diagnosis of pulmonary embolism. The test does, however, have an excellent negative predictive value (99%). A negative test result performed by ELISA argues strongly against the diagnosis of pulmonary embolism. Latex agglutination based D-dimer testing is also available but is less reliable.

Other tests available in establishing the diagnosis of pulmonary embolism are discussed below.

Ultrasonographic Examination of the Lower Extremities

The premise behind performing ultrasound of the lower extremities in patients with pulmonary embolism is that most emboli originate within the deep venous system of the lower extremities. When a patient with suspected pulmonary embolism is found to have a deep venous thrombosis, further evaluation is unnecessary as the patient can be considered to have pulmonary embolism. It is reasonable to perform testing for deep venous thrombosis even when symptoms and signs of deep venous thrombosis are absent.

It is important to realize, however, that ultrasonographic examination of the lower extremities may be unremarkable in up to 66% of all patients with pulmonary embolism. One possible reason for this is that the entire thrombus may have embolized. Although venography studies are positive in nearly 70% of patients with pulmonary embolism, the invasiveness of the procedure and need for intravenous contrast limits its performance on a more widespread basis.

Ventilation-Perfusion Scanning of the Lungs (V/Q Scan)

Ventilation-perfusion scanning of the lungs should be performed in patients suspected of having pulmonary embolism, particularly when no other diagnosis for the patient's chest pain has been found. The PIOPED trial classified the results of ventilation-perfusion scanning into four possible groups:

- High probability
- Intermediate probability
- Low probability
- Normal

Intermediate and low probability scans are considered nondiagnostic. Unfortunately, most patients with pulmonary embolism have nondiagnostic scans, as shown in the following table.

Ventilation-Perfusion Results of PIOPED Study

V/Q Classification of Patients Who Had Angiography	Likelihood of Positive Angiogram (%)	Percent of all PE Cases with this Pattern (%)
High probability	88	41
Nondiagnostic	26	57
(formerly intermediate)	30	41
(formerly low)	16	16
Normal perfusion*	9	2

*Based on this data, a normal perfusion scan will miss about 2% of PE cases. Therefore, a normal ventilation-perfusion scan does not definitively exclude pulmonary embolism, but, in the absence of high clinical suspicion, provides a strong argument against the diagnosis. Many clinicians choose not to pursue further evaluation in patients with normal ventilation-perfusion scans.

The clinician should recognize several pitfalls in the use of the ventilation-perfusion scan. Although universal criteria for the interpretation of ventilation-perfusion scans have been proposed, not all radiologists agree upon these proposed criteria. In addition, errors in interpretation may occur with radiologists who are not experienced in the reading of these scans.

It is also important to realize that the results of the ventilation-perfusion scan should always be interpreted in light of the clinical suspicion for pulmonary embolism. It is this combination that should be used to guide further evaluation. When the clinical likelihood for pulmonary embolism is high, a high probability scan provides strong evidence for the diagnosis, often obviating the need for a more definitive test such as pulmonary angiography. When the clinical likelihood for pulmonary embolism is low, a normal scan strongly argues against the diagnosis of pulmonary embolism. Angiography, if performed in this group, will be negative in 95% of patients. Although a normal scan does not exclude the diagnosis, in the presence of a low clinical likelihood for pulmonary embolism, it should prompt the clinician to consider other possibilities for the patient's symptoms.

CT Scan

Spiral CT scan has been shown to have moderate to high sensitivity in the detection of emboli in the main, lobar, or segmental vessels. Furthermore, it is quite specific in the diagnosis. Subsegmental emboli, however, may not be visualized with spiral CT scan.

Transthoracic Echocardiography

In the patient presenting with signs and symptoms compatible with pulmonary embolism, echocardiographic findings of right ventricular hypokinesis and/or dilatation provides support for the diagnosis of pulmonary embolism, particularly when these findings cannot be explained by another disease process. These findings are more typical of massive pulmonary embolism and may be absent in minor events. The clinician should realize, however, that other conditions such as acute COPD exacerbations may present with similar findings.

Although an uncommon finding, echocardiographic demonstration of thrombus in the right atrium, ventricle, or proximal pulmonary artery argues strongly for the diagnosis of pulmonary embolism.

Pulmonary Angiography

Although it is an invasive test, pulmonary angiography remains the most reliable test for the diagnosis of pulmonary embolism. Findings consistent with pulmonary embolism include the following:

- Intraluminal filling defect
- Blockage of flow (dye cut-off)

The absence of these findings should prompt the clinician to determine if the procedure was performed properly. It is important to ensure that the entire pulmonary arterial tree was well visualized. Even an adequately performed pulmonary angiogram, however, may miss emboli present in very small arteries.

Pulmonary embolism is diagnosed with almost 100% certainty when the angiogram reveals one or both of the findings listed above. When the angiogram is negative, pulmonary embolism can be excluded with over 90% certainty.

The following table summarizes the advantages and disadvantages of the imaging methods currently used in the diagnosis of pulmonary embolism.

Feature	Transthoracic Echocardiography	V/Q Scan	Pulmonary Angiography	Spiral CT Scan
Widely available	+++	+++	++	++
Noninvasive	+++	++	—	++
Low interobserver variability	++	++	++	++
Well tolerated	+++	++	+	++
Detects massive PE	+++	++	+++	+++
Detects peripheral PE	—	+	+++	++
Low cost	+++	++	+	+

+++ very good; ++ satisfactory; + poor; — does not apply

Adapted from *Cardiology*, Crawford MH and DiMarco JP (eds), St Louis, MO: Mosby, 2001, 5.18.7.

End of Section.

STEP 11: *Does the Patient Have Esophageal Perforation?*

Plain radiographs should be followed by gastrograffin and/or barium esophagography in patients suspected of having esophageal perforation. It is recommended that these studies be performed in both the upright and lateral decubitus positions. In cases where the clinician suspects free perforation into the lung or a thoracoesophageal fistula, many experts recommend not using barium because of the risk of mediastinal inflammation. In patients at high risk for aspiration, barium is preferred over gastrograffin because the latter has been implicated in the development of pulmonary edema.

It is important to realize that a negative gastrograffin study in the patient with signs and symptoms suggestive of esophageal perforation does not exclude the diagnosis. In these cases, the clinician should consider performing barium studies. Even when both procedures are performed, there is a false-negative rate between 10% and 36%. CT scan may be performed in these cases or when gastrograffin and barium studies cannot be done. Thoracentesis is another option available to the clinician. Pleural fluid analysis revealing any of the following features is strongly suggestive of esophageal perforation:

- Acidic pH
- Elevated salivary amylase
- Undigested food
- Purulent foul-smelling material

REFERENCES

Adams JE, Abendschein DR, and Jaffe AS, "Biochemical Markers of Myocardial Injury: Is MB Creatine Kinase the Choice for the 1990s?" *Circulation*, 1993, 88(2):750-63 (review).

Anderson DR and Wells PS, "D-Dimer for the Diagnosis of Venous Thromboembolism," *Curr Opin Hematol*, 2000, 7(5):296-301.

Autore C, Agati L, Piccininno M, et al, "Role of Echocardiography in Acute Chest Pain Syndrome," *Am J Cardiol*, 2000, 86(4A):41G-42G.

Barton ED, "Tension Pneumothorax," *Curr Opin Pulm Med*, 1999, 5(4):269-74.

Braverman AC, "Aortic Dissection," *Curr Opin Cardiol*, 1997, 12(4):389-90.

Chizner M, *Classic Teachings in Cardiology*, Cedar Grove, NJ: Laennec Publishing, 1996, 859.

"Clinical Policy: Critical Issues in the Evaluation and Management of Adult Patients Presenting With Suspected Acute Myocardial Infarction or Unstable Angina. American College of Emergency Physicians," *Ann Emerg Med*, 2000, 35(5):521-5.

Cardiology, Crawford MH and DiMarco JP (eds), St Louis, MO: Mosby, 2001, 1.12.6.

deFilippi CR and Runge MS, "Evaluating the Chest Pain Patient. Scope of the Problem," *Cardiol Clin*, 1999, 17(2):307-26.

Dmowski AT and Carey MJ, "Aortic Dissection," *Am J Emerg Med*, 1999, 17(4):372-5.

Kline JA, Johns KL, Colucciello SA, et al, "New Diagnostic Tests for Pulmonary Embolism," *Ann Emerg Med*, 2000, 35(2):168-80.

Kontos MC and Jesse RL, "Evaluation of the Emergency Department Chest Pain Patient," *Am J Cardiol*, 2000, 85(5A):32B-39B.

Lee TH and Goldman L, "Evaluation of the patient With Acute Chest Pain," *N Engl J Med*, 2000, 342(16):1187-95.

Lemke T and Jagminas L, "Spontaneous Esophageal Rupture: A Frequently Missed Diagnosis," *Am Surg*, 1999, 65(5):449-52.

Ma G and Jacoby I, "Spontaneous Esophageal Rupture," *J Emerg Med*, 2000, 18(2):257-8.

Penttila I, Penttila K, and Rantanen T, "Laboratory Diagnosis of Patients With Acute Chest Pain," *Clin Chem Lab Med*, 2000, 38(3):187-97.

Pretre R and Von Segesser LK, "Aortic Dissection," *Lancet*, 1997, 349(9063):1461-4.

Reeder GS, "Contemporary Diagnosis and Management of Unstable Angina," *Mayo Clin Proc*, 2000, 75(9):953-7.

Riedel M, "Acute Pulmonary Embolism 1: Pathophysiology, Clinical Presentation, and Diagnosis," *Heart*, 2001, 85(2):229-40.

Sahn SA and Heffner JE, "Spontaneous Pneumothorax," *N Engl J Med*, 2000, 342(12):868-74.

"The Urokinase Pulmonary Embolism Trial: A National Cooperative Study," *Circulation*, 1973, 47(2 Suppl):II1-108.

"Urokinase-Streptokinase Embolism Trial: Phase 2 Results. A Cooperative Study," *JAMA*, 1974, 229(12):1606-13.

CHEST PAIN (ACUTE)

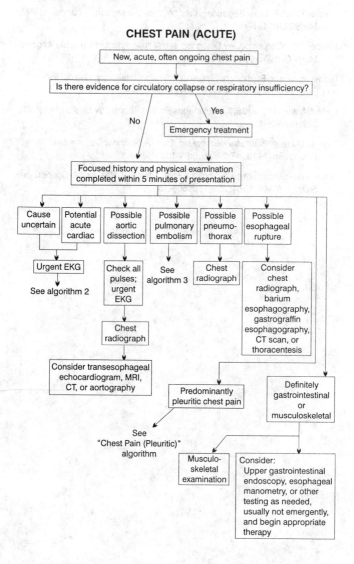

New, acute, often ongoing chest pain

Is there evidence for circulatory collapse or respiratory insufficiency?

Yes → Emergency treatment

No

Focused history and physical examination completed within 5 minutes of presentation

- Cause uncertain → Urgent EKG → See algorithm 2
- Potential acute cardiac
- Possible aortic dissection → Check all pulses; urgent EKG → Chest radiograph → Consider transesophageal echocardiogram, MRI, CT, or aortography
- Possible pulmonary embolism → See algorithm 3
- Possible pneumothorax → Chest radiograph
- Possible esophageal rupture → Consider chest radiograph, barium esophagography, gastrograffin esophagography, CT scan, or thoracentesis

Predominantly pleuritic chest pain → See "Chest Pain (Pleuritic)" algorithm

Definitely gastrointestinal or musculoskeletal

- Musculoskeletal examination
- Consider: Upper gastrointestinal endoscopy, esophageal manometry, or other testing as needed, usually not emergently, and begin appropriate therapy

Modified and adapted with permission from Goldman L, "Chest Discomfort and Palpitation," *Harrison's Principles of Internal Medicine,* 14th ed, Fauci AS, Braunwald E, Isselbacher KI, et al (eds), New York, NY: McGraw-Hill, 1998, 61.

CHEST PAIN (ACUTE)
(continued)

(Algorithm 2)

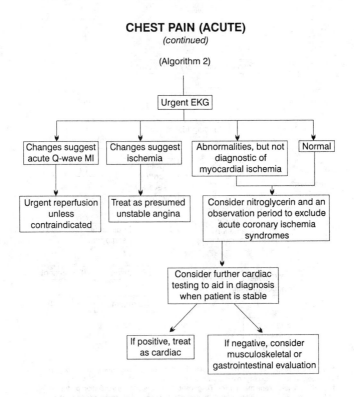

Modified and adapted with permission from Goldman L, "Chest Discomfort and Palpitation," *Harrison's Principles of Internal Medicine*, 14th ed, Fauci AS, Braunwald E, Isselbacher KI, et al (eds), New York, NY: McGraw-Hill, 1998, 61.

CHEST PAIN (ACUTE)
(continued)

(Algorithm 3)

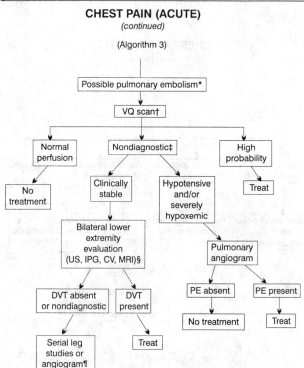

*When PE is suspected and the risk of bleeding deemed low, it is appropriate to begin anticoagulation while diagnostic testing is underway.

†A perfusion scan alone may suffice. Diagnostic alternatives to the ventilation perfusion (VQ) scan, include spiral computed tomography (CT) and magnetic resonance imaging (MRI). These are being used increasingly, and also require institutional and reader expertise and further validation in well designed trials.

‡Patients with low probability VQ scans and low clinical suspicion are unlikely to have PE. Others require further evaluation. There are several options when the VQ scan (or spiral CT or lung MRI) is nondiagnostic. Pulmonary angiography is the appropriate approach if the patient is unstable. Otherwise, leg studies can be performed. If spiral CT or lung MRI is performed, a negative result should be interpreted together with the level of clinical suspicion. Although these techniques appear to be sensitive, additional studies (pulmonary angiography or leg studies) should be performed as deemed appropriate.

§A positive test is useful. The sensitivity for compression ultrasound (US) and impedance plethysmography (IPG) is low in asymptomatic patients, and negative or nondiagnostic studies require additional data. MRI appears sensitive in this setting, but no level 1 data exists. The role of D-dimer testing in clinical algorithms is not clearly established, but recent data from a few centers suggest that the sensitivity of certain assays may help exclude VTE when combined with other diagnostic test results. General recommendations that can be extrapolated to all centers cannot be made at present.

¶Negative serial IPG in this setting has been associated with excellent outcome without anticoagulation at certain centers.

Adapted with permission from "The Diagnostic Approach to Acute Venous Thromboembolism," *Am J Respir Crit Care Med*, 1999, 160(3):1043-66.

CHEST PAIN (PLEURITIC)

STEP 1: *Does the Patient Have Pleuritic Chest Pain?*

Pleuritic chest pain is defined as pain that is worsened or precipitated by inspiration. The typical features of pleuritic chest pain are listed in the following box.

Typical Features of Pleuritic Chest Pain	
Worsened or precipitated by inspiration	"Sticking" or "stabbing"
	Brief, shallow respirations
Sharp	

If the patient does not have pleuritic chest pain, proceed to the chapter on Chest Pain (Acute) *on page 53.*

If the patient has pleuritic chest pain, ***Proceed to Step 2.***

STEP 2: *What are the Causes of Pleuritic Chest Pain?*

The causes of pleuritic chest pain are listed in the following box.

Causes of Pleuritic Chest Pain	
Abdominal abscess	Pericarditis*
Intrahepatic	Pleuritis*
Subdiaphragmatic	Pneumonia*
Chest wall pain*	Pneumothorax*
Connective tissue disease	Postpericardiotomy syndrome
Dressler's syndrome	Pulmonary embolism*
Drug-induced	Tuberculosis
Malignancy	

*Common cause

Proceed to Step 3

STEP 3: *Are There Any Clues in the Patient's History That Point to the Etiology of the Pleuritic Chest Pain?*

Clues in the patient's history that point to the etiology of the patient's pleuritic chest pain are listed in the following table.

Historical Clue	Condition Suggested
Pain worse when lying down Pain relieved with sitting up	Pericarditis
Risk factors for pulmonary embolism	Pulmonary embolism
Pain with movement of chest	Chest wall pain
History of connective tissue disease	Connective tissue disease (eg, SLE, rheumatoid arthritis)
Skin rash Arthritis Raynaud's phenomenon	Connective tissue disease (eg, SLE, rheumatoid arthritis)
History of cancer	Primary lung cancer Bronchopleural fistula Pericarditis (malignant) Pulmonary embolism Esophageal rupture due to esophageal cancer
History of recent cardiac surgery or trauma	Postpericardiotomy syndrome
History of recent MI	Dressler's syndrome Pulmonary embolism
Medication history	Drug-induced (eg, hydralazine, procainamide, nitrofurantoin, methysergide)
Postoperative	Pulmonary embolism Chest wall pain (incisional) Atelectasis predisposing to pneumonia
Post-thoracotomy	Chest wall pain (incisional) Empyema Bronchopleural fistula
Abdominal surgery	Intra-abdominal abscess Empyema (with upper quadrant surgery)
Hemoptysis	Pulmonary embolism Pneumonia Tuberculosis
Recent chest trauma	Rib fracture Other conditions associated with chest trauma
Young individual with no medical problems	Viral pleurisy Pneumonia Chest wall pain Pericarditis
Intravenous drug abuse	Infective endocarditis with septic emboli

Proceed to Step 4

STEP 4: *Are There Any Clues in the Patient's Physical Examination That Point to the Etiology of the Pleuritic Chest Pain?*

Clues in the patient's physical examination that point to the etiology of the patient's pleuritic chest pain are listed in the following table.

Physical Examination Finding	Condition Suggested
Fever	Nonspecific
High fever with shaking chills	Pneumonia Pericarditis (purulent) Tuberculosis Empyema Subphrenic abscess
Pericardial friction rub	Pericarditis
Decreased breath sounds Hyperresonance to percussion	Pneumothorax
Pleural friction rub	Pleuritis
Lower extremity tenderness confined to the calf muscles or over the course of the deep veins Lower extremity edema, principally unilateral	Deep venous thrombosis (pulmonary embolism)
Arthritis	Connective tissue disease

Proceed to Step 5

STEP 5: *Is the Pleuritic Chest Pain Due to a Life-Threatening Condition?*

Although most cases of pleuritic chest pain are due to benign conditions, the clinician must ensure that a potentially life-threatening cause is not present. The life-threatening causes of pleuritic chest pain include the following:

- Pulmonary embolism
- Pneumothorax
- Pericarditis
- Pneumonia

In the remainder of this step, the key elements in the history and physical examination that should prompt consideration of these serious causes are considered.

Pulmonary Embolism

Over 600,000 cases of pulmonary embolism occur every year in the United States. Because the symptoms and signs of pulmonary embolism are nonspecific, in many of these cases, the diagnosis is missed, only to be made at the time of autopsy.

Most often, pulmonary embolism develops when thrombi travel from the deep venous system to the pulmonary arterial tree, causing obstruction of blood flow. Approximately 70% of patients have a clot that can be demonstrated in the lower extremities by venography. Although most cases are due to thrombi originating in the deep venous system of the lower extremities, approximately 10% are thought to arise elsewhere. The majority of these originate in the upper extremity veins, especially in patients with indwelling central venous catheters.

In many cases, risk factors for venous thromboembolism are present. These risk factors are considered in the following box.

Risk Factors for Deep Venous Thrombosis and Pulmonary Embolism	
Acute myocardial infarction	Lupus anticoagulant
Antithrombin III deficiency	Malignancy
Behcet's disease	Obesity
Congestive heart failure	Oral contraceptive use
Dysfibrinogenemia	Polycythemia vera
Essential thrombocytosis	Postoperative
Estrogen replacement (high dose)	Postpartum
Hemolytic anemia	Pregnancy
Heparin-induced thrombocytopenia	Protein C deficiency
History of deep venous thrombosis	Protein S deficiency
History of pulmonary embolism	Resistance to activated protein C
Homocysteinuria	Trauma
Immobilization	Venography
Indwelling central venous catheters	Venous pacemakers

The classic triad of dyspnea, chest pain, and hemoptysis is seen in <20% of patients. No features of the chest pain are diagnostic for pulmonary embolism. While some patients present with pleuritic chest pain, others may manifest with a retrosternal heaviness that mimics what is considered classic for acute myocardial infarction. Symptoms encountered in patients proven to have pulmonary embolism by angiography are listed in the following table.

Symptom	Percent (%)
Dyspnea	93
Chest pain, pleuritic	74
Apprehension	59
Cough	53
Hemoptysis	30
Sweating	27
Chest pain, nonpleuritic	14
Syncope	13

Adapted from "The Urokinase Pulmonary Embolism Trial: A National Cooperative Study," *Circulation*, 1973, 47(2 Suppl):II1-108; also from "Urokinase-Streptokinase Embolism Trial: Phase 2 Results," *JAMA*, 1974, 229(12):1606-13.

Signs present in those proven to have pulmonary embolism by angiography are listed in the following table.

Sign	Percent (%)
Tachypnea >16/minute	92
Rales	58
Accentuated second heart sound	53
Tachycardia >100/minute	44
Fever >37.8°C	43
Diaphoresis	36
S3 or S4 gallop	34
Thrombophlebitis	32

(continued)

Sign	Percent (%)
Lower extremity edema	24
Cardiac murmur	23
Cyanosis	19

Adapted from "The Urokinase Pulmonary Embolism Trial: A National Cooperative Study," *Circulation*, 1973, 47(2 Suppl):II1-108; also from "Urokinase-Streptokinase Embolism Trial: Phase 2 Results," *JAMA*, 1974, 229(12):1606-13.

Because the signs and symptoms of pulmonary embolism are nonspecific, further evaluation is certainly indicated, especially in the setting of risk factors for venous thromboembolism. The clinician should realize, however, that not all patients have an apparent predisposition at the time of diagnosis.

Pneumothorax

Pneumothorax is defined as the presence of free air between the visceral and parietal pleura. The causes of pneumothorax can be categorized into spontaneous and iatrogenic types, as shown in the following box.

Causes of Pneumothorax	
Spontaneous	
Primary	
Secondary	
Asthma	Interstitial lung disease
Chronic obstructive pulmonary disease	Lymphangioleiomyomatosis
Cystic fibrosis	Marfan syndrome
Histiocytosis X	Pleural malignancy
Infection	Sarcoidosis
Bacterial	Trauma
Pneumocystis carinii pneumonia	Tuberous sclerosis
Tuberculosis	
Iatrogenic	
Chest compression	Positive pressure ventilation
Intercostal nerve block	Subclavian cannulation
Needle aspiration (lung biopsy)	Transbronchial biopsy

The typical patient who develops a primary spontaneous pneumothorax is a young male smoker between 20-40 years of age. Although not all patients are symptomatic, most describe the sudden onset of unilateral chest pain (often pleuritic) and shortness of breath. The symptoms of secondary spontaneous pneumothorax are essentially the same. In contrast to primary spontaneous pneumothorax, these patients can precipitously decline because the pneumothorax occurs in the setting of an existing pulmonary disease. This underlying pulmonary disease limits these patients' pulmonary reserve.

When mediastinal shift and compression of the contralateral lung occurs because of the progressive accumulation of air under pressure, a tension pneumothorax is said to be present. The symptoms of tension pneumothorax are similar to that encountered in uncomplicated spontaneous pneumothorax but may be exaggerated.

Physical examination findings consistent with primary spontaneous pneumothorax include hyperresonance to percussion and decreased breath sounds. The signs of secondary spontaneous pneumothorax are the same. In some of these patients, however, the underlying lung disease (eg, COPD) may mask some of the physical examination findings of pneumothorax (eg, breath sounds may be reduced in both pneumothorax and COPD).

Patients with tension pneumothorax usually appear quite ill and may be noted to be in severe cardiovascular and respiratory distress. These patients are often agitated, restless, and cyanotic. Vital signs may reveal tachycardia, tachypnea, and hypotension. The hallmarks of tension pneumothorax include jugular venous distention, absent breath sounds on the ipsilateral side, and hyperresonance to percussion. It is important to realize that hypotension is not invariably present, especially in those who are presenting early in the disease course.

Pericarditis

Pericarditis should clearly be a consideration in patients who describe pleuritic chest pain that is worse when recumbent and better when sitting up. The pain is classically located in the retrosternal region. Not uncommonly, there is radiation of the pain to the neck or shoulder. Particularly characteristic of pericarditis is pain over the trapezius ridge. The causes of acute pericarditis are listed in the following box.

Causes of Acute Pericarditis	
Aortic dissection	Malignancy#
Connective tissue disease	Medication-induced
Dressler's syndrome*	Myxedema
Idiopathic	Postmyocardial infarction
Infection	Radiation§
Bacterial†	Trauma
Fungal	Uremia
Tuberculosis‡	
Viral	
Other	

*Dressler's syndrome occurs weeks to months after a myocardial infarction. It needs to be differentiated from the pericarditis that occurs within the first week after a myocardial infarction (postmyocardial infarction pericarditis). Dressler's syndrome is characterized by fever, pericarditis, and pleuritis.

†Patients with bacterial pericarditis are usually acutely ill with signs and symptoms of a severe systemic infection.

‡Most patients with tuberculous pericarditis describe an insidious illness characterized by pleuritic chest pain, fever, cough, shortness of breath, night sweats, and weight loss.

#Cancers of the lung, breast, skin, leukemia, and lymphoma are the major considerations in patients with neoplastic pericarditis.

§Acute radiation pericarditis typically occur with irradiation of a mediastinal tumor that is close to the pericardium. There is a delayed form of radiation pericarditis that usually occurs within one year of therapy. In these cases, it may be difficult to differentiate radiation pericarditis from that due to malignancy.

Physical examination may reveal the presence of a pericardial friction rub. Most pericardial friction rubs are biphasic or triphasic. The term "triphasic" refers to the presence of the rub during atrial systole, ventricular systole, and ventricular diastole. A minority of rubs are monophasic. When monophasic, it may be difficult to differentiate a rub from a murmur. The classic rub is described as scratchy, high-pitched, and grating in nature. It is important to realize, however, that the absence of a rub does not exclude the diagnosis. In fact, in many cases, the rub is intermittently present. It is also important to auscultate throughout the precordium as pericardial friction rubs may only be audible in certain areas.

Pneumonia

The reader is referred to Step 4 (history), Step 5 (physical examination), Step 6 (chest radiographic findings), and Step 7 in the "Shortness of Breath" chapter *on page 455* for further information regarding pneumonia.

If the history and physical examination are consistent with pulmonary embolism, pneumothorax, or pericarditis, ***Proceed to Step 6.***

If the history and physical examination are not consistent with pulmonary embolism, pneumothorax, pneumonia, or pericarditis, ***Proceed to Step 10.***

STEP 6: *What are the EKG Findings?*

In this step, the EKG findings that should prompt the clinician to consider pulmonary embolism, pneumothorax, or pericarditis are considered.

Pulmonary Embolism

EKG abnormalities are present in 87% of patients with pulmonary embolism. The EKG abnormalities may be suggestive but are never diagnostic of pulmonary embolism. Tachycardia and nonspecific EKG findings are the most common abnormalities noted. Other findings that may be appreciated are listed in the following table.

EKG Abnormalities Noted in Pulmonary Embolism	
Atrial fibrillation	Right axis deviation
Nonspecific ST-T wave abnormalities	Right bundle branch block
Normal	SIQIIITIII pattern*
P. pulmonale	Tachycardia

*Refers to deep S wave in lead I and Q wave and T wave inversion in lead III

Pneumothorax

On occasion, patients with pneumothorax, particularly the spontaneous type, may present with EKG abnormalities mimicking that seen in patients with anterior myocardial infarctions. In these cases, the R waves may be absent in the precordial leads.

Pericarditis

EKG abnormalities are identified in over 90% of patients with acute pericarditis. Diffuse ST segment elevation is the hallmark of acute pericarditis. It is important to realize, however, that ST segment elevation is not specific for acute pericarditis. Other causes of ST segment elevation include acute myocardial infarction, left ventricular aneurysm, and early repolarization.

If serial EKGs are obtained, many patients (50%) will have progression of EKG abnormalities through a series of stages. These stages are described in the following box.

Stages in the EKG Over Time in Patients With Acute Pericarditis
Stage I
ST elevation
Concave upward
In all leads except aVR and V1
Upright T waves
Stage II
ST segment returns to baseline
T wave flattening
Stage III*
T wave inversion
Stage IV†
T wave normalization

*In contrast to acute myocardial infarction, the ST segment elevation of acute pericarditis returns to baseline before T wave inversion occurs.

†In some patients, the T wave abnormalities may persist for weeks or months.

PR segment depression may also be appreciated in patients with acute pericarditis. Reduced voltage may be noted with large effusions. Although most patients have sinus tachycardia, this is a nonspecific finding. Other atrial arrhythmias are uncommon but, if present, should prompt consideration of underlying heart disease. Ventricular tachycardia, AV block, and bundle branch block are not typical features of pericarditis. The presence of these arrhythmias warrants consideration of myocardial ischemia or myocarditis.

Proceed to Step 7

STEP 7: *What are the Chest Radiographic Findings?*

In this step, the chest radiographic findings that should prompt consideration of pulmonary embolism, pneumothorax, and pericarditis are discussed.

Pulmonary Embolism

Chest radiographic abnormalities are commonly encountered in patients with pulmonary embolism. Unfortunately, the findings are nonspecific. These findings are listed in the following box.

Chest Radiographic Findings Suggestive of Pulmonary Embolism	
Atelectasis	Normal†
Elevated hemidiaphragm*	Pleural effusion
Focal infiltrates	

*Nearly 50% of all patients will have an elevated hemidiaphragm at the time of presentation.

†At the time of presentation, normal chest radiographs are noted in approximately 30% of patients.

There are several radiographic findings that, although rare, are considered classic for pulmonary embolism. Westermark's sign refers to focal pulmonary oligemia. Hampton's hump, a finding suggestive of pulmonary infarction, is said to be present when a triangular, pleural-based density (with apex pointing to the hilum) is appreciated next to the diaphragm.

Pneumothorax

In patients with primary spontaneous pneumothorax, the chest radiograph usually confirms the diagnosis. On occasion, the chest radiograph may be unrevealing in the patient suspected of having pneumothorax. In these cases, the clinician may wish to obtain a chest radiograph in complete expiration. This film will make the pneumothorax more apparent.

Secondary spontaneous pneumothorax can also be confirmed by chest radiography. In patients with tension pneumothorax, the acuity of the presentation does not usually allow the clinician to confirm the diagnosis by obtaining a chest film. In these cases, the clinician often has to treat the patient presumptively because a delay in treatment may adversely affect the patient's outcome. If obtained, the chest radiograph will reveal complete lung collapse along with mediastinal shift.

Pericarditis

Pericarditis that is accompanied by the accumulation of significant amounts of fluid may cause enlargement of the cardiac silhouette. Although a water bottle shape of the cardiac silhouette should prompt concern for a pericardial effusion, this finding is not specific and may be seen in patients with dilated cardiomyopathy. Separation of the epicardial fat pad from the outer border of the heart is a more specific sign and is better appreciated on the lateral chest radiograph. However, this sign is present in only 15% of patients with pericardial effusion.

Nearly 25% of patients with acute pericarditis have an associated pleural effusion. When present, the effusion is typically left-sided. The chest radiograph may also provide clues to the etiology of the acute pericarditis (eg, findings consistent with aortic dissection, tuberculosis, malignancy). In Dressler's syndrome, transient pulmonary infiltrates may be present.

If the patient has a pneumothorax, *Stop Here*.

If the initial evaluation is consistent with pulmonary embolism, *Proceed to Step 8.*

If the initial evaluation is consistent with pericarditis, *Proceed to Step 9.*

If the initial evaluation is not consistent with pulmonary embolism, pneumothorax, or pericarditis, *Proceed to Step 10.*

STEP 8: *Does the Patient Have Pulmonary Embolism?*

Laboratory test abnormalities that have been appreciated in patients with pulmonary embolism are listed in the following box.

Laboratory Test Abnormalities Noted in Pulmonary Embolism	
Leukocytosis*	Arterial hypoxemia#
Elevated liver function tests	Arterial hypocapnia#
Polycythemia†	+ plasma D-dimer§
Thrombocytopenia/thrombocytosis‡	

*The white blood cell count may be elevated to as high as 20 X 10^9 cells/L. A normal white blood cell count, however, is not uncommon.

†Pulmonary embolism does not lead to an increase in the hemoglobin/hematocrit. Polycythemia is, however, a well recognized risk factor for venous thromboembolism.

‡Most patients with pulmonary embolism have normal platelet counts. Thrombocytosis is a risk factor for pulmonary embolism (ie, essential thrombocytosis). Thrombocytopenia should raise concern for the possibility of heparin-induced thrombosis.

#In the past, arterial blood gas analysis revealing arterial hypoxemia and hypocapnia were considered hallmarks of pulmonary embolism. The PIOPED study showed that many patients with pulmonary embolism have normal PaO2 and PaCO2 levels. The alveolar-arterial oxygen difference also has limited utility in the diagnosis of pulmonary embolism.

§A positive D-dimer test is present in most patients with pulmonary embolism. However, the test is not specific, with positive test results being appreciated in many different conditions including acute myocardial infarction, pneumonia, and other systemic diseases. Therefore, a positive result provides very little diagnostic information in the diagnosis of pulmonary embolism. The test does, however, have an excellent negative predictive value (99%). A negative test result performed by ELISA argues strongly against the diagnosis of pulmonary embolism. Latex agglutination based D-dimer testing is also available but is less reliable.

Other tests available in establishing the diagnosis of pulmonary embolism are discussed below.

Ultrasonographic Examination of the Lower Extremities

The premise behind performing ultrasound of the lower extremities in patients with pulmonary embolism is that most emboli originate within the deep venous system of the lower extremities. When a patient with suspected pulmonary embolism is found to have a deep venous thrombosis, further evaluation is unnecessary as the patient can be considered to have pulmonary embolism. It is reasonable to perform testing for deep venous thrombosis even when symptoms and signs of deep venous thrombosis are absent.

It is important to realize, however, that ultrasonographic examination of the lower extremities may be unremarkable in up to 66% of all patients with pulmonary embolism. One possible reason for this is that the entire thrombus may have embolized. Although venography studies are positive in nearly 70% of patients with pulmonary embolism, the invasiveness of the procedure and need for intravenous contrast limits its performance on a more widespread basis.

Ventilation-Perfusion Scanning of the Lungs (V/Q Scan)

Ventilation-perfusion scanning of the lungs should be performed in patients suspected of having pulmonary embolism, particularly when no other diagnosis for the patient's chest pain has been found. The PIOPED trial classified the results of ventilation-perfusion scanning into four possible groups:

- High probability
- Intermediate probability
- Low probability
- Normal

Intermediate and low probability scans are considered nondiagnostic. Unfortunately, most patients with pulmonary embolism have nondiagnostic scans, as shown in the following table.

V/Q Classification of Patients Who Had Angiography	Likelihood of Positive Angiogram (%)	Percent of all PE Cases With This Pattern (%)
High probability	88	41
Nondiagnostic	26	57
(formerly intermediate)	30	41
(formerly low)	16	16
Normal perfusion*	9	2

*Based on this data, a normal perfusion scan will miss about 2% of PE cases. Therefore, a normal ventilation-perfusion scan does not definitively exclude pulmonary embolism, but, in the absence of high clinical suspicion, provides a strong argument against the diagnosis. Many clinicians choose not to pursue further evaluation in patients with normal ventilation-perfusion scans.

The clinician should recognize several pitfalls in the use of the ventilation-perfusion scan. Although universal criteria for the interpretation of ventilation-perfusion scans have been proposed, not all radiologists agree upon these proposed criteria. In addition, errors in interpretation may occur with radiologists who are not experienced in the reading of these scans.

It is also important to realize that the results of the ventilation-perfusion scan should always be interpreted in light of the clinical suspicion for pulmonary embolism. It is this combination that should be used to guide further evaluation. When the clinical likelihood for pulmonary embolism is high, a high probability scan provides strong evidence for the diagnosis, often obviating the need for a more definitive test such as pulmonary angiography. When the clinical likelihood for pulmonary embolism is low, a normal scan strongly argues against the diagnosis of pulmonary embolism. Angiography, if performed in this group, will be negative in 95% of patients. Although a normal scan does not exclude the diagnosis, in the presence of a low clinical likelihood for pulmonary embolism, it should prompt the clinician to consider other possibilities for the patient's symptoms.

CT Scan

Spiral CT scan has been shown to have moderate to high sensitivity in the detection of emboli in the main, lobar, or segmental vessels. Furthermore, it is quite specific in the diagnosis. Subsegmental emboli, however, may not be visualized with spiral CT scan.

Transthoracic Echocardiography

In the patient presenting with signs and symptoms compatible with pulmonary embolism, echocardiographic findings of right ventricular hypokinesis and/or dilatation provides support for the diagnosis of pulmonary embolism, particularly when these findings cannot be explained by another disease process. These findings are more typical of massive pulmonary embolism and may be absent in minor events. The clinician should realize, however, that other conditions such as acute COPD exacerbations may present with similar findings.

Although an uncommon finding, echocardiographic demonstration of thrombus in the right atrium, ventricle, or proximal pulmonary artery argues strongly for the diagnosis of pulmonary embolism.

Pulmonary Angiography

Although it is an invasive test, pulmonary angiography remains the most reliable test for the diagnosis of pulmonary embolism. Findings consistent with pulmonary embolism include the following:

- Intraluminal filling defect
- Blockage of flow (dye cut-off)

The absence of these findings should prompt the clinician to determine if the procedure was performed properly. It is important to ensure that the entire pulmonary arterial tree was well visualized. Even an adequately performed pulmonary angiogram, however, may miss emboli present in very small arteries.

Pulmonary embolism is diagnosed with almost 100% certainty when the angiogram reveals one or both of the findings listed above. When the angiogram is negative, pulmonary embolism can be excluded with over 90% certainty.

The following table summarizes the advantages and disadvantages of the imaging methods currently used in the diagnosis of pulmonary embolism.

Feature	Transthoracic Echocardiography	V/Q Scan	Pulmonary Angiography	Spiral CT Scan
Widely available	+++	+++	++	++
Noninvasive	+++	++	−	++
Low interobserver variability	++	++	++	++
Well tolerated	+++	++	+	++
Detects massive PE	+++	++	+++	+++
Detects peripheral PE	−	+	+++	++
Low cost	+++	++	+	+

+++ = very good; ++ = satisfactory; + = poor; − = does not apply

Adapted from *Cardiology*, Crawford MH and DiMarco JP (eds), 2001, St Louis, MO: Mosby Co, 5.18.7.

End of Section.

STEP 9: *What is the Etiology of the Acute Pericarditis?*

The diagnosis of acute pericarditis is established when characteristic EKG findings are present in a patient with signs and symptoms compatible with acute pericarditis. Once the diagnosis has been established, the clinician should focus efforts on the following:

- Identifying the cause of the acute pericarditis
- Performing an echocardiogram to identify patients with a pericardial effusion who may be at risk for hemodynamic compromise

Identifying the cause of the acute pericarditis requires a thorough history and physical examination. The clinical presentation may provide clues to the etiology which can then be confirmed by appropriate laboratory testing. Laboratory tests that may be indicated in the patient with acute pericarditis are listed in the following box.

Laboratory Tests That May Help to Establish the Etiology of the Acute Pericarditis	
ANA	Fungal serology
Antistreptolysin O	Heterophil antibodies
Blood cultures	HIV
BUN	Rheumatoid factor
Cold agglutinins	TSH
Creatinine	Viral serology (acute and convalescent sera)

Of note, CK-MB levels may be elevated in acute pericarditis. This may be due to myocarditis, myopericarditis, or ischemia.

Echocardiography is indicated for the detection and quantification of pericardial fluid. Although many patients will not have pericardial fluid demonstrated by echocardiography, it is necessary to identify those patients that do. These latter patients may be at increased risk for hemodynamic compromise (eg, cardiac tamponade). In these patients, serial echocardiography may be necessary.

End of Section.

STEP 10: *Does the Patient Have a Benign Cause of the Pleuritic Chest Pain?*

A clinical presentation that is not consistent with pulmonary embolism, pneumothorax, pneumonia, or pericarditis should prompt consideration of the benign causes of pleuritic chest pain. In particular, it is worthwhile to consider viral pleuritis and chest wall pain, two common causes of pleuritic chest pain. These conditions will be discussed in the remainder of this step.

Viral Pleuritis

Although individuals of all ages may develop viral pleuritis, it tends to be more common in young adults. The pleuritic chest pain is typically accompanied by other symptoms suggestive of a viral illness. These symptoms may include cough, chills, myalgias, arthralgias, malaise, fatigue, and headache. Fever, if present, is usually low-grade. Heart and lung examination is typically unremarkable. In some patients, a pleural friction rub may be appreciated.

Chest Wall Pain

Pleuritic chest pain that is clearly related to movement should prompt the clinician to consider chest wall pain. Chest wall or musculoskeletal pain may be the manifestation of a number of conditions including rib fracture and costochondritis. Tenderness to light palpation over the chest wall is characteristic. It is important to realize, however, that deep palpation can produce tenderness in patients with pleuritis.

If the patient clearly has chest wall pain, *Stop Here.*

If the patient does not have chest wall pain, *Proceed to Step 11.*

> ## STEP 11: *Does the Patient Have Viral Pleurisy or Pulmonary Embolism?*

It is not unusual for the patient with pleuritic chest pain whose clinical presentation is not suggestive of pulmonary embolism, pneumothorax, pneumonia, or pericarditis to be diagnosed presumptively with viral pleurisy. Several studies, however, have shown that clinical findings are not entirely reliable in differentiating pulmonary embolism from viral pleurisy based upon the history and physical examination. Most authorities agree that viral pleurisy should be a diagnosis of exclusion in the patient presenting with pleuritic chest pain.

One study examined the clinical presentation of patients with both pulmonary embolism and viral pleurisy. These investigators determined that pulmonary embolism was more likely if patients had any of the following clinical features:

- Risk factors for or history of venous thromboembolism
- Physical examination findings consistent with phlebitis
- Pleural effusion demonstrated on chest radiograph

In the presence of any of these clinical features, these investigators recommend further evaluation for pulmonary embolism.

If the patient has clinical features suggestive of pulmonary embolism, *Proceed to Step 5.*

If the patient does not have clinical features suggestive of pulmonary embolism or another disease associated with pleuritic chest pain, consider the diagnosis of idiopathic or viral pleurisy.

REFERENCES

Bone RC, *Pulmonary and Critical Care Medicine*, St Louis, MO: Mosby Yearbook, 1998.

Branch WT Jr and McNeil BJ, "Analysis of the Differential Diagnosis and Assessment of Pleuritic Chest Pain in Young Adults," *Am J Med*, 1983, 75:671-9.

Heart Disease: A Textbook of Cardiovascular Medicine, 5th ed, Braunwald E (ed), Philadelphia, PA: WB Saunders Co, 1997.

Principles and Practice of Infectious Diseases, 5th ed, Mandell GL, Bennett JE, and Dolin R (eds), Philadelphia, PA: Churchill Livingstone, 2000.

CHEST PAIN (PLEURITIC)

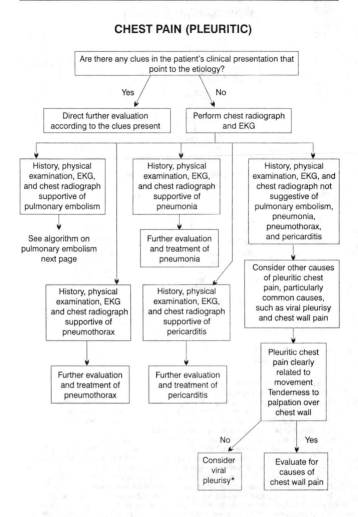

*Clinical findings from the history, physical examination, EKG, and chest radiograph are not entirely reliable in differentiating viral pleurisy from pulmonary embolism. Most authorities agree that viral pleurisy should be a diagnosis of exclusion in patients presenting with pleuritic chest pain. These patients should be evaluated for pulmonary embolism if any of the following criteria are met:
   - Risk factors for or history of venous thromboembolism
   - Physical examination findings consistent with phlebitis
   - Pleural effusion demonstrated on chest radiograph

CHEST PAIN (PLEURITIC)
(continued)

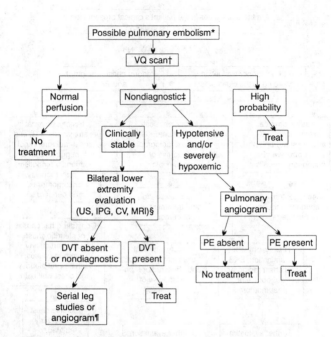

*When PE is suspected and the risk of bleeding deemed low, it is appropriate to begin
  anticoagulation while diagnostic testing is underway.
†A perfusion scan alone may suffice. Diagnostic alternatives to the ventilation perfusion
  (VQ) scan, include spiral computed tomography (CT) and magnetic resonance imaging
  (MRI). These are being used increasingly, and also require institutional and reader
  expertise and further validation in well designed trials.
‡Patients with low probability VQ scans and low clinical suspicion are unlikely to have PE.
  Others require further evaluation. There are several options when the VQ scan (or spiral
  CT or lung MRI) is nondiagnostic. Pulmonary angiography is the appropriate approach if
  the patient is unstable. Otherwise, leg studies can be performed. If spiral CT or lung MRI
  is performed, a negative result should be interpreted together with the level of clinical
  suspicion. Although these techniques appear to be sensitive, additional studies
  (pulmonary angiography or leg studies) should be performed as deemed appropriate.
§A positive test is useful. The sensitivity for compression ultrasound (US) and impedance
  plethysmography (IPG) is low in asymptomatic patients, and negative or nondiagnostic
  studies require additional data. MRI appears sensitive in this setting, but no level 1 data
  exists. The role of D-dimer testing in clinical algorithms is not clearly established, but
  recent data from a few centers suggest that the sensitivity of certain assays may help
  exclude VTE when combined with other diagnostic test results. General
  recommendations that can be extrapolated to all centers cannot be made at present.
¶Negative serial IPG in this setting has been associated with excellent outcome without
  anticoagulation at certain centers.

Adapted with permission from "The Diagnostic Approach to Acute Venous Thromboembolism,
Am J Respir Crit Care Med, 1999, 160(3):1043-66.

CONFUSION

STEP 1: *What Type of Confusion Does the Patient Have?*

Confusion is a commonly encountered problem, especially with advancing age. However, confusion is an imprecise term, meaning different things to different clinicians. While psychoses and affective disorders such as depression may present with confusion, the major considerations are delirium and dementia. This approach will focus on the identification of these disorders in the confused patient followed by a discussion on determining the etiology of the disorder.

Proceed to Step 2

STEP 2: *Does the Patient Have Delirium or Dementia?*

Delirium and dementia are the major causes of impaired cognition. The first step in the evaluation of the confused patient is to determine whether the patient has delirium or dementia. Recognition of these disorders will be discussed below followed by a summary table highlighting the key features that help to differentiate delirium from dementia.

Delirium

Delirium is a commonly encountered problem on the medical and surgical wards. It is estimated that delirium is present in up to 40% of older adults at the time of hospital admission. It may develop in another 25% to 60% during the hospitalization.

Too often, delirium is not diagnosed. In other cases, delirium is misdiagnosed. And in some cases, considerable time elapses before the diagnosis is made. In one study, delirium was not recognized by clinicians in 67% of the cases. In many of these instances, clinicians mistakenly felt that the change in cognition or behavior was due to the patient's age, dementia, or other mental condition.

It is essential for the clinician to recognize delirium because of its seriousness. In some patients, the mental status changes characteristic of delirium are the only symptoms of an underlying disease. The development of delirium prolongs the hospital stay, placing affected patients at higher risk of complications. The mortality rate increases significantly in patients with delirium, both in the hospital and after discharge. Complications of delirium that may have grave consequences for the patient are listed in the following box.

Complications of Delirium
Aspiration pneumonia
Decubitus ulcer
Deep venous thrombosis
Fracture
Injury from inappropriate removal
Arterial lines
Endotracheal tubes
Intravenous lines
Nasogastric tubes
Seizure
Subdural hematoma

Many patients with delirium die during the hospitalization, emphasizing the importance of appropriate management of these patients. This, however, requires the clinician to first recognize that delirium is truly present.

Criteria have been developed to aid the clinician in the diagnosis of delirium. Most widely used is the criteria from the Diagnostic and Statistical Manual of Mental Disorders (DSM IV), which are listed in the following box.

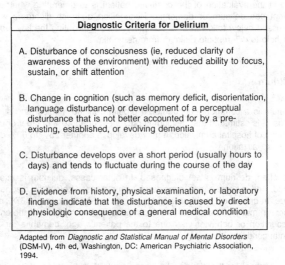

Diagnostic Criteria for Delirium

A. Disturbance of consciousness (ie, reduced clarity of awareness of the environment) with reduced ability to focus, sustain, or shift attention

B. Change in cognition (such as memory deficit, disorientation, language disturbance) or development of a perceptual disturbance that is not better accounted for by a pre-existing, established, or evolving dementia

C. Disturbance develops over a short period (usually hours to days) and tends to fluctuate during the course of the day

D. Evidence from history, physical examination, or laboratory findings indicate that the disturbance is caused by direct physiologic consequence of a general medical condition

Adapted from *Diagnostic and Statistical Manual of Mental Disorders* (DSM-IV), 4th ed, Washington, DC: American Psychiatric Association, 1994.

The Confusion Assessment Method may also be used in the diagnosis of delirium. The sensitivity of the criteria is between 94% and 100% while the specificity ranges from 90% to 95%. The criteria are listed in the following box.

Confusion Assessment Method*
Feature 1. Acute onset and fluctuating course
This feature is usually obtained from family member or nurse and is shown by positive responses to the following questions:
• Is there evidence of an acute change in mental status from the patient's baseline?
• Did the (abnormal) behavior fluctuate during the day, that is, tend to come and go, or increase or decrease in severity?
Feature 2. Inattention
This feature is shown by a positive response to the following question:
• Did the patient have difficulty focusing attention, for example, being easily distractible, or have difficulty keeping track of what was being said?
Feature 3. Disorganized thinking
This feature is shown by positive response to the following question:
• Was the patient's thinking disorganized or incoherent such as rambling or irrelevant conversation, unclear or illogical inflow of ideas, or unpredictable and switching from subject to subject?
Feature 4. Altered level of consciousness
This feature is shown by any answer other than "alert" to the following question:
• Overall, how would you rate this patient's level of consciousness (alert [normal], vigilant [hyperalert], lethargic [drowsy, easily aroused], stupor [difficult to arouse], or coma [unarousable])?

*To satisfy the diagnosis of delirium, criteria 1 and 2 and either 3 or 4 (or both) must be present.

Adapted from Inouye SK, van Dyck CH, Alessi CA, et al, "Clarifying Confusion: The Confusion Assessment Method. A New Method for Detection of Delirium," *Ann Intern Med*, 1990, 113(12):941-8.

Dementia

Five percent of individuals >65 years of age have dementia. This percentage rises to between 35% and 50% in patients >85 years of age. Establishing the diagnosis of dementia can be challenging. In some, the diagnosis is missed. In other cases, confused patients are falsely labeled as having dementia. Key to the proper evaluation and management of dementia is recognition of the illness.

Most patients with dementia do not present complaining of memory loss. In most cases, it is a family member that brings the cognitively impaired patient to clinical attention. Even when a family member prompts consideration of dementia, there is often a delay in the patient's presentation. In many instances, this delay is due to the family mistakenly attributing the cognitive changes to normal "aging." Normal "aging" may be accompanied by mild changes in memory. In addition, with advancing age, there may be a change in the rate of information processing. However, these changes are not sufficiently severe that they impact upon the patient's functional status. This is the key difference between dementia and normal "aging."

Clinicians also play a role in delaying the diagnosis. Studies have shown that clinicians fail to detect dementia in 21% to 72% of affected patients. For most clinicians, performing an assessment of the mental status is not routine. Mental status assessment should, however, be a consideration in all patients >75 years of age. It should also be performed in any patient, regardless of age, who has difficulty with certain activities. Examples of these activities are listed in the following table.

Activity	Example
Learning and retaining new information	Trouble remembering events
Handling complex tasks	Trouble with checkbook, cooking
Reasoning ability	Inability to deal with unexpected events
Spatial ability and orientation	Getting lost in familiar places
Language	Word finding
Behavior	Less initiative More irritable Depressed

Adapted from Costa PT, Williams TF, Somerfield M, et al, *Early Identification of Alzheimer's Disease and Related Dementias*, Washington, DC: US Department of Health and Human Services, Agency for Health Care Policy and Research, 1996, Clinical Practice Guideline: No. 19. Also adapted from Knopman DS, "The Initial Recognition and Diagnosis of Dementia," *Am J Med*, 1998, 104(4A):2S-12S.

The clinician should perform a cognitive test in any patient suspected of having dementia. Most widely used in the United States is the Mini-Mental State Examination (MMSE) which is shown below.

The Mini-Mental State Examination

Maximum Score	Patient's Score	Questions
5		"What is the (year) (season) (date) (day) (month)?"
5		"Where are we?" Name of (state) (county) (city or town) (place, such as hospital or clinic) (specific location, such as floor or room)
3		The examiner names three unrelated objects clearly and slowly, then asks the patient to name all three of them. The patient's response is used for scoring. The examiner repeats them until the patient learns all of them, if possible.
5		"Begin with 100 and count backwards by subtracting seven. Stop at 65." (five responses)
3		If the patient learned the three objects above, ask the patient to recall them now.
2		The examiner shows the patient two simple objects, such as a wrist watch and a pencil, and asks the patient to name them.
1		"Repeat the phrase, 'No ifs, ands, or buts.'"
3		The examiner gives the patient a piece of blank paper and asks him or her to follow the three-step command: "Take the paper in your right hand, fold it in half, and put it on the floor."
1		On a blank piece of paper, the examiner prints the command "Close your eyes," in letters large enough for the patient to see clearly, then asks the patient to read it and follow the command.
1		"Make up and write a sentence about anything." This sentence must contain a noun and a verb.

(continued)

Maximum Score	Patient's Score	Questions
1		The examiner gives the patient a blank piece of paper and asks him or her to draw this symbol. All 10 angles must be present and two must intersect.

Total possible = 30	Patient's total =	If total score is 23 or below, further evaluation may be indicated.

Instructions: Score one point for each correct response within each question or activity.

The maximum score attainable on the MMSE is 30. A score <24 should prompt the clinician to consider dementia or delirium. Using 24 as a cutoff, the sensitivity and specificity of the MMSE is 87% and 82%, respectively. It is important to realize, however, that the test lacks sensitivity in patients with mild dementia. In addition, spuriously low scores may be noted in the groups listed in the following box.

Groups in Which the MMSE Score May be Spuriously Low	
Ethnic minorities	Poor language skills
Impaired vision	Poor motor function
Low educational level	

Of particular importance is correlation of the MMSE score with the patient's clinical presentation. A diagnosis of dementia is probable when both the patient's history and MMSE score are concordant. In some cases, however, the history and the MMSE score may be discordant. The following box describes the clinical significance of discordance between the history and the MMSE score.

History is suggestive of dementia but mental status examination is normal	
Mild dementia	Depression
High intelligence or education	Misinterpretation on part of informants

Mental status examination is suggestive of dementia but history is normal	
Acute confusional state (eg, delirium)	Inadequate recognition by family
Very low intelligence or education	

When the history and mental status examination are discordant, the clinician may consider performing neuropsychological testing. The usual scenario is a patient who is concerned about their cognitive function but mental status assessment is normal or near normal. As shown in the box above, this may be due to, among other possibilities, mild dementia or high intelligence or education. In these patients, neuropsychological testing may reveal subtle cognitive deficits not apparent during routine mental status assessment. Alternatively, the clinician may elect to re-evaluate these patients at six month intervals in an effort to demonstrate progressive cognitive decline.

Distinguishing Delirium from Dementia

The key features that help to differentiate delirium from dementia are considered in the following table.

Delirium	Dementia
Abrupt, precise onset with an identifiable date	Gradual onset that cannot be dated
Acute illness, generally lasting days to weeks	Chronic illness that characteristically progresses over years
Usually reversible, often completely	Generally irreversible and often chronically progressive
Disorientation early	Disorientation later in the illness, often after months or years
Variability from moment to moment, hour to hour, throughout the day	Generally stable from day to day (unless delirium develops)
Prominent physiologic changes	Less prominent physiologic changes
Clouded, altered and changing level of consciousness	Consciousness not clouded until terminal stage
Strikingly short attention span	Attention span not characteristically reduced
Disturbed sleep-wake cycle with hour to hour variation	Disturbed sleep-wake cycle with day-night reversal, not hour to hour variation
Marked psychomotor changes (hyperactive or hypoactive)	Psychomotor changes characteristically occurring late in the illness (unless depression develops)

Adapted from Ham RJ, "Confusion, Dementia, and Delirium," Ham RJ, and Sloane PD (eds), *Primary Care Geriatrics: A Case-Based Approach*, 3rd ed, St. Louis, MO: Mosby, 1997, 106-7; also adapted from Espino DV, Jules-Bradley AC, Johnston CL, et al, "Diagnostic Approach to the Confused Elderly Patient," *Am Fam Phys*, 1998, 57(6):1358-66 (review).

It is important to realize that dementia and delirium often coexist. In fact, dementia is a risk factor for delirium. When both coexist, treatment of the delirium often results in an improvement in the patient's cognition.

If the patient has delirium, **Proceed to Step 3**.

If the patient has dementia, **Proceed to Step 10**.

If it is unclear whether the patient has delirium or dementia, it is best to approach the patient as having delirium. **Proceed to Step 3**.

STEP 3: *What are the Causes of Delirium?*

The many causes of delirium are listed in the following box.

Causes of Delirium	
Dehydration	Metabolic disturbances
Endocrine disorders	Acidosis
Adrenal insufficiency	Hepatic encephalopathy
Hyperparathyroidism	Hypercarbia
Hypothyroidism / hyperthyroidism	Hypercalcemia
Infection	Hypoglycemia / hyperglycemia
Intoxication / withdrawal	Hyponatremia / hypernatremia
Alcohol	Hypoxemia
Barbiturates	Uremia
Benzodiazepines	Postoperative
Opiates	Primary CNS disorder
Others	Abscess
Medications	Epilepsy (postical)
	Head injury
	Increased intracranial pressure
	Meningitis / encephalitis
	Stroke
	Subarachnoid hemorrhage
	Subdural hematoma

It is important to realize that the cause of the delirium is often multifactorial.

Proceed to Step 4

STEP 4: *What are the Important Elements of the History That May Help the Clinician Determine the Etiology of the Delirium?*

Once the presence of delirium has been confirmed, the clinician should perform a focused history. A detailed history is often difficult or even impossible in the patient with delirium. This is especially true if the patient is delusional, agitated, or hallucinating. It is helpful to be calm while questioning the patient. In general, it is best to ask questions that can be answered with brief responses. In most cases, however, the patient is only able to provide a limited history. As a result, it is important to query family members and caregivers.

In the patient presenting with delirium, it is important to review the following:

- Previous medical diagnoses/past medical history
- Medications (including over-the-counter)
- Use of alcohol
- Use of illicit drugs
- Occupational exposures to toxic agents

Historical clues that may point to the etiology of the delirium are listed in the following table.

Historical Clue	Condition Suggested
Recent head trauma	Subdural hematoma
Recent surgery	Postoperative delirium
Recently stopped drinking	Alcohol withdrawal
Recently stopped benzodiazepine or other sedative	Drug withdrawal
Fever/chills	Infection
Seizure	Epilepsy (postictal)
Heavy intake of alcohol	Alcohol intoxication
History of liver disease	Hepatic encephalopathy
History of kidney disease	Uremia
History of cardiac or pulmonary condition	Acidosis Hypercarbia Hypoxia
Recent use of drugs (eg, opiates, sedatives, hallucinogens, or other drugs)	Drug intoxication
Headache	Primary CNS disorder

Proceed to Step 5

> **STEP 5: What are the Important Elements of the Physical Examination That May Help the Clinician Determine the Etiology of the Delirium?**

Particular attention should be focused on the following elements of the physical examination:

- Vital signs

    The vital signs may reveal fever, which may suggest the presence of infection. It is important to realize, however, that the absence of fever does not exclude infection. Hypothermia should prompt consideration of myxedema, hypoglycemia, and barbiturate intoxication. Tachypnea warrants consideration of a cardiopulmonary disorder associated with hypoxia.

- Volume status

    Signs of dehydration include poor skin turgor, absence of axillary sweat, dry mucous membranes, and orthostatic hypotension.

- Sources of infection

    Pneumonia, urinary tract infection, skin, and soft tissue infection are the more common infectious causes of delirium.

- Neurologic findings

    The clinician should try to determine if there are any focal findings on neurological exam.

Clues in the physical examination that may point to the etiology of the delirium are listed in the following table.

Physical Examination Finding	Condition Suggested
Fever	Anticholinergic drug ingestion Infection Other causes of delirium
Flapping tremor (asterixis)	Hepatic encephalopathy Other metabolic causes of delirium Uremia
Focal neurologic deficits	Primary CNS disorder
Jaundice	Hepatic encephalopathy
Papilledema	Primary CNS disorder (increased intracranial pressure)

Proceed to Step 6

STEP 6: *What Laboratory Tests Should Be Ordered in the Patient With Delirium?*

Once the history and physical examination have been performed, the clinician should then obtain certain laboratory tests. The laboratory tests that should be obtained in every patient with delirium are listed in the following box.

Laboratory Tests Routinely Indicated in Patients with Delirium	
BUN	Electrolytes
CBC with differential	Calcium
Creatinine	Sodium
Glucose	Liver function tests
	Urinalysis

It is reasonable to perform the above tests when the etiology of the delirium is unclear. In addition, an EKG and CXR should be done as well. Not uncommonly, delirium may be the initial presentation of an acute myocardial infarction in the elderly patient. The CXR may identify an infiltrate consistent with pneumonia or identify another cardiopulmonary disorder in the hypoxemic or hypercarbic patient. It is also reasonable to determine drug levels when patients are on medications that require periodic monitoring of levels. It is important to realize, however, that delirium may be due to the medication even when the drug levels are within the normal range. Examples of medications that can cause delirium even when the levels are normal include lithium, digoxin, and quinidine.

Proceed to Step 7

STEP 7: *Are There Any Other Laboratory Tests or Studies That Need to b e Performed in the Evaluation of the Patient With Delirium?*

When the etiology of the delirium remains unclear after history, physical examination, and routine laboratory tests, the clinician should consider performing further testing. Based upon the patient's clinical presentation, further testing may include any of the following:

- Ammonia level

- Arterial blood gas

- Magnesium

- Thyroid function tests

- Toxicology screen

- Vitamin B_{12} level

In addition, the clinician should perform brain imaging in delirious patients who have focal neurological deficits or evidence of head trauma on physical examination. A significantly impaired level of consciousness also warrants consideration of brain imaging.

Lumbar puncture is indicated when bacterial meningitis is a distinct possibility. It is important to realize that older patients do not always present with the classic symptoms of fever, headache, and nuchal rigidity. Not all patients with fever, however, require lumbar puncture. If infection is a concern and there is an obvious source of infection outside of the CNS, lumbar puncture is probably not required. It should, however, be performed in the febrile patient with no apparent focus of infection.

It is also important to realize that fever is not always present in the older patient with infection. As a result, lumbar puncture should also be a consideration in any septic-appearing patient without an obvious source of infection.

Proceed to Step 8

STEP 8: *Is the Delirium Medication-Induced?*

Medications cause or contribute to delirium in up to 40% of cases. As such, the clinician should review the medication list including any over-the-counter and herbal preparations. In addition, it is important to be aware of medications that may have been prescribed by other clinicians. It is also worthwhile to ascertain if the patient has taken any medications prescribed to other family members. Many clinicians like to have family members or caregivers bring the entire contents of the medicine cabinet in for review. Although any medication can cause delirium, the clinician should be familiar with the common offenders, which are listed in the following box.

Medications Commonly Causing Delirium	
Antianxiety agents	Antipsychotics
Antibiotics	Benzodiazepines
Anticholinergics	Cardiovascular agents
Anticonvulsants	ACE inhibitors
Carbamazepine	Antiarrhythmics
Dilantin	β-blockers
Phenobarbital	Clonidine
Primidone	Digoxin
Valproic acid	Methyldopa
Antidepressants	Corticosteroids
Doxepin	NSAIDs
Tricyclic antidepressants	Opiate analgesics
Antihistamines	Psychostimulants
Antiparkinsonian agents	Sympathomimetics
Amantadine	Miscellaneous
Benztropine	Cimetidine
Bromocriptine	Theophylline
Levodopa	
Pergolide	
Selegiline	

Potential offenders should be discontinued or their dosage should be decreased. It is also important to realize that the withdrawal of certain medications such as sedative/hypnotics can also result in delirium.

Proceed to Step 9

STEP 9: *What Should be Done When the Etiology of the Delirium Remains Unclear or the Patient Does Not Improve Despite Treatment of the Cause?*

When the cause remains unclear, it is important to perform serial examinations of the patient. Of particular importance is another review of the medication list. All medications that are not necessary should be discontinued. Others that are necessary should have the dosage reduced.

In the patient who fails to improve despite identification and treatment of the cause, the clinician should realize that there may be a delay in improvement after removal or treatment of the cause. While it is true that most patients with delirium improve within days after correction of the cause, in some patients, it may take weeks for the patient to completely recover. It is reasonable to consider neurology consultation in these difficult cases.

End of Section.

> ### STEP 10: *Does the Patient have Depression Rather Than Dementia?*

Depression and dementia may be difficult to differentiate from one another, particularly in the elderly. In this age group, it is not uncommon for depression to present with the cognitive impairment that is characteristic of dementia. The term pseudodementia is often said to be present when the depressed patient presents with cognitive impairment suggestive of dementia. About 10% of patients with progressive impairment in cognition have improvement with treatment for depression. As a result, it behooves the clinician to make this distinction.

Memory loss can be a feature of both depression and dementia. However, the depressed patient tends to complain of memory loss while the demented patient usually does not. In most cases of dementia, it is the patient's family that brings the memory problem to clinical attention. Poor effort on cognitive testing is more suggestive of depression. In contrast, patients with dementia try hard during cognitive testing but often provide incorrect answers. These and other features used to differentiate between depression and dementia are listed in the table below.

Depression	Dementia
Abrupt onset	Insidious onset
Short duration	Long duration
Previous psychiatric history (including undiagnosed depressive episodes)	No psychiatric history
Complains of memory loss	Often unaware of memory loss
"I don't know" answers	Near-miss answers
Fluctuating cognitive loss	Stable cognitive loss (although loss is progressive over time)
Equal memory loss for recent and remote events	Memory loss greatest for recent events
Depressed mood (if present) occurs first	Memory loss occurs first

Adapted from Wells CE, "Pseudodementia," *Am J Psychiatry*, 1979, 136(7):895-900; also adapted from Espino DV, Jules-Bradley AC, Johnston CL, et al, "Diagnostic Approach to the Confused Elderly Patient," *Am Fam Phys*, 1998, 57(6):1358-66 (review).

Because it can be extremely difficult to differentiate between depression and dementia, the clinician may elect to try a therapeutic trial of antidepressant medication, particularly when considerable uncertainty exists. It is not warranted in all patients, however, because antidepressant therapy has the potential, as with any psychoactive agent, to worsen the cognitive impairment. Alternatively, the clinician may choose to perform neuropsychological testing to distinguish depression from dementia.

It is also important to realize that depression and dementia can coexist. In fact, depression develops in 30% to 40% of patients with Alzheimer's disease at some point in the course of the illness.

If the patient has depression, *Stop Here*.

If the patient has dementia, *Proceed to Step 11*.

If the patient has both depression and dementia, *Proceed to Step 11*.

STEP 11: *What are the Causes of Dementia?*

The causes of dementia are extensive. Despite this, a handful of diagnoses account for most cases of dementia. About 60% to 80% of elderly patients with dementia have Alzheimer's disease. Another 10% to 20% have vascular or multi-infarct dementia. Parkinson's disease and frontotemporal dementia are other considerations, accounting for about 5% of cases. Approximately 15% of cases are due to reversible causes. There are many conditions that may be associated with reversible dementia. These will be considered in Step 14.

Proceed to Step 12

STEP 12: *Are There Any Clues in the Patient's History That Point to the Etiology of the Dementia?*

Clues in the patient's history that may point to the etiology of the dementia are listed in the following table.

Historical Clue	Condition Suggested
History of Parkinson's disease	Dementia related to Parkinson's disease
Change in social demeanor and language early in the course of the dementia	Frontotemporal dementia (eg, Pick's disease)
Risk factors for vascular dementia: Hypertension Diabetes mellitus Cigarette smoking Heavy alcohol use	Vascular dementia
History of stroke	Vascular dementia
Stepwise progression of cognitive, motor, and sensory deficits	Vascular dementia
History of HIV	HIV-associated dementia Also consider: Toxoplasmosis Cryptococcal meningitis Primary CNS lymphoma CMV encephalitis Progressive multifocal leukoencephalopathy
History of liver disease	Hepatic encephalopathy
History of kidney disease	Uremia
History of treated or untreated syphilis	Neurosyphilis
Offending medication	Medication-induced dementia
Long-term hemodialysis	Dialysis encephalopathy
History of radiation therapy to the brain	Radiation-induced dementia
Diarrhea	Whipple's disease
History of head trauma	Subdural hematoma

(Continued)

(continued)

Historical Clue	Condition Suggested
Triad of dementia, gait apraxia, and urinary incontinence	Normal pressure hydrocephalus
Long-standing heavy alcohol use	Alcohol-related dementia
Risk factors for HIV	HIV-associated dementia

Proceed to Step 13

STEP 13: *Are There Any Clues in the Patient's Physical Examination That Point to the Etiology of the Dementia?*

Clues in the physical examination that point to the etiology of the dementia are listed in the following table.

Physical Examination Clue	Condition Suggested
Resting tremor	Dementia related to Parkinson's disease
Shuffling gait	Dementia related to Parkinson's disease
Bradykinesia	Dementia related to Parkinson's disease
Disorder of vertical eye movements (impaired downward gaze)	Progressive supranuclear palsy
Stooped posture	Dementia related to Parkinson's disease
Hyperextended posture	Progressive supranuclear palsy
Myoclonus	Creutzfeldt-Jakob disease
Focal neurological deficits	Vascular dementia Argues against Alzheimer's disease Other subcortical dementias
Gait abnormality	Parkinson's disease Vascular dementia Normal pressure hydrocephalus Progressive supranuclear palsy Other subcortical dementias
Cogwheel rigidity	Dementia related to Parkinson's disease
Chorea	Huntington's chorea

Proceed to Step 14

STEP 14: *Is the Dementia Due to a Reversible Cause?*

On average, fewer than 15% of patients with dementia have a reversible cause. The reversible causes of dementia are listed in the following box.

Reversible Causes of Dementia		
Alcoholism (chronic)	Infection	Neurosyphilis
Connective tissue	AIDS	Normal pressure
diseases	Chronic meningitis	hydrocephalus
Systemic lupus	Tuberculosis	Nutritional
erythematosus	Fungal	Vitamin B_{12}
Temporal arteritis	Parasitic	deficiency
Rheumatoid vasculitis	Lyme neuroborelliosis	Thiamine deficiency
Sarcoidosis	Mass lesions	Pellagra
TTP	Tumor	Whipple's disease
Granulomatous	Subdural hematoma	Miscellaneous
angiitis	Medications	Obstructive sleep
Endocrine disorders	Metabolic disorders	apnea
Adrenal insufficiency	Electrolyte	Chronic obstructive
Hyperparathyroidism	abnormalities	pulmonary disease
Hyperthyroidism	Hepatic	Congestive heart
Hypothyroidism	encephalopathy	failure
	Hypoxemia	Radiation-induced
	Renal failure	dementia
		Dialysis dementia

Adapted from Arnold SE and Kumar A, "Reversible Dementias," *Med Clin N Am*, 1994, 77(1):215-30.

The identification of one of the above disorders is important because appropriate therapy can then be directed at the primary disorder. With treatment, the patient's cognitive impairment may stabilize. In others, there may be reversal, either partial or complete, of the intellectual decline. Just how extensive an evaluation should be searching for one of the above causes is a matter of some debate. The steps that follow focus on laboratory testing and imaging tests that will allow the clinician to identify the majority of the reversible causes of dementia listed in the box above.

Proceed to Step 15

STEP 15: *What are the Results of the Laboratory Tests?*

The American Academy of Neurology recommends routinely performing the tests in the following box in the evaluation of every patient with dementia.

Routine Laboratory Tests Indicated in Every Patient with Dementia	
BUN	Liver function tests
Calcium	Serum vitamin B_{12}
CBC	Syphilis serology
Creatinine	Thyroid function tests (TSH, free T_4
Electrolytes	or free thyroxine index)
Glucose	

Tests that are not considered routine but that may be indicated in certain situations are listed in the following box.

Laboratory Tests That May be Indicated in the Evaluation of Dementia	
CXR	24-hour urine for heavy metals
ESR	Toxicology screen
HIV	Urinalysis

Of note, testing for HIV should be performed in any patient with risk factors for HIV. Up to 20% of patients with HIV develop dementia. However, most patients with HIV dementia are known to have HIV prior to the diagnosis. Dementia as the initial presentation of HIV would be particularly unusual.

Proceed to Step 16

STEP 16: *Should the Patient Have a CT Scan or MRI of the Head?*

In recent years, the use of CT scan or MRI of the head has become routine in the evaluation of dementia patients. The principal role of neuroimaging in patients with dementia is to exclude structural causes such as infarction, neoplasm, hydrocephalus, and subdural hematoma. Once identified, the proper management of these structural causes of dementia has the potential to lead to an improvement in or even resolution of the cognitive impairment. There is controversy, however, as to whether all patients with dementia require neuroimaging.

Some authorities maintain that neuroimaging should be obtained once in the evaluation of all cases of dementia. Recognizing that the yield of these imaging tests are low, these investigators maintain that the low yield may be acceptable in these patients, particularly if a potentially life-threatening cause such as subdural hematoma can be identified. In addition, proponents of neuroimaging in all patients with dementia also argue that silent cerebrovascular disease may be detected, leading to more aggressive treatment of risk factors for vascular dementia. With more aggressive therapy, the progression of the dementia could potentially be slowed down.

Other experts propose that neuroimaging should not be performed in all patients with dementia. Most of these authorities do agree, however, that CT scan or MRI of the head should be performed in most patients with dementia. They argue that patients with the following characteristics may forego neuroimaging:

- No features suggestive of structural CNS lesion on history
- Physical exam, particularly neurological assessment, is normal
- Onset and progression of cognitive impairment is consistent with Alzheimer's disease

Clear indications for neuroimaging are listed in the following box.

Indications for Neuroimaging in the Patient with Dementia	
Atypical presentation of dementia	Rapidly progressive dementia
Focal neurologic symptoms or signs	Seizure
Headache	Systemic disease that affects the
History of head trauma	brain (eg, HIV, SLE)
Incontinence	

Neuroimaging may reveal findings consistent with the following diagnoses:

- Subdural hematoma

    A history of head trauma is not always elicited in patients with chronic subdural hematoma. While many of these patients may present with focal neurological deficits along with an alteration in the level of consciousness secondary to increased intracranial pressure, cognitive decline may be the only manifestation in some patients.

- Brain tumor

    For many years, clinicians have recognized that brain tumors, particularly those that affect the frontal or temporal lobes, can present with dementia. In these locations, there may be no focal neurological deficits suggestive of a mass lesion.

- Normal pressure hydrocephalus (NPH)

    Normal pressure hydrocephalus accounts for less than 2% of all dementia cases. It is characterized by the triad of gait abnormality, urinary incontinence, and dementia. Ventricular enlargement that is disproportionate to cerebral atrophy is the hallmark neuroimaging abnormality.

- Vascular dementia

    Features suggestive of vascular dementia include the following:

    - Abrupt onset

    - Step-wise deterioration

    - Symptomatic improvement following acute event

    - Onset of cognitive deficit associated with stroke

Physical examination revealing focal neurologic deficits consistent with stroke are also supportive of vascular dementia. In patients with a history and physical examination suggestive of vascular dementia, neuroimaging may reveal evidence of infarcts.

In other patients, however, neuroimaging may reveal infarcts that were clinically silent. Especially difficult to decide in these cases is whether the infarction noted on neuroimaging is enough to satisfy the diagnosis of vascular dementia. Estimating the volume of tissue infarcted may be helpful to determine if the infarction noted is the primary cause of the dementia.

Volume of Tissue Infarcted	Likelihood of Vascular Dementia
>100 mL	Vascular dementia invariably present
50-100 mL	Vascular dementia usually present
10-50 mL	Likelihood of vascular dementia depends on location of infarct*
<10 mL	Vascular dementia rarely present

*When the total infarct volume is between 10-50 mL, the clinician should consider the location of the lesion. Lesions located in the medial thalamus, caudate, and hippocampus are more likely to cause dementia.

Finally, the clinician should realize that some patients with dementia have more than one cause. For example, it is not uncommon for Alzheimer's disease and vascular dementia to coexist. Therefore, the demonstration of infarcts on neuroimaging does not exclude other causes of dementia.

If the CT or MRI reveals the etiology of the dementia, **_Stop Here_**.

If the CT or MRI does not reveal the etiology of the dementia, **Proceed to Step 17**.

STEP 17: *Does the Patient Need to Have a Lumbar Puncture?*

Lumbar puncture should not be a routine part of the dementia evaluation. The indications for lumbar puncture are listed in the following box.

Indications for Lumbar Puncture in Patients with Dementia	
Acute or subacute onset (<8 weeks)	Meningeal signs
Fever	Presentation consistent with NPH
History of metastatic cancer	Rapidly progressive dementia
Immunosuppression	Reactive syphilis serology
Meningeal enhancement on imaging tests	Suspected CNS vasculitis
	Younger patient (<55 years)

Prior to performing lumbar puncture, it is important to ensure that there are no contraindications to the procedure.

If lumbar puncture is indicated and it reveals the etiology of the dementia, **Stop Here**.

If lumbar puncture is indicated but it does not reveal the etiology of the dementia, **Proceed to Step 18**.

If lumbar puncture is not indicated, **Proceed to Step 18**.

STEP 18: *Is the Cognitive Decline Related to a Medication?*

One of the most common forms of reversible dementia is drug-induced cognitive impairment. While medications may be the sole cause of the dementia in some, in other cases, patients with pre-existing dementia may have worsening cognition secondary to a medication. Medications that commonly cause cognitive impairment are listed in the following box.

Medications that Commonly Cause or Exacerbate Dementia	
Anticholinergic agents	Opiate analgesics
Anticonvulsants	Psychotropic agents
Dilantin	Benzodiazepines
Phenobarbital	Lithium
Antihistamines	Neuroleptics
Antihypertensive agents	Psychostimulants
Clonidine	Tricyclic antidepressants
Diuretics	Miscellaneous
Methyldopa	Antibiotics
Propranolol	Antineoplastic agents
Antiparkinsonian agents	Cimetidine
Bromocriptine	Corticosteroids
Levodopa	Ergot
Pergolide	Metoclopramide
Cardiovascular agents	Oral contraceptives
Digoxin	
Procainamide	
Quinidine	

Discontinuation of the suspect medication followed by an improvement in cognition supports the diagnosis of drug-induced cognitive dysfunction.

If the patient has drug-induced cognitive dysfunction, **Stop Here**.

If the patient does not have drug-induced cognitive dysfunction, **Proceed to Step 19**.

> **STEP 19: What are the Likely Etiologies in Patients Who Do Not Have a Reversible Cause of Dementia?**

If no reversible cause is identified, the clinician should focus on determining if the dementia is cortical, subcortical, or mixed. Features of cortical and subcortical dementia are listed in the following table.

	Cortical Dementia	Subcortical Dementia
Aphasia	Often present	Not present
Apraxia	Often present	Not present
Agnosia	Often present	Not present
Focal motor or sensory deficits	Usually not present unless advanced disease	Usually present
Gait **Posture** **Tone**	Usually normal	Often abnormal
Involuntary movements (eg, tremor, chorea, athetosis, dystonia)	Not present	Often present

By classifying the dementia as cortical or subcortical, the clinician can narrow the differential diagnosis listed in the following box.

Irreversible Dementias in Adults	
Alzheimer's disease	Parkinson's disease
Creutzfeldt-Jakob disease	Pick's disease
Hereditary metabolic diseases	Progressive supranuclear palsy
Huntington's chorea	Vascular dementia
Lewy body variant of Alzheimer's disease	

Causes of cortical dementia include Alzheimer's disease and Pick's disease. Subcortical dementia may be due to Parkinson's disease, progressive supranuclear palsy, and Huntington's chorea. Of note, vascular dementia may be cortical (eg, multiple large cortical infarcts), subcortical (eg, lacunar states or Binswanger's disease), or mixed.

Alzheimer's disease and vascular dementia, the two major causes of dementia, are discussed in further detail below. It is important to realize that the two may coexist.

Alzheimer's Disease

In the United States, nearly four million people have Alzheimer's disease. Criteria for the diagnosis of Alzheimer's disease have been proposed by the following groups:

- American Psychiatric Association's *Diagnostic and Statistical Manual of Mental Disorders* (DSM-IV)

- National Institute of Neurologic and Communicative Disorders and Stroke-Alzheimer's Dementia and Related Disorders Association (NINCDS-ADRDA) Work Group

- Eisdorfer and Cohen Research Diagnostic Criteria (ECRDC)

The NINCDS-ADRDA criteria has the highest sensitivity (92%) while the DSM-IV criteria has the highest specificity (80%). The NINCDS-ADRDA criteria are listed in the following box.

NINCDS-ADRDA Criteria for the Diagnosis of Alzheimer's Disease

Criteria for the clinical diagnosis of probable Alzheimer's disease
- Establishment of dementia by clinical examination, documented by a cognitive screening measure, and confirmed with neuropsychological tests
- Deficits in two or more areas of cognition
- Progressive worsening of memory and other cognitive functions
- No disturbance of consciousness
- Onset between ages 40 and 90 years, most often after age 65
- Absence of other potential causes of cognitive impairment

The diagnosis of probable Alzheimer's disease is supported by
- Progressive deterioration of specific cognitive functions such as language (aphasia), motor skills (apraxia), and perception (agnosia)
- Impaired activities of daily living and altered patterns of behavior
- Family history of similar disorders, particularly if neuropathologically confirmed
- Laboratory results of
  1) Normal lumbar puncture as evaluated by standard techniques
  2) Normal pattern or nonspecific EEG changes, such as increased slow wave activity
  3) Evidence of cerebral atrophy on CT with progression documented by serial observation

Other clinical features consistent with probable Alzheimer's disease, after exclusion of other causes of dementia
- Plateaus in the course of progression of the disease
- Associated symptoms of depression, insomnia, incontinence, delusions, illusions, hallucinations, catastrophic verbal, emotional, or physical outburst, sexual disorders, and weight loss
- Other neurologic abnormalities in some patients, especially those with more advanced disease, including motor signs such as increased muscle tone, myoclonus, or gait disorder
- Seizures in advanced disease
- CT normal for age

Features that make the diagnosis of probable Alzheimer's disease uncertain or unlikely
- Sudden, apoplectic onset
- Focal neurologic findings such as hemiparesis, sensory loss, visual field deficits, and incoordination early in the course of the illness
- Seizures or gait disturbances at the onset of symptoms or very early in the course of the illness

---

...Criteria for the Diagnosis of Alzheimer's Disease *(continued)*

Diagnosis of possible Alzheimer's disease

- May be made on the basis of the dementia syndrome; in the absence of other neurologic, psychiatric, or systemic disorders sufficient to cause dementia; and in the presence of variations in the onset, presentation, or clinical course

- May be made in the presence of a second systemic or brain disorder sufficient to produce dementia but not considered to be the cause of the dementia

- Should be used in research studies when a single, gradually progressive, severe cognitive deficit is identified in the absence of another identifiable cause

Criteria for diagnosis of definite Alzheimer's disease

- Clinical criteria for probable Alzheimer's disease
- Histopathologic evidence obtained from biopsy or autopsy

Adapted from McKhann G, Drachman D, Folstein M, et al, "Clinical Diagnosis of Alzheimer's Disease: Report of the NINCDS-ADRDA Work Group Under the Auspices of the Department of Health and Human Services Task Force on Alzheimer's Disease," *Neurology*, 1984, 34(7):939-44.

Vascular Dementia

In most populations, cerebrovascular disease is the second most common cause of dementia. Often present in patients with vascular dementia are atherosclerotic risk factors such as hypertension and diabetes mellitus. A history of transient ischemic attacks or stroke is not uncommon. Vascular dementia often progresses in a stepwise manner, characterized by acute episodes of confusion accompanied by focal neurologic signs and symptoms. Criteria have been proposed for vascular dementia but have not yet been widely accepted. The NINDS-AIREN criteria for vascular dementia is shown in the following box.

NINDS-AIREN Criteria for Vascular Dementia

- Dementia defined by cognitive decline from a previously higher level of functioning and manifested by impairment of memory and of two or more cognitive domains; deficits should be severe enough to interfere with activities of daily living not due to physical effects of stroke alone.

- Cerebrovascular disease, defined by the presence of focal signs on neurologic examination, such as hemiparesis, lower facial weakness, Babinski sign, sensory deficit, hemianopsia, and dysarthria consistent with stroke (with or without history of stroke), and evidence of relevant cerebrovascular disease by brain imaging (CT or MRI) including multiple large-vessel infarcts or a single strategically-placed infarct (angular gyrus, thalamus, basal forebrain, or PCA or ACA territories), as well as multiple basal ganglia and white matter lacunes or extensive periventricular white matter lesions, or combinations thereof.

- A relationship between the above two disorders, manifested or inferred by the presence of one or more of the following:

   1) Onset of dementia within three months following a recognized stroke

   2) Abrupt deterioration in cognitive functions; or fluctuating, stepwise progression of cognitive deficits

Adapted from Roman GC, Tatemichi TK, Erkinjunttii T, et al, "Vascular Dementia: Diagnostic Criteria for Research Studies. Report of the NINDS-AIREN International Workshop," *Neurology*, 1993, 43(2):250-60.

REFERENCES

Arnold SE and Kumar A, "Reversible Dementias," *Med Clin N Am*, 1994, 77(1):215-30.

Brown TM, "Drug-Induced Delirium," *Semin Clin Neuropsychiatry*, 2000, 5(2):113-24.

Casey DA, DeFazio JV, Vansickle K, et al, "Delirium. Quick Recognition, Careful Evaluation, and Appropriate Treatment," *Postgrad Med*, 1996, 100(1):121-4, 128, 133-4.

Chan D and Brennan NJ, "Delirium: Making the Diagnosis, Improving the Prognosis," *Geriatrics*, 1999, 54(3):28-30, 36, 39-42.

Costa PT, Williams TF, Somerfield M, et al, *Early Identification of Alzheimer's Disease and Related Dementias*, Washington, DC: US Department of Health and Human Services, Agency for Health Care Policy and Research, 1996, Clinical Practice Guideline: No. 19.

Diagnostic and Statistical Manual of Mental Disorders (DSM-IV), 4th ed, Washington, DC: American Psychiatric Association, 1994.

Espino DV, Jules-Bradley AC, Johnston CL, et al, "Diagnostic Approach to the Confused Elderly Patient," *Am Fam Phys*, 1998, 57(6):1358-66 (review).

Geldmacher DS and Whitehouse PJ, "Differential Diagnosis of Alzheimer's Disease," *Neurology*, 1997, 48(5 Suppl 6):S2-9.

Ham RJ, "Confusion, Dementia, and Delirium," Ham RJ, Sloane PD, eds, *Primary Care Geriatrics: A Case-Based Approach*, 3rd ed, St. Louis, MO: Mosby, 1997, 106-7.

Inouye SK, "Delirium in Hospitalized Older Patients," *Clin Geriatr Med*, 1998, 14(4):745-64.

Inouye SK, van Dyck CH, Alessi CA, et al, "Clarifying Confusion: The Confusion Assessment Method. A New Method for Detection of Delirium," *Ann Intern Med*, 1990, 113(12):941-8.

Jacobson SA, "Delirium in the Elderly," *Psychiatr Clin North Am*, 1997, 20(1):91-110.

Johnson J, "Identifying and Recognizing Delirium," *Dement Geriatr Cogn Disord*, 1999, 10(5):353-8.

Karlsson I, "Drugs that Induce Delirium," *Dement Geriatr Cogn Disord*, 1999, 10(5):412-5.

Knopman DS, "The Initial Recognition and Diagnosis of Dementia," *Am J Med*, 1998, 104(4A):2S-12S; discussion 39S-42S.

Lerner DM and Rosenstein DL, "Neuroimaging in Delirium and Related Conditions," *Semin Clin Neuropsychiatry*, 2000, 5(2):98-112.

McKhann G, Drachman D, Folstein M, et al, "Clinical Diagnosis of Alzheimer's Disease: Report of the NINCDS-ADRDA Work Group Under the Auspices of the Department of Health and Human Services Task Force on Alzheimer's Disease," *Neurology*, 1984, 34(7):939-44.

Moore AR and O'Keeffe ST, "Drug-Induced Cognitive Impairment in the Elderly," *Drugs Aging*, 1999, 15(1):15-28.

Murphy BA, "Delirium," *Emerg Med Clin North Am*, 2000, 18(2):243-52.

"Practice Parameter for Diagnosis and Evaluation of Dementia. (Summary Statement) Report of the Quality Standards Subcommittee of the American Academy of Neurology," *Neurology*, 1994, 44(11):2203-6.

Roman GC, Tatemichi TK, Erkinjunttii T, et al, "Vascular Dementia: Diagnostic Criteria for Research Studies. Report of the NINDS-AIREN International Workshop," *Neurology*, 1993, 43(2):250-60.

Trzepacz PT, "Delirium. Advances in Diagnosis, Pathophysiology, and Treatment," *Psychiatr Clin North Am*, 1996, 19(3):429-48.

Vanneste JA, "Diagnosis and Management of Normal-Pressure Hydrocephalus," *J Neurol*, 2000, 247(1):5-14.

Wells CE, "Pseudodementia," *Am J Psychiatry*, 1979, 136(7):895-900.

CONSTIPATION

STEP 1: *What is Constipation?*

Constipation is a common complaint among patients visiting their primary care physician. It has been noted in up to 26% and 34% of men and women, respectively, >65 years of age. Because constipation means different things to different people, it is necessary to ascertain exactly what the patient presenting with constipation is experiencing. Most often, it refers to a change in bowel habits, which may include any of the following:

- Decrease in the frequency of defecation
- Alteration in the consistency of the stool (eg, hard stool)
- Excessive straining during defecation

Most individuals defecate at least 3 times/week. As such, a frequency of defecation ≤2 times/week is considered by many to satisfy the definition of constipation. Other individuals who complain of constipation do not report a decrease in the frequency of defecation. Rather, they complain of excessive straining during defecation or a change in the consistency of the stool (eg, hard stool).

The lack of a precise definition has contributed to the uncertainty regarding the incidence, pathogenesis, and treatment of constipation. In an effort to address these issues, an international group of experts has proposed the following definition for constipation:

- Stool frequency ≤2 times/week

   Studies have shown that the frequency of bowel movements in most healthy people range from 3 bowel movements/day to 3 bowel movements/week. Having <3 bowel movements/week does not invariably indicate the presence of constipation. For some patients, having 1-2 bowel movements/week is their baseline. No further evaluation is needed in these individuals, especially if complaints of bloating or painful defecation are absent.

- Sensation of incomplete evacuation at least 25% of the time

- Excessive straining during defecation at least 25% of the time

- Passage of lumpy or hard stool at least 25% of the time

Constipation is said to be present if two or more of the above have been present for at least three months.

Proceed to Step 2

STEP 2: *What are the Results of the Bowel Diary?*

Misconceptions regarding normal bowel habits are quite common. Studies have shown that patients often underestimate their bowel movement frequency. Prior to undertaking an evaluation for constipation, it may be worthwhile to have the patient keep a two week bowel diary so that the presence of constipation can be confirmed.

If the patient does not have constipation, ***Stop Here***.

If the patient has constipation, ***Proceed to Step 3***.

STEP 3: *What are the Causes of Constipation?*

The causes of constipation are listed in the following box.

Causes of Constipation	
Neurologic	Connective tissue disease
Spinal cord lesions	Scleroderma
Cauda equina tumor	Amyloidosis
Tabes dorsalis	Mixed connective tissue disease
Brain tumor	
Parkinson's disease	Endocrine / metabolic
Shy-Drager syndrome	Diabetes mellitus
Multiple sclerosis	Hypothyroidism
Autonomic neuropathy	Panhypopituitarism
Hirschsprung's disease	Pheochromocytoma
Chagas disease	Glucagonoma
Cerebrovascular events	Hypokalemia
Prior pelvic surgery	Hypercalcemia
Ganglioneuromatosis	Pregnancy
Neurofibromatosis	
Intestinal pseudo-obstruction	Irritable bowel syndrome
Psychogenic (depression)	Miscellaneous
	Dehydration
Structural disorders	Inadequate fiber intake
Anorectal	Immobility
Fissure	Dementia
Hemorrhoids	
Prolapse	Medications
Rectocele	
Colon carcinoma	
Colonic stricture	

Proceed to Step 4

STEP 4: *Are There Any Clues in the Patient's History That Point to the Etiology of the Constipation?*

Clues in the patient's history that may point to the etiology of the constipation are listed in the following table.

Historical Clue	Condition Suggested
Weight loss	Colon or rectal cancer
Weight gain	Hypothyroidism
Low fiber intake	Associated with constipation
Sedentary lifestyle	Predisposes to constipation
Constipation follows institution of a new medication	Constipation secondary to medication use
Constipation resolves following discontinuation of suspect medication	Constipation secondary to medication use
Fatigue Sleepiness Slow speech Cold intolerance Decreased appetite	Hypothyroidism
Polyuria	Hypercalcemia Diabetes mellitus

Blood in stool	Anal disease
	  Hemorrhoid
	  Fissure
	Colon or rectal cancer

Recent change in bowel habits	Mandates an evaluation for structural or organic etiology
Fecal incontinence	Neurologic disorder associated with constipation Fecal impaction
Currently pregnant	Constipation common in pregnancy
Pain with defecation	Suggests anal or perianal inflammatory disorder
Bowel movements accompanied by excessive mucus	Irritable bowel syndrome
Laxative use (chronic)	Sensitivity of rectal defecatory reflexes are impaired with laxative abuse
Perineal splinting* Digital disimpaction Assuming unusual positions during defecation	Pelvic outlet dysfunction
Constipation present for several years	Functional disorder
History of malignancy	Hypercalcemia

*Perineal splinting refers to the use of manual perineal support to facilitate defecation.

Proceed to Step 5

STEP 5: *Are There Any Clues in the Physical Examination That Point to the Etiology of the Constipation?*

Clues in the patient's physical examination that may point to the etiology of the constipation are listed in the following table.

Physical Examination Finding	Condition Suggested
Abdominal mass	Colon cancer Retained stool
Dry skin Hoarseness Delayed relaxation phase of deep tendon reflexes Loss of 1/3 of eyebrows Slow speech Bradycardia Puffy face	Hypothyroidism
Rectal mass	Rectal cancer Fecal impaction
Fissure or hemorrhoids noted on rectal examination	May be caused by constipation or lead to constipation
Absence of anal wink*	Suggests disease affecting the terminal spinal cord and cauda equina (S-2 to S-5)
Gaping or asymmetric anal opening	Neurologic disorder impairing sphincter function
Shiny, tight skin Pinched nose Telangiectasias Sclerodactyly	Scleroderma

*The anal reflex or wink is said to be present if contraction of the external anal sphincter is noted following pinprick of the perianal area.

Proceed to Step 6

STEP 6: *Does the Patient Have Any Alarm Features?*

The challenge that the clinician faces in the patient presenting with constipation is differentiating benign constipation from that which is due to a more serious problem. Making this distinction begins with consideration of whether or not the patient has alarm symptoms. The alarm symptoms to consider are listed in the following box.

Alarm Symptoms in the Patient Presenting with Constipation	
Age >45 years	Recent change in bowel habit
Weight loss	Severe pain
Evidence of blood loss	Nocturnal pain
Anemia	Pain localized to rectum
Hematochezia	Pain persisting after defecation
Melena	Family history of colorectal cancer
Occult blood loss	

If the patient does not have alarm symptoms, **Proceed to Step 7**.

If the patient has alarm symptoms, **Proceed to Step 15**.

> **STEP 7: *Does the Patient Have Medication-Induced Constipation?***

A thorough medication history is essential in the patient presenting with constipation. Medications that are associated with constipation are listed in the following box.

Medications Associated with or Causing Constipation	
Anticholinergic	Opiate analgesics
Antidepressants	Miscellaneous
Monoamine oxidase inhibitors	Aluminum antacids
Tricyclic antidepressants	Calcium (antacids, supplements)
Antihistamines	Cholestyramine
Antiparkinsonian	Ferrous sulfate
Antipsychotics	Sucralfate
Phenothiazines	Vinca alkaloids
Anticonvulsants	
Antihypertensives	
β-blockers	
Calcium channel blockers	
Clonidine	
Diuretics	

The resolution of the constipation following discontinuation of the suspect medication establishes the diagnosis of medication-induced constipation.

If the patient has medication-induced constipation, ***Stop Here.***

If the patient does not have medication-induced constipation, ***Proceed to Step 8.***

> **STEP 8: *Does the Patient Have a Neurologic Disorder?***

Diseases of both the central and peripheral nervous systems are associated with constipation. In these conditions, the patient usually has a known neurological condition. Rarely is constipation the initial manifestation of an occult neurological condition. The neurological diseases associated with constipation are listed in the box in Step 3.

If the constipation is due to a neurologic disorder, ***Stop Here.***

If the constipation is not due to a neurologic disorder, ***Proceed to Step 9.***

> **STEP 9: *Does the Patient Have a Metabolic or Endocrine Disorder?***

Endocrine and metabolic disorders that are associated with constipation are listed in the box in step 3. The constipation associated with diabetes mellitus is thought to be due to autonomic neuropathy. Hypothyroidism predisposes to constipation because of impaired colonic motility. On occasion, the constipation may be so severe that patients present with life-threatening megacolon. An alteration in hormone levels may be the basis of the constipation that frequently occurs during pregnancy. Even in the absence of signs and symptoms suggestive of a metabolic/endocrine disorder, the clinician should obtain the following tests:

- TSH
- Potassium level
- Calcium level
- Fasting glucose level
- Pregnancy test (if indicated)

If the constipation is caused by a metabolic/endocrine disorder, **Stop Here**.

If the constipation is not caused by a metabolic/endocrine disorder, **Proceed to Step 10.**

STEP 10: *Does the Patient Have a Connective Tissue Disorder?*

Patients with scleroderma and amyloidosis may complain of constipation. The mechanism of the constipation involves both nerve involvement and muscle fibrosis. The diagnosis of scleroderma is usually known when the patient presents with constipation. In other cases, signs and symptoms suggestive of scleroderma are present.

If the constipation is caused by a connective tissue disease, **Stop Here**.

If the constipation is not caused by a connective tissue disease, **Proceed to Step 11**.

STEP 11: *Does the Patient Have Cancer?*

Constipation is frequently reported in patients with cancer. One or more of the following may be responsible for the constipation in patients with cancer:

- Decreased oral intake
- Immobility
- Invasion of pelvic or spinal nerves that coordinate colonic function
- Mechanical obstruction by tumor
- Narcotic analgesics
- Paraneoplastic syndrome

If the constipation is caused by cancer, **Stop Here**.

If the constipation is not caused by cancer, **Proceed to Step 12**.

STEP 12: *Does the Patient Have Irritable Bowel Syndrome?*

With exclusion of the more serious causes of constipation, the clinician should consider the irritable bowel syndrome. Over 20% of the U.S. population is thought to have the irritable bowel syndrome. In 1978, investigators reported six symptoms that were more common in patients with irritable bowel syndrome than in those with other gastrointestinal conditions. These symptoms, now known as the Manning criteria, are listed in the following box.

Manning Criteria for Irritable Bowel Syndrome
Feeling of incomplete evacuation
Abdominal distention
Mucus in the stools
Pain relief after defecation
More frequent stools after onset of pain
Looser stools after onset of pain

Adapted from Manning AP, Thompson WG, Heaton KW, et al," Towards Positive Diagnosis in Irritable Bowel," *Br Med J,* 1978, 2(6138):653-4.

The sensitivity and specificity of the Manning criteria in distinguishing irritable bowel syndrome from organic disease is 58% and 74%, respectively. In 1989, Thompson and colleagues developed a set of criteria that has gained widespread acceptance in the diagnosis of irritable bowel syndrome. These criteria, known as the Rome criteria, are listed in the following box.

Rome Criteria for Irritable Bowel Syndrome
Two or more of the following, at least 25% of the time
Altered stool form
Altered stool frequency
Altered stool passage
Bloating or feeling of abdominal distention
Passage of mucus
and/or
Abdominal pain or discomfort which is
Associated with a change in the frequency of bowel movements
and/or
Relieved with defecation

Adapted from Thompson WG, Dotevall G, Drossman DA, et al, "Irritable Bowel Syndrome: Guidelines for the Diagnosis," *Gastroenterol Int,* 1989, 2:92-5.

Other symptoms that commonly occur in patients with irritable bowel syndrome are listed in the following box.

Other Symptoms Commonly Appreciated in Patients with Irritable Bowel Syndrome	
Dyspepsia	Nausea/vomiting
Headache	Palpitations
Insomnia	Sexual impairment
Loss of concentration	Urinary frequency
Lower back pain	Urinary urgency

Establishing the diagnosis of irritable bowel syndrome requires determination of whether the patient's symptoms fulfill the criteria listed above. In addition, the clinician should exclude organic disease. Extensive diagnostic tests are not always required in the patient presenting with symptoms consistent with irritable bowel syndrome. In those suspected of having irritable bowel syndrome, a full diagnostic evaluation is recommended, however, in the following patients:

- Age >50 years
- Signs of organic disease
- Severe symptoms
- Change in symptoms
- New onset of symptoms

In the younger patient with mild, chronic symptoms and no signs of organic disease, the evaluation may be kept to a minimum.

If the constipation is caused by irritable bowel syndrome, **Stop Here**.

If the constipation is not caused by irritable bowel syndrome, **Proceed to Step 13**.

STEP 13: *What Simple Treatment Measures or Pharmacologic Agents Should be Recommended?*

Once gastrointestinal and systemic causes of constipation have been excluded, the clinician is left with a chronically constipated patient who likely has an idiopathic cause. While functional testing of the colon is available, most patients with chronic idiopathic constipation respond to simple therapy. Initially, the clinician should recommend the following:

- Adequate fluid intake
- Bowel retraining
- Increased intake of fiber
- Institution of exercise

Some patients may respond to these lifestyle modifications. In others, however, constipation continues to be a problem. The clinician should consider pharmacologic therapy in this group of patients. Since there is no consensus on which agent should be initially started, the clinician should individualize therapy.

If the constipation is controlled by simple or pharmacologic therapy, **Stop Here.**

If the constipation is refractory or difficult to control with pharmacologic therapy, **Proceed to Step 14.**

STEP 14: *Should the Patient Have Functional Testing Performed?*

Further evaluation of colonic and anorectal function should be considered in the patient who fails to respond to simple therapeutic measures. These patients are considered to have severe idiopathic constipation. Prior to performing functional studies, these patients should have either colonoscopy or the combination of flexible sigmoidoscopy and barium enema to exclude a structural abnormality.

Once a structural cause has been excluded, further evaluation depends on the patient's symptoms. In those patients complaining of decreased frequency of defecation, a colonic transit study should be performed. In this study, the colonic transit time of ingested radiopaque markers is measured by serial abdominal x-rays. In a normal study, 80% of the ingested markers should be excreted by the fifth day. Some patients found to have normal motility on the colonic transit time study have irritable bowel syndrome. Those who are found to have an abnormal transit time are considered to have colonic inertia.

Anorectal testing should be performed in patients who complain of excessive straining or digital extraction of stool. These tests may include the balloon expulsion test, anorectal manometry, and defecography.

End of Section.

> **STEP 15:** *What Testing Should be Performed in the Patient With Alarm Features?*

Structural colonic abnormalities such as colon or rectal cancer must be excluded when alarm features are present in the patient with constipation. Most gastroenterologists recommend colonoscopy over the combination of flexible sigmoidoscopy and barium enema if any of the following alarm features are present:

- Age >45 years
- Weight loss
- Evidence of blood loss (anemia, hemoccult positive stools, melena, hematochezia)
- Family history of colon or rectal cancer

In those who do not have any of the above features, it is reasonable to perform flexible sigmoidoscopy. Both flexible sigmoidoscopy and colonoscopy are excellent in identifying colonic lesions that narrow or occlude the bowel.

The need to perform a barium enema in addition to flexible sigmoidoscopy should be individualized. The addition of the barium enema allows the clinician to assess the colon that is not accessible to the flexible sigmoidoscope.

Barium enema, however, should never be done alone in the evaluation of the constipated patient with alarm features. Subtle mucosal abnormalities may be missed. In addition, the distal 15-20 cm of the colon are not adequately visualized radiographically. Barium enema is also unable to demonstrate melanosis coli, the black leopard-like spotting of the colonic mucosa seen in patients abusing anthraquinone laxatives.

Barium enema is more useful when there is concern that the constipation may be due to extrinsic compression of the colon from malignancy.

REFERENCES

Barloon TJ and Lu CC, "Diagnostic Imaging in the Evaluation of Constipation in Adults," *Am Fam Phys*, 1997, 56(2):513-20.

De Bosset V, Gonvers JJ, Vader JP, et al, "Appropriateness of Colonoscopy: Lower Abdominal Pain or Constipation," *Endoscopy*, 1999, 31(8):637-40.

Halligan S and Bartram CI, "The Radiological Investigation of Constipation," *Clin Radiol*, 1995, 50(7):429-35.

Manning AP, Thompson WG, Heaton KW, et al, "Towards Positive Diagnosis in Irritable Bowel," *Br Med J*, 1978, 2(6138):653-4.

Prather CM and Ortiz-Camacho CP, "Evaluation and Treatment of Constipation and Fecal Impaction in Adults," *Mayo Clin Proc*, 1998, 73(9):881-6.

Schaefer DC and Cheskin LJ, "Constipation in the Elderly," *Am Fam Phys*, 1998, 58(4):907-14.

Schmulson MW and Chang L, "Diagnostic Approach to the Patient With Irritable Bowel Syndrome," *Am J Med*, 1999, 107(5A):20S-26S.

Soffer EE, "Constipation: An Approach to Diagnosis, Treatment, Referral," *Cleve Clin J Med*, 1999, 66(1):41-6.

Thompson WG, Dotevall G, Drossman DA, et al, "Irritable Bowel Syndrome: Guidelines for the Diagnosis," *Gastroenterol Int*, 1989, 2:92-5.

Wilson JA, "Constipation in the Elderly," *Clin Geriatr Med*, 1999, 15(3):499-510.

CONSTIPATION

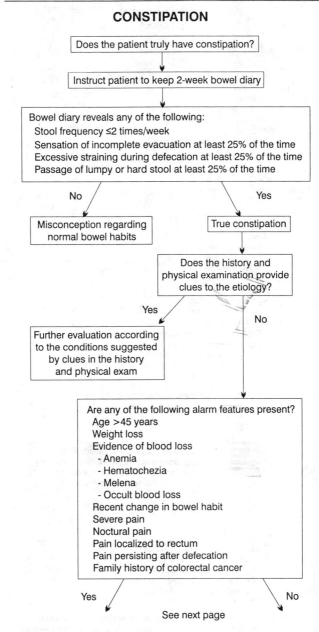

Does the patient truly have constipation?

Instruct patient to keep 2-week bowel diary

Bowel diary reveals any of the following:
Stool frequency ≤2 times/week
Sensation of incomplete evacuation at least 25% of the time
Excessive straining during defecation at least 25% of the time
Passage of lumpy or hard stool at least 25% of the time

No → Misconception regarding normal bowel habits

Yes → True constipation

Does the history and physical examination provide clues to the etiology?

Yes → Further evaluation according to the conditions suggested by clues in the history and physical exam

No →

Are any of the following alarm features present?
Age >45 years
Weight loss
Evidence of blood loss
  - Anemia
  - Hematochezia
  - Melena
  - Occult blood loss
Recent change in bowel habit
Severe pain
Noctural pain
Pain localized to rectum
Pain persisting after defecation
Family history of colorectal cancer

Yes   No

See next page

CONSTIPATION
(continued)

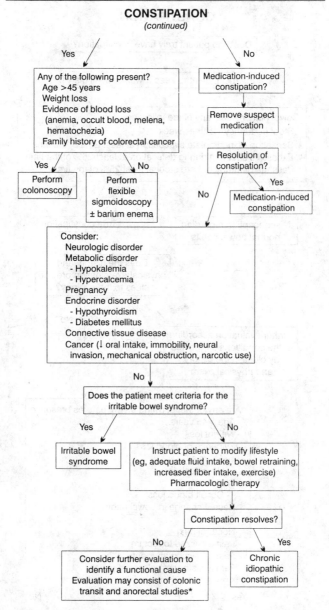

Yes

Any of the following present?
Age >45 years
Weight loss
Evidence of blood loss
(anemia, occult blood, melena,
hematochezia)
Family history of colorectal cancer

Yes → Perform colonoscopy

No → Perform flexible sigmoidoscopy ± barium enema

No → Medication-induced constipation?

Remove suspect medication

Resolution of constipation?

Yes → Medication-induced constipation

No →

Consider:
Neurologic disorder
Metabolic disorder
- Hypokalemia
- Hypercalcemia
Pregnancy
Endocrine disorder
- Hypothyroidism
- Diabetes mellitus
Connective tissue disease
Cancer (↓ oral intake, immobility, neural
invasion, mechanical obstruction, narcotic use)

No →

Does the patient meet criteria for the irritable bowel syndrome?

Yes → Irritable bowel syndrome

No → Instruct patient to modify lifestyle
(eg, adequate fluid intake, bowel retraining,
increased fiber intake, exercise)
Pharmacologic therapy

Constipation resolves?

No → Consider further evaluation to
identify a functional cause
Evaluation may consist of colonic
transit and anorectal studies*

Yes → Chronic idiopathic constipation

*Before pursuing a functional cause, patients with constipation that is
difficult to control with lifestyle modifications and pharmacologic therapy
should have colonscopy or flexible sigmoidoscopy with barium enema to
exclude a structural cause.

COUGH (CHRONIC)

STEP 1: *What are the Causes of Chronic Cough?*

Although there is some debate about how best to define chronic cough, most authorities define chronic cough as a cough that persists for over 3 weeks. It is the fifth most common symptom that prompts patients to seek medical care. The causes of chronic cough are listed in the following box.

Causes of Chronic Cough

ACE inhibitor
Asthma
Bronchiectasis
Chronic bronchitis
Chronic fungal infection
Congestive heart failure
Cystic fibrosis
Foreign body
Gastroesophageal reflux disease (GERD)
Impacted cerumen
Interstitial lung disease
Lung cancer
Occupational (inhalation of bronchial irritants)
Postinfectious cough
Postnasal drip syndrome
Pressure from intrathoracic mass
   Mediastinal lymphadenopathy
   Thoracic aneurysm
   Thyromegaly
Psychogenic
Tuberculosis

Proceed to Step 2

STEP 2: *Are There Any Clues in the Patient's History That Point to the Etiology of the Chronic Cough?*

In approximately 70% of cases, the history provides clues to the etiology of the chronic cough. Historical clues that may suggest the etiology of the chronic cough are listed in the following table.

Historical Clue	Condition Suggested
Sensation of something dripping down the throat Nasal discharge Frequent need to clear the throat	Postnasal drip syndrome
Episodic symptoms of wheezing and shortness of breath	Asthma
Heartburn Regurgitation Sour taste in the mouth	GERD
Smoker who expectorates phlegm on most days during periods that span at least 3 months for more than 2 successive years	Chronic bronchitis
Recent institution of ACE inhibitor	Cough due to ACE inhibitor therapy
Smoker	Chronic bronchitis Lung cancer*
History of weight loss	Lung cancer* Tuberculosis
High risk of tuberculosis exposure	Tuberculosis
Night sweats	Tuberculosis
Nocturnal cough or wheezing	Congestive heart failure Asthma
Smoker with new or recent change in cough	Lung cancer*
Orthopnea PND	Congestive heart failure
Hemoptysis	Tuberculosis Lung cancer* Bronchiectasis
Fever	Tuberculosis
Cough gets better on vacation	Occupational exposure to irritants (dust, fumes)

*One concern for both clinicians and patients is the possibility of lung cancer. However, <2% of cases of chronic cough are due to lung cancer. Lung cancer is mainly a concern in any patient with a current or past smoking history. A new cough or any recent change in a smoker should prompt concern for the possibility of lung cancer. Hemoptysis is also concerning for lung cancer. Since cough is more commonly appreciated in lung cancer patients having cancers affecting the larger airways, physical examination may reveal localized wheezing.

If the patient has hemoptysis, proceed to the chapter on Hemoptysis *on page 299.*

If there are clues in the history that point to the etiology of the chronic cough, the evaluation should be tailored accordingly.

If there are no clues in the history that point to the etiology of the chronic cough, *Proceed to Step 3.*

STEP 3: *What are the Most Common Causes of Chronic Cough?*

It is important to realize that studies of patients with chronic cough have determined that the following conditions are responsible for 95% of cases:

- ACE inhibitor
- Asthma
- Chronic bronchitis
- GERD
- Postnasal drip syndrome

Proceed to Step 4

STEP 4: *Does the Patient Need a CXR?*

A CXR is recommended in almost all patients with chronic cough. The only exceptions to this rule are young nonsmokers and pregnant women. The chest x-ray may reveal an etiology in the 5% of patients who do not have one of the common causes of chronic cough listed in Step 3. Findings noted on the CXR may be classified as follows:

- Normal
- Abnormal but findings are consistent with an old and unrelated process
- Abnormal and findings are not consistent with an old and unrelated process

A normal CXR argues for the diagnosis of one of the common causes of chronic cough such as postnasal drip syndrome, asthma, gastroesophageal reflux disease, chronic bronchitis, and cough due to ACE inhibitor therapy. An abnormal CXR that reveals findings consistent with an old and unrelated process should also prompt the clinician to consider these same causes. An abnormal CXR (findings not consistent with an old and unrelated process) should prompt the clinician to evaluate the diseases suggested by the radiographic findings.

If the CXR is normal, *Proceed to Step 5*.

If the CXR is abnormal but reveals findings consistent with an old and unrelated process, *Proceed to Step 5*.

If the CXR is abnormal and reveals findings not consistent with an old and unrelated process, the clinician should tailor the work up to the diseases suggested by the radiographic findings.

STEP 5: *Is the Patient Taking an ACE Inhibitor?*

A nonproductive cough develops in 3% to 20% of patients started on ACE inhibitor therapy. There is no relationship between the dose of the ACE inhibitor and the development of cough. Although most cases of ACE inhibitor-induced cough begin within the first few weeks of therapy, cases have been reported in which the cough did not start until six months after the institution of the ACE inhibitor.

Before embarking on an extensive evaluation of the patient having a chronic cough, ACE inhibitor therapy should be discontinued. The great majority of cough due to ACE inhibitor therapy resolves during the four weeks that follow the discontinuation of the medication. Persistence of the cough in these patients or chronic cough in the patient not taking an ACE inhibitor mandates further evaluation.

If the patient has a cough due to ACE inhibitor therapy, **Stop Here**.

If the patient does not have a cough due to ACE inhibitor therapy, **Proceed to Step 6**.

STEP 6: *Does the Patient Have Chronic Bronchitis?*

Chronic bronchitis is the major consideration in the smoker having a chronic cough. It is defined as the expectoration of phlegm on most days during at least three months for over two consecutive years in a patient who has no other etiology for the cough. A clear or white sputum is typical of the productive cough that occurs in chronic bronchitis. Supportive of chronic bronchitis are physical examination findings of wheezing or rhonchi.

A chronic cough in a smoker with a normal chest film should not be evaluated further until the response to smoking cessation is known. A smoker's cough should improve considerably or resolve during the four weeks that follow smoking cessation. A cough that has improved but not resolved suggests that the cough is partially due to chronic bronchitis. In these patients, the cough is likely to be multifactorial and the clinician should consider some of the other common causes of chronic cough, which will be discussed in the following steps.

Not uncommonly, smokers are reluctant to stop smoking. In these patients, it may be useful to obtain pulmonary function tests. Documentation of obstructive deficits may be just the impetus the smoker needs to stop smoking. In addition, the information is useful in not only assessing the response to therapy but also prognosis.

If the cough resolves with cessation of smoking, **Stop Here**.

If the cough improves but does not resolve with cessation of smoking, **Proceed to Step 7**.

If the cough does not resolve with cessation of smoking, **Proceed to Step 7**.

STEP 7: *Does the Patient Have the Postnasal Drip Syndrome?*

The postnasal drip syndrome is the most common cause of chronic cough. In adults, sinusitis is the most common cause of the postnasal drip syndrome accounting for 30% to 60% of cases. Less common causes include the different forms of rhinitis (allergic, postinfectious, vasomotor, nonallergic, environmental-irritant-induced, and drug-induced). Postnasal drip syndrome should be suspected if any of the features listed in the following box are present.

Features of Postnasal Drip Syndrome
Nasal discharge
Need to clear the throat frequently
Sensation of something dripping down the throat

A cobblestone appearance of the pharyngeal mucosa supports the diagnosis. Mucoid or mucopurulent secretions may be noted on inspection of the nasopharynx.

It is important to realize, however, that the above features are absent in some patients with the postnasal drip syndrome. As a result, it is the response to therapy that often provides the definitive diagnosis. Therefore, patients should receive empiric treatment for the postnasal drip syndrome based upon the etiology of the postnasal drip syndrome. Recommendations for therapy are listed in the following table.

Cause of Postnasal Drip Syndrome	Recommended Treatment
Allergic rhinitis	Avoidance of offending allergens
	Loratadine, 10 mg once daily
Chronic bacterial sinusitis*	Antibiotic directed against *H. influenzae, S. pneumoniae*, and oral anaerobes
	Dexbrompheniramine plus pseudoephedrine for 3 weeks
	Oxymetazoline for 5 days
Nonallergic rhinitis*	Dexbrompheniramine plus pseudoephedrine for 3 weeks or
	Ipratropium (0.06%) nasal spray for 3 weeks
Vasomotor rhinitis	Ipratropium (0.06%) nasal spray for 3 weeks and then as needed

*After resolution of the cough, patients should be prescribed a 3-month course of nasal corticosteroids

Adapted from Irwin RS and Madison JM, "Review Articles: Primary Care: The Diagnosis and Treatment of Cough," *N Engl J Med*, 2000, 343(23):1715-21.

If the cough resolves with treatment for the postnasal drip syndrome, ***Stop Here***.

If the cough does not resolve with treatment for the postnasal drip syndrome, ***Proceed to Step 8***.

STEP 8: *Does the Patient Have Asthma?*

If the cough persists despite appropriate treatment for the postnasal drip syndrome, the clinician should consider asthma, the second most common cause of chronic cough. While many patients with asthma have episodic wheezing and shortness of breath along with the cough, cough may be the only symptom of asthma in 28% to 57% of patients. This form of asthma is known as cough-variant asthma. Clues to the diagnosis are a history of atopy or other family members with asthma. Asthma should also be a consideration when chronic cough begins after the institution of β-blocker medication.

Pulmonary function test results consistent with obstructive airways disease support the diagnosis of asthma. In particular, documentation of reversible airway obstruction (ie, 15% to 20% improvement in FEV1) is very supportive of the diagnosis. The clinician, however, should realize that the test may be falsely positive. In fact, false-positive test results occur in 33% of patients with chronic cough.

Standard pulmonary function tests may not reveal the diagnosis of cough-variant asthma in all cases. Therefore, when asthma remains a consideration, it is worthwhile to perform a bronchoprovocation test using methacholine. Because this test has a negative predictive value of 100%, a negative result excludes the diagnosis. Unfortunately, false-positive test results may occur in up to 22% of patients. As a result, a positive test result should not be considered diagnostic of asthma unless there is clear improvement in the cough with asthma therapy.

If the cough resolves with treatment for asthma, *Stop Here*.

If the cough does not resolve with treatment for asthma, *Proceed to Step 9*.

STEP 9: *Does the Patient Have Gastroesophageal Reflux Disease?*

In patients whose cough persists despite treatment for postnasal drip syndrome and asthma, attention should focus on the possibility of gastroesophageal reflux disease (GERD). Chronic cough occurring in combination with heartburn and regurgitation strongly supports the diagnosis of GERD.

However, some patients with GERD may only complain of chronic cough. In up to 40% of patients with GERD, chronic cough is the sole manifestation of the illness. Although testing such as 24-hour esophageal pH monitoring is available to establish the diagnosis in these patients, most authorities prefer to make the diagnosis of GERD if the cough resolves with appropriate therapy. Therapy for GERD may include any of the following:

- Discontinuation of medications that may worsen GERD

- Gastric acid suppression therapy

   Gastric-acid suppression therapy, preferably with high doses of proton-pump inhibitors (omeprazole 80 mg/day), should be instituted in these patients.

- Modification of diet and lifestyle

- Prokinetic therapy

A prolonged course of therapy (at least eight weeks) may be necessary for resolution of the cough.

If the cough resolves with treatment for GERD, *Stop Here*.

If the cough does not resolve with treatment for GERD, *Proceed to Step 10*.

STEP 10: *What are Some Considerations When the Etiology of the Chronic Cough Remains Unclear?*

When the chronic cough persists despite therapy for the common causes, the clinician should consider the possibilities listed in the following box.

Common Pitfalls in Managing the Most Common Causes of Chronic Cough

Asthma

- Failing to recognize that it can present as a syndrome of cough and phlegm
- Failing to recognize that inhaled medication may exacerbate cough
- Assuming that a positive result of methacholine challenge alone is diagnostic of asthma

Gastroesophageal Reflux Disease

- Failing to recognize that it can present as a syndrome of cough and phlegm
- Failing to recognize that "silent" reflux disease can be the cause of cough and that it may take 2-3 months of intensive medical therapy before cough starts to improve and, on average, 5-6 months before cough resolves
- Assuming that cough cannot be due to GERD because cough remains unchanged when gastrointestinal symptoms improve
- Failing to recognize that cough may fail to improve with the most intensive medical therapy and that the adequacy of therapy and the need for surgery can be assessed by means of 24-hour monitoring of esophageal pH
- Failing to recognize the effects of coexisting diseases (eg, obstructive sleep apnea or coronary artery disease) or their treatment (eg, nitrates)
- Failing to treat adequately coexisting causes of cough that perpetuate the cycle of cough and reflux

Postnasal Drip Syndrome

- Failing to recognize that it can present as a syndrome of chronic cough and phlegm
- Assuming that all H_1 antagonists are the same
- Failing to consider sinusitis because it is not obvious
- Failing to consider allergic rhinitis and failing to recommend the avoidance of allergens because the symptoms are perennial

Postnasal Drip, Asthma, and GERD

- Failing to consider that more than one of these conditions may be contributing simultaneously to cough
- Failing to consider these common conditions because of another "obvious" cause (eg, chronic interstitial pneumonia)

Adapted from Irwin RS and Madison JM, "Review Articles: Primary Care: The Diagnosis and Treatment of Cough," *N Engl J Med*, 2000, 343(23):1715-21.

Avoiding the above pitfalls often results in the resolution of the cough.

If the cough resolves, ***Stop Here.***

If the cough does not resolve, ***Proceed to Step 11.***

STEP 11: *What are Considerations in the Patient Whose Cough Persists?*

It is reasonable to consult a pulmonary specialist when the etiology of the chronic cough continues to remain elusive. The pulmonary specialist may recommend one of the following tests.

High Resolution CT Scan of the Lungs

High resolution CT scan of the lungs may be useful in the diagnosis of bronchiectasis. The hallmark of bronchiectasis is cough that is usually productive of mucopurulent sputum. With exacerbations of bronchiectasis, the cough may become purulent. It is important to realize, however, that a dry cough is reported in some patients. Although the physical examination may be unremarkable, some patients may have bilateral rhonchi, crackles, or wheezes. Although CXR may reveal findings consistent with bronchiectasis, in some, the CXR may be unrevealing. More sensitive and specific in the diagnosis of bronchiectasis is high resolution chest CT scanning.

In addition, CT scan is more sensitive in the diagnosis of other lung pathology including, for example, interstitial lung disease. In approximately 10% of interstitial lung disease cases, the CXR may be normal.

Pulmonary Function Tests

Pulmonary function testing may be useful in establishing a diagnosis of obstructive lung disease. The CXR is normal in many patients with obstructive lung disease. The diagnosis rests upon the history, physical examination, and pulmonary function tests.

In the patient with a normal CXR, pulmonary function tests that reveal a restrictive pattern should prompt the clinician to consider interstitial lung disease.

Bronchoscopy

When cough remains unexplained despite a thorough evaluation, bronchoscopy should be considered. Of concern to both the clinician and the patient is the possibility of lung cancer. Lung cancer can be present in patients with chronic cough who have a normal CXR. In these cases, the lung cancer is entirely endobronchial. Bronchoscopy should be more of a consideration if the patient has any of the following characteristics:

1. Age >40 years
2. History of hemoptysis
3. Smoker

Even in these patients, however, the yield of bronchoscopy is low. In the absence of these features, bronchoscopy may still be performed, particularly for reassurance in those who are concerned about the possibility of lung cancer.

Echocardiography

Another consideration is congestive heart failure. In patients with known congestive heart failure, the presence of chronic cough may be a manifestation of suboptimal treatment. In these patients, EKG and echocardiogram may be warranted.

If the etiology of the chronic cough is elucidated, **Stop Here.**

If the etiology of the chronic cough is not elucidated, **Proceed to Step 12.**

STEP 12: *Does the Patient Have a Psychogenic Cough?*

When the etiology remains unclear despite a thorough evaluation, the clinician should consider the possibility that the chronic cough has a psychogenic origin. Although it is a rare cause of chronic cough, it should be suspected when any of the features listed in the following box are present.

Features Suggestive of Psychogenic Cough
Coexisting anxiety or depression is present
Cough abates with relief of stress
Cough is apparent in public but inapparent when patient thinks he or she is alone
Cough recurs with stress

Psychogenic cough can be a difficult diagnosis to make. It should always be considered a diagnosis of exclusion.

REFERENCES

Burns MW, "Chronic Cough. Diagnostic and Management Options," *Aust Fam Physician*, 1996, 25(2):161-2, 166-7.

Harding SM and Richter JE, "The Role of Gastroesophageal Reflux in Chronic Cough and Asthma," *Chest*, 1997, 111(5):1389-402 (review).

Irwin RS and Madison JM, "Review Articles: Primary Care: The Diagnosis and Treatment of Cough," *N Engl J Med*, 2000, 343(23):1715-21.

Irwin RS and Richter JE, "Gastroesophageal Reflux and Chronic Cough," *Am J Gastroenterol*, 2000, 95(8 Suppl):S9-14 (review).

Lawler WR, "An Office Approach to the Diagnosis of Chronic Cough," *Am Fam Phys*, 1998, 58(9):2015-22 (review).

Patrick H and Patrick F, "Chronic Cough," *Med Clin North Am*, 1995, 79(2):361-72.

Philip EB, "Chronic Cough," *Am Fam Phys*, 1997, 56(5):1395-404 (review).

Tan RA and Spector SL, "Chronic Cough," *Compr Ther*, 1997, 23(7):467-71 (review).

COUGH (CHRONIC)

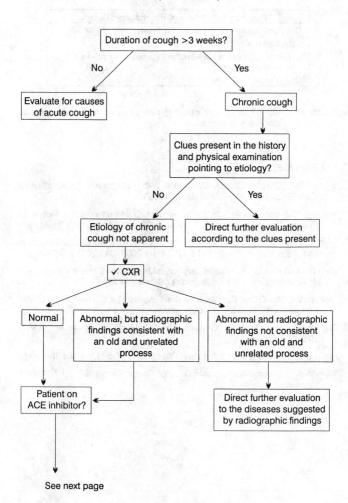

COUGH (CHRONIC)
(continued)

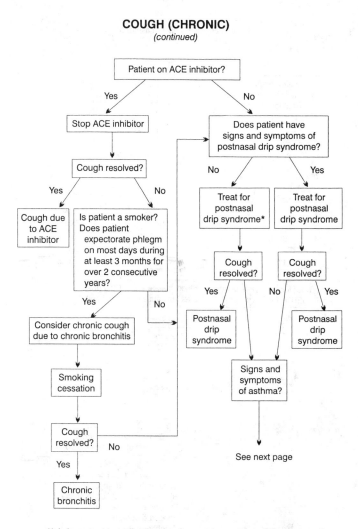

*It is important to realize that the signs and symptoms of the postnasal drip syndrome may be absent in some patients. In these patients, it is the response to therapy that will allow the clinician to establish the diagnosis.

COUGH (CHRONIC)
(continued)

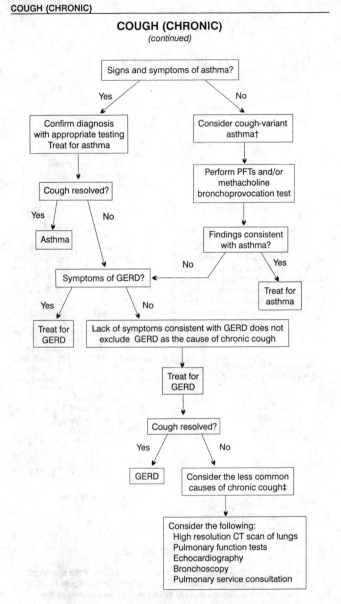

†In some patients with asthma, chronic cough may be the only symptom.
This is known as cough-variant asthma.
‡It is also worthwhile to consider the common pitfalls in establishing the
etiology of chronic cough (see Step 10 in the preceding text).

DIARRHEA (ACUTE)

STEP 1: *What is Acute Diarrhea?*

A diarrheal illness of less than two weeks duration is considered to be the definition of acute diarrhea. Chronic diarrhea is defined as diarrhea that lasts at least one month. That which falls between acute and chronic diarrhea is considered to be persistent diarrhea. This chapter will focus on the approach to the patient presenting with acute diarrhea.

Worldwide, diarrheal illnesses are the second leading cause of death. Even in developed countries such as the United States, diarrhea accounts for significant morbidity and mortality. In fact, in the United States alone, diarrhea is responsible for 1.5 million outpatient visits a year. Although most cases of acute diarrhea can be treated on an outpatient basis, over 450,000 patients are hospitalized every year with gastroenteritis, the most common cause of acute diarrhea. This accounts for 1.5% of all adult hospitalizations.

Proceed to Step 2

STEP 2: *What are the Causes of Acute Diarrhea?*

The causes of acute diarrhea are listed in the following box.

Causes of Acute Diarrhea	
Infection	Parasitic
Bacterial	*Cryptosporidium*
Aeromonas	*Cyclospora*
Bacillus cereus	*Entamoeba histolytica*
Campylobacter	*Giardia lamblia*
Chlamydia	*Isospora belli*
Clostridium difficile	*Microsporidium*
Clostridium perfringens	Others
Escherichia coli	**Noninfectious**
Neisseria gonorrhoeae	Acute radiation sickness
Plesiomonas	Appendicitis
Salmonella	Chemical poisons
Shigella	Arsenic
Staphylococcus aureus	Cadmium
Treponema pallidum	Lead
Vibrio	Mercury
Yersinia	Diverticulitis
Viral	Fecal impaction
Adenovirus	Inflammatory bowel disease
Astrovirus	Ischemic bowel disease
Calicivirus	Medications
Coronavirus	Mushroom intoxication
Cytomegalovirus	
Herpes simplex virus	
Norwalk	
Rotavirus	

Proceed to Step 3

STEP 3: *Are There Any Clues in the Patient's History That Point to the Etiology of Acute Diarrhea?*

Clues in the patient's history that point to the etiology of acute diarrhea are listed in the following table.

Historical Clue	Condition Suggested
Recent antibiotic use	*C. difficile* infection Other causes of antibiotic-associated diarrhea
Recently started new medication*	Medication-related diarrhea
Recent ingestion of undercooked ground beef or unpasteurized apple cider	Enterohemorrhagic *E. coli* (EHEC)
Diarrhea developing at least 72 hours after hospitalization	*C. difficile* infection Noninfectious causes Medication-related diarrhea Tube feedings Others Argues strongly against parasitic cause
Light-headedness or dizziness with standing Decreased urine output Weakness Thirst	Symptoms of dehydration
Male homosexual practicing anal intercourse†	*Neisseria gonorrhoeae* Herpes simplex virus *Chlamydia trachomatis* *Treponema pallidum*
Recent travel to developing countries	Traveler's diarrhea
Sore throat	*Yersinia enterocolitica* *Neisseria gonorrhoeae*
Recent excessive ingestion of chewing gum or sodas	Medication-related diarrhea (sorbitol)
History of prolonged bed rest, analgesic use, or recent constipation	Fecal impaction
History of peripheral vascular disease History of coronary artery disease Oral contraceptive use Bacterial endocarditis Prosthetic valve	Risk factors for ischemic bowel disease
Predominantly vomiting	Food poisoning Viral gastroenteritis
Manifestations of dysentery: Passage of bloody stools Small volume stools Passage of mucus Tenesmus	*Shigella* *C. jejuni* *Salmonella* *Aeromonas* *Vibrio parahaemolyticus* *Yersinia enterocolitica* *E. coli* (enteroinvasive or enterohemorrhagic) *Entamoeba histolytica*
History of inflammatory bowel disease	Relapse of inflammatory bowel disease
Acute diarrhea affecting two or more persons who have shared a meal	Food poisoning

(continued)

Historical Clue	Condition Suggested
Neurologic symptoms and signs in patient with acute diarrhea	Ciguatera fish poisoning
	Neurotoxic shellfish poisoning
	Paralytic shellfish poisoning
Tenesmus	Proctocolitis

*Although any medication can cause diarrhea, the medications more commonly associated with acute diarrhea include antacids, antibiotics, antihypertensives, antineoplastic agents, diuretics, lactulose, metoclopramide, quinidine, sorbitol, and theophylline.

†Male homosexuals are also at risk for acute diarrhea due to any agent that is spread by fecal-oral transmission. In addition, those who have AIDS are also susceptible to pathogens not commonly encountered in immunocompetent hosts.

Epidemiologic clues to the etiology of infectious diarrhea are listed in the following table.

Vehicle	Classic Pathogen
Water (including foods washed in such water)	*Cryptosporidium*
	Giardia
	Norwalk virus
	Vibrio cholerae
Poultry	*Campylobacter*
	Salmonella
	Shigella
Beef, unpasteurized fruit juice	Enterohemorrhagic *E. coli*
Seafood and shellfish*	Hepatitis A, B, and C
	Salmonella species
	Vibrio cholerae
	Vibrio parahaemolyticus
	Vibrio vulnificus
Cheese, milk	*Listeria* species
Eggs	*Salmonella* species
Mayonnaise-containing food and cream pies	Staphylococcal and clostridial food poisonings
Fried rice	*Bacillus cereus*
Fresh berries	*Cyclospora* species
Canned vegetables or fruits	*Clostridium* species
Animal-to-person (pets and livestock)	*Campylobacter*
	Cryptosporidium
	Giardia
	Salmonella
Daycare center	*Campylobacter*
	C. difficile
	Cryptosporidium
	Giardia
	Shigella
	Viruses
Hospital, antibiotics, or chemotherapy	*C. difficile*
Swimming pool	*Cryptosporidium*
	Giardia

*Also includes fish poisonings such as scombroid, ciguatera, paralytic, diarrhetic, and neurotoxic disease

Adapted from Park SI and Giannella RA, "Approach to the Adult Patient With Acute Diarrhea," *Gastroenterol Clin North Am*, 1993, 22(3):482-97 (review); also from Yamada T, Alpers DH, Owyang C, et al (eds), *Textbook of Gastroenterology*, 3rd ed, Philadelphia, PA: Lippincott-Raven, 1999.

Proceed to Step 4

> **STEP 4:** *Are There Any Clues in the Patient's Physical Examination That Point to the Etiology of Acute Diarrhea?*

Clues in the patient's physical examination that point to the etiology of the acute diarrhea are listed in the following table.

Physical Examination Finding	Condition Suggested
Absence of axillary sweat Diminished skin turgor Dry mucous membranes Postural hypotension Tachycardia	Volume depletion/dehydration
Fever*	Suggests invasive pathogen
Distention Hypoactive bowel sounds	Consider toxic megacolon (due to invasive pathogen or noninfectious condition)
Peritoneal signs or rigidity	Toxic megacolon or perforation
Anal fissure or fistula	Crohn's disease
Jaundice	Malaria
Skin rash	Rocky Mountain spotted fever *Salmonella typhi* (rose spots) Toxic shock syndrome *Vibrio vulnificus* (hemorrhagic bullae) Viral gastroenteritis
Bradycardia	Typhoid fever
Constricted pupils	Cholinesterase inhibitor poisoning

Shigella, Salmonella, C. jejuni, C. difficile, Aeromonas, and viruses are the major causes of febrile diarrhea.

After a thorough history and physical examination, the clinician may be able to elicit features in the clinical presentation that suggest infection of either the small or large intestine, as shown in the following table.

	Small Intestinal Pathogen	Large Intestinal Pathogen
Abdominal pain	Midabdominal	Lower abdominal or rectal
Stool volume	Large	Small
Stool consistency	Usually watery (rare blood)	Often mucoid or bloody
Stool for occult blood	Rarely positive	Often positive
Tenesmus	Absent	Often present

Determining the location of the enteric infection is a useful way of narrowing the differential diagnosis of acute infectious diarrhea. The predilection of pathogens for the large or small intestine is described in the following box.

Predilection of Pathogens for Large or Small Intestine	
Small intestine	Large intestine
Cryptosporidium	*Aeromonas*
Cyclospora	*Campylobacter*
E. coli (enteropathogenic)	*C. difficile*
E. coli (enterotoxigenic)	Cytomegalovirus
Giardia lamblia	*E. coli* (enterohemorrhagic)
Isospora belli	*E. coli* (enteroinvasive)
Microsporidia	*E. histolytica*
Norwalk	*Plesiomonas*
Rotavirus	*Shigella*
Vibrio cholerae	

There are, however, certain pathogens that can involve both the lower small intestine and colon. These organisms include *Salmonella* and *Yersinia.* In most of these cases, the diarrheal illness is characterized by watery stools. Bloody diarrhea, however, does occur in some cases.

Proceed to Step 5

STEP 5: *Should Laboratory Tests be Obtained in the Patient Presenting With Acute Diarrhea?*

Although there are many causes of acute diarrhea, infection is the leading etiology. Over 90% of patients with acute infectious diarrhea have a mild illness that readily improves with time. In fact, most patients have improved or recovered within five days. In these patients, laboratory evaluation to determine the etiologic organism is not recommended for the following reasons:

- Laboratory testing is expensive
- Test results are often unrevealing
- Testing does not affect treatment
- Testing does not affect outcome

The clinician's goal is to identify features in the patient's clinical presentation that suggest severe illness. Those patients having a severe acute diarrheal illness require further testing. In these patients, it is reasonable to send blood for determination of BUN, creatinine, electrolytes, CBC, and liver function tests. Blood cultures should be performed in clinically septic patients. The indications for fecal leukocyte testing, stool cultures for bacteria, ova and parasite examination, and proctosigmoidoscopy are discussed in the steps that follow.

Proceed to Step 6

STEP 6: *Should Testing for Fecal Leukocytes be Performed?*

Since most cases of acute diarrhea due to infection are self-limited illnesses, fecal leukocyte testing should only be performed in certain situations. Indications for fecal leukocyte testing are listed in the following box.

Indications for Fecal Leukocyte Testing
Moderate or severe diarrhea*
Profuse watery diarrhea with dehydration
Passage of very small volume stools containing blood or mucus
Temperature >38.5°C or 101.3°F
≥6 unformed stools/24 hours
Duration >48 hours
Severe abdominal pain in patient >50 years of age
Diarrhea in elderly patient ≥70 years of age
Immunocompromised patient

*A diarrheal illness that forces a change in a patient's normal activities is referred to as moderate diarrhea. Severe diarrhea is said to be present when the illness confines the patient to bed.

The clinician should consider inflammatory causes of acute diarrhea when numerous fecal leukocytes are noted. Although the presence of fecal leukocytes is not specific for infection, this finding in the patient having clinical manifestations consistent with infectious diarrhea should prompt the clinician to consider invasive pathogens. These pathogens as well as other causes of acute diarrhea associated with fecal leukocytes in the stool are listed in the following box.

Causes of Acute Diarrhea Associated with Fecal Leukocytes in the Stool
Infection
Aeromonas
Campylobacter
Clostridium difficile
E. coli
Enterohemorrhagic (EHEC)
Enteroinvasive (EIEC)
Salmonella
Shigella
Vibrio (noncholera species)
Yersinia enterocolitica
Inflammatory bowel disease

Significant numbers of fecal leukocytes are not found in patients with viral gastroenteritis, parasitic diarrhea, and enterotoxigenic diarrhea (eg, enterotoxigenic *E. coli*, cholera). The clinician must ensure that there is no delay in the processing of the stool specimen for fecal leukocytes as the cells may lyse readily.

Proceed to Step 7

STEP 7: *Should Stool Cultures be Performed?*

It is not cost-effective to obtain a stool culture in every patient presenting with acute diarrhea, especially since the isolation rate of a pathogenic organism is about 3% to 20% in an unselected population. The diagnostic yield of stool culture is improved if the clinician takes the time to elicit certain features in the patient's clinical presentation. The features that should prompt the clinician to obtain stool cultures are listed in the following box.

Indications for Stool Culture in Patients with Acute Diarrhea	
AIDS-related diarrhea	Persistent diarrhea
Bloody stools	Severe diarrhea
+ fecal leukocytes	Temperature >38.5°C or 101.3°F (oral)
+ occult blood in stool	

Laboratories differ as to the pathogens that are tested when stool cultures are requested. In fact, most laboratories will routinely process stool specimens for *Shigella*, *Salmonella*, and *Campylobacter*. If other organisms are possibilities, it behooves the clinician to communicate these concerns with the laboratory. When the stool culture reveals the growth of a known gastrointestinal pathogen in a patient presenting with acute diarrhea, the clinician can be reasonably confident that the organism identified is the etiologic agent.

A history of recent antibiotic therapy should raise concern for the possibility of *C. difficile* infection. Other risk factors include recent hospitalization, daycare exposure, and recent chemotherapy. The most widely used test in the diagnosis of *C. difficile* diarrhea is detection of *C. difficile* toxin in stool specimens. Toxin assays as well as other laboratory tests available in the diagnosis of *C. difficile* infection are described in the following table.

Test	Sensitivity (%)	Specificity (%)	Clinical Utility
Endoscopy	51	100	Diagnostic of pseudomembranous colitis
Culture for *C. difficile**	89-100	84-99	Highly sensitive; confirmation of organism toxicity optimal
Cell culture cytotoxin test	67-100	85-100	With clinical data, diagnostic of CDAD†
EIA toxin test	63-99	75-100	With clinical data, diagnostic of CDAD†
Latex test for *C. difficile* antigen	58-92	80-96	Less sensitive and specific than other tests; rapid results
PCR toxin gene detection	Undetermined	Undetermined	Research test

*Although *C. difficile* culture is a fairly sensitive test in the diagnosis of *C. difficile* infection, most laboratories are unable to differentiate between toxigenic and nonpathogenic strains of the organism. As a result, false-positive test results occur in up to 25% of cases.

†CDAD is an abbreviation for *Clostridium difficile*-associated disease.

Adapted from Gerding DN, Johnson S, Peterson LR, et al, "*Clostridium difficile*-Associated Diarrhea and Colitis," *Infect Control Hosp Epidemiol*, 1995, 16(8):459-77 (review); also from Mandell GL, Bennett JE, and Dolin R, *Principles and Practice of Infectious Disease*, 5th ed, New York, NY: Churchill Livingstone, 2000, 1117.

Proceed to Step 8

STEP 8: *Should an Ova and Parasite Examination be Performed?*

Not all patients with acute diarrhea require stool examination for ova and parasites. In fact, the yield of the ova and parasite examination is low (<10%) in the absence of certain clinical or epidemiologic features. Indications for ova and parasite examination are listed in the following box.

Indications for Stool Ova and Parasite Examination in Patients With Acute Diarrhea
Community waterborne outbreak
Exposure to daycare center
HIV / AIDS
Homosexual males
Persistent diarrhea (>2 weeks)
Recent travel to developing countries, Russia, Nepal, or Rocky Mountains
Stools bloody but few fecal leukocytes noted

The clinician should not examine the stool for ova and parasites in the patient who develops diarrhea while in the hospital because a parasitic cause of the diarrhea is very unlikely in this setting. The clinician should be aware of substances that can negatively impact upon the yield of stool examination for ova and parasites. These substances include bismuth, antibiotic therapy (eg, tetracycline, erythromycin), barium, laxatives, antacids, and hypertonic enemas. If possible, these substances should be avoided.

Intestinal Amebiasis

The identification of cysts and trophozoites in stool specimens establishes the diagnosis of intestinal amebiasis. The yield of the stool examination is increased if the laboratory concentrates the fecal specimens. The clinician should realize that the organism will be identified in just 33% of cases if only one stool specimen is submitted for analysis. Hence, the recommendation for ova and parasite examination of three stool specimens when parasitic causes of acute diarrhea are a consideration.

The endoscopic appearance of amebiasis does not distinguish this infection from other infectious causes of acute diarrhea. However, biopsy or scrapings of lesions (wet preparation of ulcer aspirates or biopsy specimens) noted during endoscopy may reveal findings consistent with amebiasis. In recent years, serum antiamebic antibody tests have become available. These are probably the most useful tests in the diagnosis of amebiasis. One particular antibody test, the indirect hemagglutination test, yields positive results in almost 90% of intestinal amebiasis cases.

Giardiasis

Three separate stool specimens should be examined for the trophozoites and cysts of *Giardia lamblia*. If unrevealing, the clinician may choose to perform ELISA or immunofluorescence testing of the stool for *Giardia* antigens. Unremarkable stool studies should prompt consideration of duodenal aspiration, duodenal biopsy, or the Entero-Test string to establish the diagnosis.

Other Parasitic Causes of Diarrhea

Many of the other parasitic causes of acute diarrhea require acid-fast staining of the stool to identify the organism. Modified Kinyoun's acid-fast stain and trichrome staining of the stool, especially if the stool is concentrated, can demonstrate findings consistent with *Cryptosporidium, Isospora belli*, and microsporidiosis. Microsporidiosis may also be detected by light microscopy of properly stained stool specimens. At times, however, identification of these parasitic causes of acute diarrhea may require small intestinal aspirates or, even, jejunal biopsy. Recently, monoclonal-based tests (ELISA and immuno-fluorescence stains) have been developed for the detection of many of these parasites. The clinician should inform the laboratory if these parasitic causes of acute diarrhea are considerations, especially since routine ova and para-site examination does not always include screening for these protozoal orga-nisms.

Proceed to Step 9

STEP 9: *Should Proctosigmoidoscopy be Performed?*

Indications for proctosigmoidoscopy in patients with acute diarrhea are listed in the following box.

Indications for Proctosigmoidoscopy in Acute Diarrhea
Amebiasis*
Chronic diarrhea
History of anal manipulation
HIV-positive with large bowel diarrhea or acute proctitis
Idiopathic inflammatory bowel disease
Severe antibiotic-associated diarrhea with equivocal test for *C. difficile* toxin†

*Indications for endoscopy in patients suspected of having amebiasis include the following:

- Stool ova and parasite exam is negative but serum anti-amebic antibody test is positive
- Stool ova and parasite exam is negative and immediate diagnosis is needed
- High suspicion for amebiasis but stool ova and parasite examination and serum anti-amebic antibody test are negative

†The American College of Gastroenterology has developed guidelines for the role of endoscopy in patients suspected of having *C. difficile* infection. Their recommendations for endoscopy include the following:

- Rapid diagnosis is necessary but test results are either delayed or insensitive tests were performed
- Patient has ileus and stool is not available

Adapted from Fekety R, "Guidelines for the Diagnosis and Management of *Clostridium difficile*-Associated Diarrhea and Colitis. American College of Gastroenterology, Practice Parameters Committee," *Am J Gastroenterol*, 1997, 92(5):739-50 (review); also from "Intestinal Disease Caused by *Entamoeba histolytica*," *Amebiasis: Human Infection By Entamoeba histolytica*, Ravin JI (ed), New York, NY: Wiley, 1988, 495-510.

Proceed to Step 10

STEP 10: *Has the Diarrhea Resolved?*

Most cases of acute diarrhea resolve within two weeks. Even with extensive laboratory testing, an etiologic agent is not identified in up to 40% of cases. When a diarrheal illness persists after two weeks, the patient is said to have persistent diarrhea. Common causes of persistent diarrhea are listed in the following box.

Common Causes of Persistent Diarrhea	
Bacterial diarrhea	Inflammatory bowel disease
Campylobacter	Lactase deficiency
E. coli (enteropathogenic)	Parasitic
Salmonella	*Cryptosporidium parvum*
Shigella	*Giardia lamblia*
Yersinia	*Isospora belli*
Brainerd diarrhea	*Microsporidia*
Host deficiency (ie, AIDS)	Small intestinal bacterial overgrowth

REFERENCES

Aranda-Michel J and Giannella RA, "Acute Diarrhea: A Practical Review," *Am J Med*, 1999, 106(6):670-6.

Cheney CP and Wong RK, "Acute Infectious Diarrhea," *Med Clin North Am*, 1993, 77(5):1169-96.

DuPont HL, "Guidelines on Acute Infectious Diarrhea in Adults. The Practice Parameters Committee of the American College of Gastroenterology," *Am J Gastroenterol*, 1997, 92(11):1962-75.

Farthing MJ, "Giardiasis," *Gastroenterol Clin North Am*, 1996, 25(3):493-515.

Fekety R, "Guidelines for the Diagnosis and Management of *Clostridium difficile*-Associated Diarrhea and Colitis. American College of Gastroenterology, Practice Parameters Committee," *Am J Gastroenterol*, 1997, 92(5):739-50 (review).

Gerding DN, Johnson S, Peterson LR, et al, "*Clostridium difficile*-Associated Diarrhea and Colitis," *Infect Control Hosp Epidemiol*, 1995, 16(8):459-77 (review).

Mandell GL, Bennett JE, and Dolin RA, *Principles and Practice of Infectious Disease*, 5th ed, New York, NY: Churchill Livingstone, 2000, 1117.

Park SI and Giannella R, "Approach to the Adult Patient with Acute Diarrhea," *Gastroenterol Clin North Am*, 1993, 22(3):483-97 (review).

Plevris JN and Hayes PC, "Investigation and Management of Acute Diarrhoea," *Br J Hosp Med*, 1996, 56(11):569-73.

Ravdin JI, "Intestinal Disease Caused by *Entamoeba histolytica*," *Amebiasis: Human Infection By Entamoeba histolytica*, New York, NY: Wiley, 1988, 495-510.

Talal AH and Murray JA, "Acute and Chronic Diarrhea. How to Keep Laboratory Testing to a Minimum," *Postgrad Med*, 1994, 96(3):30-2, 35-8, 43.

Textbook of Gastroenterology, 3rd ed, Yamada T, Alpers DH, Owyang C, et al (eds), Philadelphia, PA: Lippincott-Raven, 1999.

DIARRHEA (ACUTE)

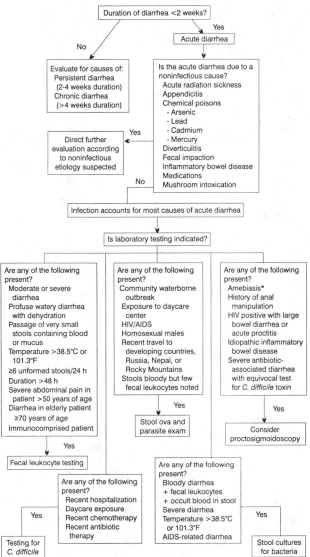

*Indications for proctosigmoidoscopy in acute diarrhea patients suspected of having amebiasis include:
- Stool ova and parasite exam is nevative but serum antiamebic antibody test is positive
- Stool ova and parasite exam is negative and immediate diagnosis is needed
- High suspicion for amebiasis but stool ova and parasite examination and serum antiamebic antibody test are negative

DYSPEPSIA

STEP 1: *What is Dyspepsia?*

Over the years, clinicians have defined dyspepsia in many different ways. These varying definitions have led to considerable confusion about what constitutes dyspepsia. In addition, the absence of a consensus definition hampered clinical research studies for years. In an effort to address these problems, an international committee defined dyspepsia as an upper abdominal discomfort or pain that may be episodic or persistent. Not uncommonly, dyspepsia is accompanied by other symptoms such as belching, heartburn, fullness, early satiety, nausea, vomiting, and anorexia. Dyspepsia occurs in about 25% of the population every year.

Proceed to Step 2

STEP 2: *What are the Causes of Dyspepsia?*

The causes of dyspepsia are listed in the following box.

Causes of Dyspepsia	
Abdominal wall pain	Irritable bowel syndrome
Biliary tract disease	Malignancy
Cholelithiasis	Gastric cancer
Sphincter of Oddi dysfunction	Esophageal cancer
Carbohydrate malabsorption	Hepatoma
Fructose	Pancreatic cancer
Lactose	Medication-induced
Sorbitol	Metabolic disorders
Chronic mesenteric ischemia	Hypercalcemia
Functional (nonulcer)	Hyperkalemia
Gastroesophageal reflux disease	Pancreatitis
Gastroparesis	Peptic ulcer disease
Infiltrative diseases of the stomach	Systemic disorders
Crohn's disease	Connective tissue disease
Sarcoidosis	Diabetes mellitus
Intestinal parasites	Thyroid and parathyroid disorders
Giardia	
Strongyloides	

Proceed to Step 3

STEP 3: *What are the Major Causes of Dyspepsia?*

Most dyspepsia cases are due to functional dyspepsia (nonulcer dyspepsia), peptic ulcer disease, and gastroesophageal reflux disease. The approximate prevalence of these major causes of dyspepsia is listed in the following table.

Condition	Approximate Prevalence
Functional or nonulcer dyspepsia	Up to 60%
Peptic ulcer disease	15% to 25%
Gastroesophageal reflux disease	5% to 15%
Gastric or esophageal cancer	<2%
Other causes	Rare

Adapted from Talley NJ, Silverstein MD, Agreus L, et al, "AGA Technical Review: Evaluation of Dyspepsia," American Gastroenterological Association, *Gastroenterology*, 1998, 114(3):582-95 (review); Fisher RS and Parkman HP, "Management of Nonulcer Dyspepsia," *N Engl J Med*, 1998, 339(19):1376-81 (review); Bazaldua OV and Schneider FD, "Evaluation and Management of Dyspepsia," *Am Fam Phys*, 1999, 60(6):1773-84, 1787-8, (review).

Proceed to Step 4

STEP 4: *Are There Any Clues in the Patient's Clinical Presentation That Point to the Etiology of the Dyspepsia?*

Unfortunately, the clinical presentation often does not allow the clinician to differentiate functional dyspepsia from the structural causes of dyspepsia. The following table describes the difficulty in distinguishing peptic ulcer disease, the leading organic cause of dyspepsia, from functional dyspepsia based on the symptoms alone.

Symptom	Duodenal Ulcer (%)	Gastric Ulcer (%)	Functional Dyspepsia (%)
Epigastric pain	70	70	70
Nocturnal pain	50-80	30-45	25-35
Food causes pain relief	20-65	5-50	5-30
Episodic pain	50-60	10-20	30-40
Belching / bloating	30-65	30-70	40-80

Adapted from Isenberg JI, Walsh JH, and Johnson LR, "Peptic Ulcer Diseases," *AGA Undergraduate Teaching Project - Unit 23*, Timonium, MD: Milner-Fenwick, Inc, 1991; also adapted from *Cecil Textbook of Medicine*, 21st ed, Goldman L and Bennett C (eds), Philadelphia, PA: WB Saunders Co, 2000.

While it is true that symptoms often do not allow the clinician to differentiate functional from structural causes of dyspepsia, at times, the history may be revealing. In some cases of dyspepsia, the clinician may be able to elicit symptoms that strongly suggest a particular disease. Steps 5 through 9 offer a discussion about some of these diseases that may be identified based upon suggestive signs or symptoms.

Proceed to Step 5

STEP 5: *Does the Patient Have Medication-Related Dyspepsia?*

Medication-related dyspepsia should be a consideration in all patients. Although any medication can potentially cause dyspepsia, the common offending agents are listed in the following box.

Common Causes of Medication-Related Dyspepsia
Antibiotics (eg, ampicillin, erythromycin)
Digoxin
Iron supplements
Potassium supplements
Theophylline

Resolution of the dyspepsia following a reduction in the dosage or discontinuation of the suspect medication supports the diagnosis of medication-related dyspepsia.

If the patient has medication-related dyspepsia, *Stop Here.*

If the patient does not have medication-related dyspepsia, *Proceed to Step 6.*

STEP 6: *Does the Patient Have Gastroesophageal Reflux Disease?*

Gastroesophageal reflux disease should be suspected when a patient presents with epigastric or retrosternal burning or discomfort. Classically, this burning sensation, known as heartburn, moves from the xiphoid region to the oropharynx.

In many cases, patients are able to identify factors that precipitate the heartburn. These factors include bending over, lifting heavy objects, straining during defecation, and running. There are certain foods that can predispose to heartburn either by decreasing pressure in the lower esophageal sphincter or irritating the esophageal mucosa directly. These foods include chocolate, onions, coffee, peppermint, spicy foods, citrus products, and tomato products.

The heartburn is usually relieved by antacids. Not uncommonly, patients with gastroesophageal reflux disease describe the regurgitation of bitter tasting liquid.

If the patient has classic features of gastroesophageal reflux disease, *Stop Here.*

If the patient does not have classic features of gastroesophageal reflux disease, *Proceed to Step 7.*

STEP 7: *Does the Patient Have the Irritable Bowel Syndrome?*

Eighty-seven percent of patients having the irritable bowel syndrome report dyspepsia. As such, the clinician should recognize the features of the irritable bowel syndrome. The hallmark of the irritable bowel syndrome is an alteration in bowel habits with or without accompanying abdominal pain. In patients with the irritable bowel syndrome, no organic cause for the symptoms can be found. An international committee developed the Rome criteria, widely used in the diagnosis of the irritable bowel syndrome. The Rome criteria are listed in the following box.

Rome Criteria for the Diagnosis of Irritable Bowel Syndrome

1. Presence of at least three months of continuous or recurrent abdominal pain or discomfort relieved by defecation or associated with a change in the frequency or consistency of the stool

2. Two of the following symptoms at least 25% of the time:

   A. Altered stool frequency

   B. Altered stool form

   C. Altered stool passage

   D. Passage of mucus

   E. Bloating or distention

Adapted from Thompson WG, Dotevall G, Drossman DA, et al, "Irritable Bowel Syndrome: Guidelines for the Diagnosis," *Gastroenterol Int*, 1989, 2:92-5.

If the patient has the irritable bowel syndrome, *Stop Here.*

If the patient does not have the irritable bowel syndrome, *Proceed to Step 8.*

STEP 8: *Does the Patient Have Biliary Tract Disease?*

Biliary tract disease is another consideration in the patient presenting with dyspepsia. Biliary colic develops when a stone transiently obstructs the cystic or common bile duct. This pain has been termed biliary colic, which is really a misnomer in that the pain is usually steady. It is characterized by a gradual onset, building slowly to a plateau and then gradually resolving over a period of one to five hours. Most often, patients describe right upper quadrant pain but, in some, the pain is localized to the epigastrium or left upper quadrant. A classic feature of biliary pain is radiation of the pain to the right shoulder or subscapular region. Not uncommonly, the pain is accompanied by nausea and vomiting.

Gallstones may be found in 1% to 3% of all patients with dyspepsia. However, in the absence of the characteristic history described above, the clinician should not assume that gallstones are the cause of the dyspepsia. Too often, cholecystectomy is performed in patients with vague dyspeptic symptoms, with the feeling that the symptoms are due to the gallstones detected during imaging. In the majority of these patients, the dyspeptic symptoms persist after cholecystectomy.

When dyspepsia develops after a cholecystectomy, the clinician should consider the possibility of sphincter of Oddi dysfunction, which is an abnormality of sphincter of Oddi contractility. Most often, these patients present with right upper quadrant or epigastric pain. Lasting up to several hours in duration, the pain is usually constant. In some patients, the pain radiates to the back or shoulder. Accompanying symptoms in some patients include nausea and vomiting. The diagnosis should be pursued if some of the more common causes of upper abdominal pain such as peptic ulcer disease have been excluded.

If the patient has biliary tract disease, *Stop Here.*

If the patient does not have biliary tract disease, *Proceed to Step 9.*

STEP 9: *Does the Patient Have Carbohydrate Malabsorption?*

Lactase deficiency affects over 50% of the world's population. It tends to have a predilection for African American, Native American, Mediterranean, Asian, and Mexican American populations. Affected individuals develop abdominal pain, bloating, flatulence, and diarrhea after ingesting lactose-containing products (eg, milk). The symptoms of lactase deficiency may not always occur soon after the ingestion of lactose-containing products, making the diagnosis difficult at times. In fact, in some patients, symptoms may develop only hours later. Supportive of the diagnosis is the resolution of symptoms after the institution of a low lactose diet. The gold standard for the diagnosis of lactase deficiency is breath hydrogen testing.

Lactose is just one of the major carbohydrates found in the diet. Deficiency of other enzymes involved in carbohydrate metabolism usually manifests in infancy or childhood.

Two other sugars, fructose and sorbitol, also deserve mention here. Even when enzyme function is intact, the ingestion of fructose- or sorbitol-containing products can cause symptoms of bloating, abdominal pain, flatulence, and diarrhea. Fructose is found in fruits and soft drinks. Sorbitol is found in fruits and chewing gum. As little as two cans of soda or four sticks of chewing gum may be enough to precipitate symptoms. The diagnosis is supported by the resolution of symptoms after avoidance of products containing fructose or sorbitol.

If the patient has carbohydrate malabsorption, *Stop Here.*

If the patient does not have carbohydrate malabsorption, *Proceed to Step 10.*

STEP 10: *Does the Patient Need to Have an Upper Endoscopy?*

Upper endoscopy is recommended in dyspeptic patients if any of the following criteria are met:

- Patient >45 years of age
- Patient <45 years of age having alarm symptoms

Alarm symptoms are listed in the following box.

Alarm Symptoms in the Patient Presenting with Dyspepsia	
Anemia	Palpable mass
Anorexia	Protracted vomiting
Dysphagia	Unexplained weight loss (>3 kg)
Melena	

It is also reasonable to proceed with upper endoscopy in any patient who is overly concerned that the symptoms may be due to malignancy. At this time, upper endoscopy is clearly the diagnostic procedure of choice in these patients, having an accuracy of approximately 90%. In contrast, the accuracy of double-contrast barium radiography in the evaluation of dyspepsia is only 65%. One limitation of barium radiography is that it does not allow the clinician to obtain a biopsy.

If the patient is >45 years of age, *Proceed to Step 11.*

If the patient is <45 years of age but has alarm symptoms, *Proceed to Step 11.*

If the patient is <45 years of age and has no alarm symptoms, *Proceed to Step 13.*

STEP 11: *What are the Results of the Upper Endoscopy?*

Patients >45 years of age should have an upper endoscopy since this group is at higher risk for malignancy. Any patient with alarm symptoms should have an upper endoscopy irrespective of age. An upper endoscopy will allow the clinician to distinguish structural from functional causes of dyspepsia. A normal upper endoscopy in the patient presenting with dyspepsia argues for functional or nonulcer dyspepsia.

If the patient has a structural cause of the dyspepsia, *Stop Here.*

If the patient does not have a structural cause of the dyspepsia, *Proceed to Step 12.*

STEP 12: *Does the Patient Have Functional Dyspepsia?*

While normal endoscopic findings in the patient with dyspepsia suggest a functional etiology, the clinician should consider several other possibilities. Of note, gastroesophageal reflux disease, a major cause of dyspepsia, is not excluded in patients who have a macroscopically normal esophageal mucosa. More sensitive and specific for demonstrating the presence of gastroesophageal reflux disease is mucosal biopsy at the time of endoscopy. Histologic findings consistent with esophageal epithelial proliferation support the diagnosis of gastroesophageal reflux disease. Another test that may be useful in the diagnosis of gastroesophageal reflux disease when endoscopy is macroscopically unrevealing is 24-hour esophageal pH testing. In fact, there is no visible evidence of gastroesophageal reflux disease at the time of endoscopy in 50% of patients found to have GERD by 24-hour esophageal pH testing. It is important not to deem these patients as having functional dyspepsia on the results of the upper endoscopy alone.

In addition, in the presence of alarm symptoms, other possibilities need to be considered. These include the following:

Pancreatic Cancer

Poorly localized pain in the upper abdomen is not uncommon in patients with pancreatic cancer. The pain is due to either malignant biliary obstruction or perineural invasion. Malignant invasion of the retroperitoneal nerves may result in the radiation of the pain to the back. As in pancreatitis, the severity of the pain may vary with position, often increasing when supine and decreasing when leaning forward while sitting up. Imaging, preferably with CT scanning, is the initial diagnostic test of choice.

Hepatoma

Most patients with hepatoma have nonspecific symptoms of malaise, fatigue, anorexia, and weight loss. Some patients also describe upper abdominal pain, particularly right upper quadrant pain. The major risk factor for the development of hepatoma is cirrhosis. Since cirrhotic patients often have the same nonspecific symptoms, the presence of these symptoms do not discriminate between uncomplicated cirrhosis and cirrhosis complicated by hepatoma development. As a result, the clinician should consider imaging the liver with CT or ultrasound, especially when the patient has underlying cirrhosis.

Chronic Mesenteric Ischemia

Chronic mesenteric ischemia, also known as intestinal angina, is a rare disorder characterized by postprandial pain and weight loss. Most patients have sitophobia, defined as fear of eating. The characteristic patient has atherosclerotic risk factors and many have apparent atherosclerotic disease elsewhere. The pain typically occurs 30-90 minutes after eating, often lasting several hours in duration. Angiography is required to establish the diagnosis.

End of Section.

STEP 13: *Does the Patient Have H. pylori?*

In the younger patient (<45 years and no alarm symptoms) with dyspepsia, evidence-based medicine argues for *H. pylori* testing followed by treatment to eradicate the organism if the testing is positive. Noninvasive tests available for the detection of *H. pylori* include the following:

- Serology
- Urea breath test

Both of these noninvasive tests have a sensitivity and specificity exceeding 90%. Because urea breath testing tends to be expensive, most clinicians obtain serology for *H. pylori*. A positive result of either test should be followed by treatment to eradicate the organism.

If the *H. pylori* noninvasive test is positive and treatment of the *H. pylori* results in the resolution of the dyspepsia, *Stop Here.*

If the *H. pylori* noninvasive test is negative, *Proceed to Step 14.*

If the *H. pylori* noninvasive test is positive but treatment of the *H. pylori* does not result in the resolution of the dyspepsia, *Proceed to Step 15.*

STEP 14: *What are the Results of Antisecretory Therapy?*

A negative noninvasive test for *H. pylori* suggests the presence of functional dyspepsia. In these patients, it is reasonable to start antisecretory therapy with either H_2 blockers or proton pump inhibitors. Upper endoscopy is required if there is no response to antisecretory therapy within eight weeks. Upper endoscopy is also indicated if the dyspepsia returns after cessation of the antisecretory therapy.

End of Section.

STEP 15: *What are the Results of the Upper Endoscopy?*

Failure to respond to *H. pylori* therapy mandates endoscopy. Endoscopy will help determine if the patient has a structural cause of the dyspepsia. In those who do not have a structural cause, functional dyspepsia is the likely diagnosis.

REFERENCES

Agreus L and Talley NJ, "Dyspepsia: Current Understanding and Management," *Annu Rev Med*, 1998, 49:475-93.

Bazaldua OV and Schneider FD, "Evaluation and Management of Dyspepsia," *Am Fam Phys*, 1999, 60(6):1773-84, 1787-8 (review).

Cecil Textbook of Medicine, 21st ed, Goldman L and Bennett C (eds), Philadelphia, PA: WB Saunders Co, 2000.

Fisher RS and Parkman HP, "Management of Nonulcer Dyspepsia," *N Engl J Med*, 1998, 339(19):1376-81 (review).

Froehlich F, Bochud M, Gonvers JJ, et al, "Appropriateness of Gastroscopy: Dyspepsia," *Endoscopy*, 1999, 31(8):579-95 (review).

Isenberg JI, Walsh JH, and Johnson LR, "Peptic Ulcer Diseases," *AGA Undergraduate Teaching Project – Unit 23*, Timonium, MD: Milner-Fenwick, Inc, 1991.

Locke GR, "Nonulcer Dyspepsia: What It Is and What It Is Not," *Mayo Clin Proc*, 1999, 74(10):1011-4.

Pare P, "Systematic Approach Toward the Clinical Diagnosis of Functional Dyspepsia," *Can J Gastroenterol*, 1999, 13(8):647-54.

Talley NJ, Silverstein MD, Agreus L, et al, "AGA Technical Review: Evaluation of Dyspepsia," American Gastroenterological Association, *Gastroenterology*, 1998, 114(3):582-95 (review).

Thompson WG, Dotevall G, Drossman DA, et al, "Irritable Bowel Syndrome: Guidelines for the Diagnosis," *Gastroenterol Int*, 1989, 2:92-5.

DYSPEPSIA

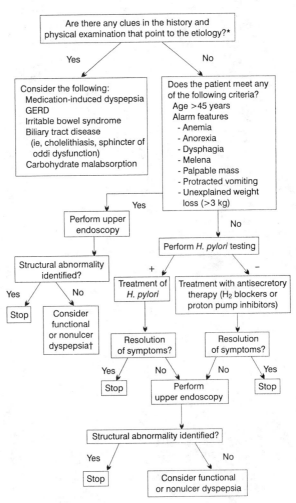

*In most cases, the clinical presentation of the patient with dyspepsia does not allow the clinician to determine the etiology. In a minority of cases, however, the clinical presentation may be classic for medication-induced dyspepsia, GERD, irritable bowel syndrome, biliary tract disease, or carbohydrate malabsorption.

†An unremarkable upper endoscopy in the patient >45 years of age and/or who has alarm features, does not unequivocally establish the diagnosis of nonulcer dyspepsia. The clinician should also consider serious causes of dyspepsia not diagnosed by upper endoscopy such as pancreatic or liver cancer, etc.

DYSPHAGIA

STEP 1: *What is Dysphagia?*

Dysphagia is defined as a difficulty in swallowing. It is present in up to 10% of adults >50 years of age. Prior to embarking on an evaluation of dysphagia, it is necessary to ensure that dysphagia is truly present. In particular, dysphagia needs to be differentiated from the following complaints:

Odynophagia

Odynophagia refers to pain on swallowing. In some cases, dysphagia and odynophagia may occur together.

Globus

Globus is a sensation of a lump, fullness, or tightness in the throat. In contrast to dysphagia, globus is often a constant sensation that does not interfere with swallowing. In fact, some patients report that globus is relieved with swallowing. In the past, this sensation of a lump was termed globus hystericus because it was believed that hysterical personality traits were more common in patients with globus. It is now known, however, that there is an increase in depression and obsessive-compulsive tendencies in this group of patients.

If the patient has globus, **Stop Here.**

If the patient has odynophagia, proceed to the chapter on Odynophagia *on page 401.*

If the patient has dysphagia, **Proceed to Step 2.**

STEP 2: *Does the Patient Have Oropharyngeal or Esophageal Dysphagia?*

Oropharyngeal Dysphagia

Oropharyngeal dysphagia, also known as transfer dysphagia, is characterized by an inability to begin the swallowing function. The signs and symptoms of oropharyngeal dysphagia are listed in the following table.

Signs and Symptoms of Oropharyngeal Dysphagia	
Aspiration	Gurgling
Choking during swallowing	Regurgitation of food into nasal
Coughing during swallowing	passages
Difficulty initiating a swallow	Associated symptoms / signs
Difficulty transporting food through	Cranial nerve dysfunction
the pharynx into throat	Dysarthria
Drooling of food or saliva	Muscular weakness in extremities
Food sticking in throat	Nasal speech
Frequent throat clearing	Recurrent pneumonia

Esophageal Dysphagia

When the passage of food through the esophagus is impaired, esophageal dysphagia is said to exist. Patients often complain of food getting stuck. At times, the patient may be able to describe where the food gets stuck. However, localization of symptoms to the neck does not always predict the site of the lesion. In fact, nearly 33% of patients with structural lesions of the distal esophagus incorrectly localized their complaint to the neck. Dysphagia that is perceived in the lower sternal area has better predictive value in terms of lesion localization than that perceived in the cervical region.

If symptoms or signs are consistent with oropharyngeal dysphagia, *Proceed to Step 3*.

If symptoms or signs are consistent with esophageal dysphagia, *Proceed to Step 7*.

STEP 3: *What are the Causes of Oropharyngeal Dysphagia?*

Oropharyngeal dysphagia occurs in conditions associated with neuromuscular abnormalities of the mouth, pharynx, or upper esophageal sphincter. The causes of oropharyngeal dysphagia are listed in the following box.

Causes of Oropharyngeal Dysphagia	
Diseases of myoneural junction	Neurologic disorders
Myasthenia gravis	Cerebrovascular accident
Eaton-Lambert syndrome	Amyotrophic lateral sclerosis
Botulism	Parkinson's disease
Medication-induced	Multiple sclerosis
Motor dysfunction	Alzheimer's disease / dementia
Myotonic dystrophy	Huntington's chorea
Oculopharyngeal muscular dystrophy	Brainstem tumor
Hypothyroidism	Paraneoplastic syndrome
Hyperthyroidism	Polio / postpolio syndrome
Steroid-induced myopathy	Wilson's disease
Dermatomyositis / polymyositis	Tabes dorsalis
Structural disorders	Head trauma
Oropharyngeal neoplasms	Cerebral palsy
Osteophytes	Guillain-Barre syndrome
Thyromegaly	Upper esophageal sphincter dysfunction
Esophageal web	Cricopharyngeal achalasia
Zenker's diverticulum	Hypertensive UES

Proceed to Step 4

STEP 4: *Are There Any Clues in the Patient's History and Physical Examination That Point to the Etiology of Oropharyngeal Dysphagia?*

While there are many causes of oropharyngeal dysphagia, establishing the etiology is usually not difficult. In most cases, the underlying etiology is readily apparent at the time of presentation. Less commonly, dysphagia may be the initial manifestation of a neuromuscular condition such as myasthenia gravis, hyperthyroidism, motor neuron disease, or Parkinson's disease.

The medication history is also important in the evaluation of oropharyngeal dysphagia. Medications that may cause or contribute to oropharyngeal dysphagia are listed in the following box.

Medications That May Cause or Contribute to Oropharyngeal Dysphagia

Medications causing xerostomia
  ACE inhibitors
  α-adrenergic blockers
  Angiotensin II receptor blockers
  Antiarrhythmics
    Disopyramide
    Mexiletine
  Anticholinergics
  Antihistamines
  Antipsychotics
  Atrovent
  Diuretics
  Opiates
Medications causing sedation, pharyngeal weakness, or dystonia
  Anticonvulsants
  Benzodiazepines
  Neuroleptics
Medications causing myopathy
  Corticosteroids
  HMG-CoA reductase inhibitors

Adapted from Boyce HW, "Drug-Induced Esophageal Damage: Diseases of Medical Progress," *Gastrointest Endosc*, 1998, 47(6):547-50 (review); Stoschus B and Allescher HD, "Drug-Induced Dysphagia," *Dysphagia*, 1993, 8(2):154-9 (review).

In the physical examination, the clinician should focus on the following:
- Mental status
- Sensory and motor function
- Deep tendon reflexes
- Cerebellar function
- Cranial nerve function (especially those that are involved in the swallowing process; ie, V, VII, IX, X, and XII)

In conjunction with the history, abnormalities of the above on physical examination may suggest a particular neuromuscular disorder. Palpation of the lips, tongue, and mouth are important in the detection of masses that may interfere with the swallowing process. A pink, well-hydrated oropharynx argues against the presence of xerostomia. Palpation of the neck may identify masses, lymphadenopathy, or goiter. Tremor and gait disturbance suggest the diagnosis of an extrapyramidal movement disorder such as Parkinson's disease. Tremor along with sweating and tachycardia should raise suspicion for hyperthyroidism. The ocular examination may reveal findings consistent with hyperthyroidism or myasthenia gravis.

Proceed to Step 5

> **STEP 5:** *Are Any Laboratory Studies Indicated in the Patient With Oropharyngeal Dysphagia?*

When the cause of the oropharyngeal dysphagia is apparent, laboratory testing is not necessary. When the etiology is unclear, laboratory testing may be helpful in the diagnosis of the following conditions:

Myasthenia Gravis

Dysphagia is a significant problem in up to 60% of patients with myasthenia gravis. In those known to have the disease, laboratory testing is not needed. However, dysphagia may be the sole presentation of the illness in up to 20% of patients. As a result, laboratory testing for myasthenia gravis is indicated when the etiology of the oropharyngeal dysphagia is not clear.

The serologic detection of acetylcholine receptor antibodies (AchR) is supportive of the diagnosis since the antibodies are present in 85% of cases. These antibodies are very specific for myasthenia gravis and many consider a positive test to be diagnostic of this condition. The test may be negative, however, in some patients with myasthenia gravis. In these patients, it may be worthwhile to perform the Tensilon (edrophonium) stimulation test. The clinician may also consider performing EMG to establish the diagnosis.

Inflammatory Myopathy

The diagnosis of inflammatory myopathy (dermatomyositis, polymyositis) is based on muscle enzyme abnormalities and characteristic findings on EMG and muscle biopsy. At the time of presentation, only 70% of patients with inflammatory myopathy have an elevated creatine phosphokinase. However, an increased creatine phosphokinase is noted at some point in the disease course in 95% of patients. Therefore, a normal creatine phosphokinase level does not exclude the diagnosis. Although elevated C-reactive protein and ESR commonly accompany creatine phosphokinase elevations in patients with inflammatory myopathy, these abnormalities are nonspecific. A positive ANA is detected in 25% of patients but is found in a higher percentage (nearly 90%) of patients who have the overlap syndrome.

Needle EMG may demonstrate features consistent with inflammatory myopathy in approximately 90% of patients. Unfortunately, the findings are not entirely specific for inflammatory myopathy. Muscle biopsy is often considered to be the gold standard in the diagnosis but it is diagnostic in only 80% of cases. In summary, the diagnosis of inflammatory myopathy can be difficult to establish but the above studies, taken together, usually allow the clinician to make the diagnosis.

Metabolic / Toxic Myopathy

Hyperthyroidism should be a consideration, particularly in the elderly. In this age group, the illness may not present with the classic signs and symptoms. As such, thyroid function tests should be performed.

Proceed to Step 6

STEP 6: *What Diagnostic Study Should be Performed in Patients With Oropharyngeal Dysphagia?*

Barium esophagography along with videofluoroscopic assessment (also known as the modified barium swallow) of the swallowing should be performed in the patient with oropharyngeal dysphagia. During this test, the swallowing process is recorded after the patient ingests barium of various consistencies. This study will reveal the type of abnormality present in patients with oropharyngeal dysphagia. Findings are usually grouped into the following:

- Inability or excessive delay in initiation of pharyngeal swallowing
- Aspiration of ingestate
- Nasopharyngeal regurgitation
- Residue of ingestate within pharyngeal cavity after swallowing

Identification of the abnormality will allow the clinician to institute effective therapy in an effort to prevent the adverse consequences of oropharyngeal dysphagia.

End of Section.

STEP 7: *What are the Causes of Esophageal Dysphagia?*

The causes of esophageal dysphagia are listed in the following box.

Causes of Esophageal Dysphagia	
Motility disorders	Intrinsic abnormalities
Achalasia	Benign stricture
Scleroderma	Peptic
Diffuse esophageal spasm	Caustic-induced
Nutcracker esophagus	Pill-induced
Extrinsic compression	Postirradiation
Mediastinal masses	Postoperative
Tumor	Ischemic
Lymphadenopathy	Esophageal carcinoma
Substernal thyroid	Esophageal diverticula
Vertebral osteophytes	Esophageal foreign body
Vascular compression	Esophageal ring (Schatzki's ring)
Aberrant right subclavian artery	Esophageal web
Left atrial enlargement	
Aortic aneurysm	

Proceed to Step 8

STEP 8: *Are There Any Clues in the Patient's Clinical Presentation That Point to the Etiology of the Esophageal Dysphagia?*

Mechanical or structural lesions account for 85% of esophageal dysphagia. The most common structural lesions identified are lower esophageal rings, strictures, and esophageal carcinoma. Approximately 15% of cases are due to motility disorders, the most common of which are achalasia, diffuse esophageal spasm, and nonspecific esophageal motility disorders. Clues in the patient's history that may point to the etiology of esophageal dysphagia are listed in the following table.

Historical Clue	Condition Suggested

Any of the following:
  Cigarette smoking
  Heavy alcohol use
  Achalasia
  Lye stricture
  Barrett's mucosa
	Risk factors for esophageal carcinoma

Solid and liquid food dysphagia from the onset	Motility disorder
Solid food dysphagia only or solid food dysphagia followed by liquid food dysphagia	Structural or mechanical lesion of the esophagus
Progressive dysphagia for few weeks or months	Esophageal carcinoma
Episodic solid food dysphagia for several years	Lower esophageal ring
History of melena	Esophageal cancer
History of sclerotherapy	Esophageal stricture
Severe weight loss*	Esophageal carcinoma
Hoarseness preceding dysphagia	Laryngeal etiology
Dysphagia precipitated or worsened by cold liquids	Esophageal motility disorder
Hoarseness following dysphagia	Esophageal carcinoma involving recurrent laryngeal nerve
Unilateral wheezing	Mediastinal mass compressing bronchus and esophagus
Chest pain	Diffuse esophageal spasm Impaction of a large food bolus in esophagus Gastroesophageal reflux disease/peptic stricture
Heartburn preceding dysphagia	Peptic stricture
Ingestion of caustic agents	Caustic-induced stricture
Ingestion of pills without water	Pill-induced stricture
Previous radiation therapy	Radiation-induced stricture
Odynophagia	Infectious esophagitis Pill-induced esophagitis Esophageal carcinoma

*Weight loss may also be seen with any etiology that interferes with the patient's ability to maintain adequate caloric intake.

Physical examination findings that may point to the etiology of the esophageal dysphagia are listed in the following table.

Physical Examination Finding	Condition Suggested
Telangiectasia Subcutaneous calcifications Sclerodactyly	Scleroderma
Hyperkeratosis of the palms and soles (tylosis palmaris et plantaris)	Risk factor for esophageal cancer
Dystrophic skin changes	Epidermolysis bullosa (associated with esophageal stricture)

(continued)

Physical Examination Finding	Condition Suggested
Leukoplakia of labial mucosa	Plummer-Vinson syndrome (esophageal web)
Lymphadenopathy	Esophageal carcinoma

Laboratory testing is usually not helpful in establishing the etiology of the esophageal dysphagia. The presence of anemia, however, is suggestive of esophageal carcinoma or web.

Proceed to Step 9

STEP 9: *Should the Patient Have an Endoscopy or a Barium Esophagogram to Evaluate the Esophageal Dysphagia?*

Most clinicians prefer to perform barium esophagography as the initial test in the evaluation of the patient with esophageal dysphagia. Barium esophagography provides information not only about structural lesions but also esophageal motility. In contrast, endoscopy provides limited information about esophageal motility. In addition, barium esophagography is superior to endoscopy in the detection of rings and webs, many of which are subtle and may be missed with endoscopy.

Despite the limitations of endoscopy, there are certain instances when endoscopy may be favored over barium esophagography. To decide whether the patient with esophageal dysphagia should have endoscopy or barium esophagography as the initial test requires consideration of the patient's presentation. In particular, the clinician should strive to answer the following questions:

- Does the patient have significant weight loss?
- Does the patient's presentation suggest esophageal carcinoma?
- Does the patient have a history of persistent heartburn?
- Does the patient's presentation suggest peptic stricture?
- Is the esophageal dysphagia acute in onset (while eating)?

An affirmative answer to any of the above questions should prompt the clinician to consider performing endoscopy as the initial test. Although barium esophagography performed in the patient with significant weight loss (suggestive of esophageal carcinoma) may reveal findings suggestive of cancer, an endoscopy will be required for biopsy and cytologic brushings.

In the patient with a history of persistent heartburn (suggestive of peptic stricture), barium esophagography may reveal findings suggestive of peptic stricture. Despite this, endoscopy will be required to definitively distinguish a peptic from malignant stricture.

The acute onset of esophageal dysphagia while eating usually suggests an impacted food bolus. Endoscopy is often necessary for direct removal of the food bolus.

If endoscopy is normal, ***Proceed to Step 10.***

If endoscopy reveals a structural abnormality of the esophagus, ***Proceed to Step 11.***

If barium esophagogram reveals a structural abnormality of the esophagus, ***Proceed to Step 11.***

If barium esophagogram reveals an abnormality of motility, *Proceed to Step 12.*

If barium esophagogram is normal, *Proceed to Step 12.*

STEP 10: *What are the Results of the Barium Esophagography?*

Normal findings during endoscopy in the patient with esophageal dysphagia should prompt the clinician to perform barium esophagography. Recall that barium esophagography is superior to endoscopy in the detection of motility abnormalities of the esophagus. In addition, subtle mucosal rings or webs may be missed with endoscopy.

If the barium esophagography reveals a structural lesion in the esophagus, *Proceed to Step 11.*

If the barium esophagogram is normal or reveals an abnormality of motility, *Proceed to Step 12.*

STEP 11: *What Structural Disorders of the Esophagus Can Lead to Dysphagia?*

Structural lesions of the esophagus may be identified either by barium esophagography or endoscopy. When structural lesions are identified by barium esophagography, the clinician must determine if endoscopy is indicated for further diagnosis. Endoscopy is usually not indicated when the following structural lesions of the esophagus are identified:

- Extrinsic compression (mediastinal mass, osteophytes, vascular compression)
- Esophageal web, ring, diverticula (unless endoscopic treatment is planned)

Endoscopy is indicated, however, when a stricture or a lesion suspicious for malignancy is identified on the radiographic study. The structural causes of esophageal dysphagia are considered below.

Peptic Stricture

Many patients with peptic stricture have a long-standing history of gastroesophageal reflux disease. In some patients, however, dysphagia may be the initial manifestation (25%). Typically, patients report that symptoms have been present for years. As affected patients become accustomed to their difficulty in swallowing solids, there is a gradual change in diet to semisolid foods. Because patients change their diets, weight loss is uncommon. Barium radiography reveals the stricture to be smooth and symmetric in appearance. The typical location of the stricture is in the lower 1/3 of the esophagus. A stricture in a more proximal location should prompt the clinician to consider the possibility of Barrett's esophagus. Because barium radiography does not allow a peptic stricture to be differentiated from malignancy, endoscopy is required for biopsy and cytology.

Other Esophageal Strictures

Other causes of esophageal stricture are listed in the following box.

Causes of Esophageal Stricture	
Bullous skin disorders	Extrinsic compression
Epidermolysis bullosa dystrophica	Infection
Pemphigoid	*Candida*
Caustic*	Tuberculosis
Chronic graft-vs-host disease	Malignancy
Crohn's disease	Peptic
Drug-induced†	Radiation‡
	Sclerotherapy

*Caustic-induced strictures may develop in the chronic phase of caustic injury. The chronic phase starts about four weeks after exposure to the caustic substance.

†Medications associated with the development of strictures include NSAIDs, tetracycline, other antibiotics, potassium, and iron preparations.

‡Radiation-induced strictures typically do not occur until at least three months have passed since the completion of radiation therapy.

Esophageal Cancer

Patients with esophageal cancer present with rapidly progressive dysphagia. Risk factors for esophageal cancer are listed in the following box.

Risk Factors for Esophageal Cancer	
Achalasia	Plummer-Vinson syndrome
Alcohol use	Radiation
Barrett's esophagus	Tobacco use
Lye ingestion / stricture	Tylosis palmaris et plantaris*

*Tylosis palmaris et plantaris is an autosomal dominant condition characterized by hyperkeratosis of the palms and soles.

Esophageal cancer patients tend to be older than patients with peptic stricture. While dysphagia is the most common symptom, other symptoms include anorexia, weight loss, odynophagia, and gastrointestinal blood loss (overt or occult). Hoarseness may result from recurrent laryngeal nerve infiltration or recurrent regurgitation.

Barium esophagography is suggestive of esophageal malignancy when a narrow, irregular stricture with mucosal ulceration is noted. Because it does not allow a histologic diagnosis, a suspicious barium esophagogram must be followed by endoscopy. During endoscopy, the clinician can not only directly visualize the lesion but can also obtain biopsy and cytologic brushings. Once the presence of an esophageal carcinoma is established, further imaging may include endoscopic ultrasound and CT scanning. Endoscopic ultrasound provides information about the esophageal wall and nearby structures. CT scanning is useful in determining the presence of distant metastases. Both are important in the staging of patients with esophageal carcinoma.

Esophageal Rings / Webs

Solid food dysphagia that is intermittent suggests an esophageal ring or web. In patients with lower esophageal or Schatzki's ring, a history of episodic dysphagia is elicited. Typically, a bolus of food will get stuck in the lower esophagus. With impaction of the bolus, the patient may experience chest pain. Because steak is often the culprit, this has been termed the "steak-house" syndrome. On occasion, the patient may be successful forcing the bolus of food through by drinking liquids. In most cases, however, the patient must regurgitate the food bolus. After regurgitation, the patient may finish the meal without trouble. Eliciting this characteristic history lends strong support to the diagnosis. Barium studies can be performed for confirmation of the diagnosis.

Extrinsic Compression

The following conditions may cause extrinsic compression of the esophagus:

- **Osteophytes**

  Hypertrophic spurs on the anterior portion of the cervical vertebrae may compress the esophagus.

- **Vascular abnormalities**

  Vascular abnormalities that may cause extrinsic compression include the following:
  1. Enlarged or distorted aortic arch (dysphagia aortica)
  2. Aberrant subclavian artery (dysphagia lusoria)

- **Mediastinal masses** (lymphadenopathy, tumor, substernal thyroid)

End of Section.

STEP 12: *Does the Patient Have a Disorder of Esophageal Motility?*

Findings noted on barium esophagography may be suggestive of a motility disorder. However, it is important to realize that a normal study does not exclude a motility disorder. Disorders of esophageal motility include the following:

- Achalasia
- Diffuse esophageal spasm
- Scleroderma
- Nutcracker esophagus
- Nonspecific esophageal motility disorders

Establishing a diagnosis of an esophageal motility disorder requires fulfillment of two criteria:

- Symptoms consistent with an esophageal motility disorder must be present

  An esophageal motility disorder is likely to be present in patients who complain of dysphagia to both solids and liquids. Intermittent solid and liquid food dysphagia is suggestive of diffuse esophageal spasm. Progressive solid and liquid food dysphagia may be consistent with either scleroderma or achalasia. In the patient with progressive solid and liquid food dysphagia, the presence of heartburn favors a diagnosis of scleroderma over achalasia. Other symptoms of esophageal motility disorders include weight loss, regurgitation, pulmonary symptoms, and chest pain.

- Abnormal esophageal motility must be demonstrated by manometry. Manometric findings in the esophageal motility disorders described above are listed in the following table.

Manometric Finding	Condition Suggested
Aperistalsis of esophageal body Incomplete relaxation of lower esophageal sphincter	Achalasia
Nonperistaltic contractions with simultaneous contraction onset	Diffuse esophageal spasm

Lower esophageal sphincter pressure
  >45 mm Hg
	Hypertensive lower esophageal
	  sphincter

Mean distal esophageal contraction >180 mm Hg	Nutcracker esophagus

Abnormal motility not consistent with
  any of the above conditions
	Nonspecific esophageal motility
	  disorder

If the esophageal manometric findings are normal, *Proceed to Step 13.*

The esophageal motility disorders are discussed in further detail below.

Diffuse Esophageal Spasm

Diffuse esophageal spasm may present with chest pain and dysphagia. The dysphagia is typically described as intermittent and nonprogressive. Chest pain is not always present but can be particularly severe. The pain is typically retrosternal and often radiates to the back. In many cases, the pain mimics angina.

Suggestive findings on barium esophagogram include corkscrew esophagus and tertiary contractions. Manometry is required to confirm the diagnosis. Manometric findings suggest that patients with diffuse esophageal spasm can be divided into two groups. Those with high-amplitude contractions tend to complain of chest pain while those with lower-amplitude contractions usually have dysphagia.

Scleroderma

Dysphagia for solids and liquids can occur in patients with scleroderma. Although esophageal involvement is rarely present at the onset of the disease, close to 80% of patients with scleroderma will develop esophageal disease later in the course of the disease. Scleroderma is characterized by abnormalities in smooth muscle function of the lower esophagus and esophageal sphincter. Heartburn is a common complaint in patients with scleroderma having esophageal dysfunction. A suggestive finding of scleroderma on barium esophagogram is a dilated esophagus. Manometric studies reveal a decrease in lower esophageal sphincter pressure and absent or diminished peristalsis.

Achalasia

Progressive dysphagia for solids and liquids is present in over 90% of patients with achalasia. The dysphagia is typically gradual in onset. In fact, the average duration of symptoms prior to diagnosis is about two years. Some patients with achalasia complain of substernal chest pain that radiates to the back. Chest pain seems to be a more common complaint early in the course of the disease, often resolving as the disease progresses.

Regurgitation of undigested food eaten hours ago is common in achalasia. Regurgitation can be worse at night and may result in aspiration and nocturnal coughing. Patients adapt to their disorder by assuming certain postures. These postures improve esophageal emptying by raising intrathoracic pressures. As such, patients may describe that straightening of the back or standing erect helps. Others may raise their arms above the head.

Findings consistent with achalasia on barium radiography include dilation of the esophageal body, poor opening of the lower esophageal sphincter with swallowing, and absent or diminished peristalsis. A smoothly tapered narrowing may be appreciated at the distal end of the esophagus. This finding is described as a "bird's-beak" appearance.

Endoscopic findings of achalasia include a dilated esophageal body and the presence of retained esophageal contents. Sustained pressure may be required to pass the endoscope through the lower esophageal sphincter.

The diagnosis of idiopathic achalasia should not be made until endoscopy excludes pseudoachalasia. A major cause of pseudoachalasia is malignancy. It is well described with tumors of the gastric cardia which may cause symptoms similar to achalasia by compressing the gastroesophageal junction or invading the myenteric plexus. Pseudoachalasia can also occur with distant tumors as a paraneoplastic phenomenon. It has been described in patients with oat cell carcinoma, gastric carcinoma, pancreatic carcinoma, and lymphoma.

End of Section.

STEP 13: *Does the Patient Have Psychogenic Dysphagia?*

Although psychogenic or factitious dysphagia has been reported, it is rare. As a result, normal results of barium esophagography, endoscopy, and manometry should prompt the clinician to review these studies. For example, inadequate distention of the esophagus during the barium study may prevent the detection of lower esophageal rings and mild strictures. A psychogenic cause should only be considered after the clinician is sure that the studies performed were adequately done.

REFERENCES

Bastian RW, "Contemporary Diagnosis of the Dysphagic Patient," *Otolaryngol Clin North Am*, 1998, 31(3):489-506 (review).

Boyce HW, "Drug-Induced Esophageal Damage: Diseases of Medical Progress," *Gastrointest Endosc*, 1998, 47(6):547-50, (review).

Broniatowski M, Sonies BC, Rubin JS, et al, "Current Evaluation and Treatment of Patients with Swallowing Disorders," *Otolaryngol Head Neck Surg*, 1999, 120(4):464-73.

de Bosset V, Gonvers JJ, Froehlich F, et al, "Appropriateness of Gastroscopy: Bleeding and Dysphagia," *Endoscopy*, 1999, 31(8):615-22 (review).

DiMarino AJ, Allen ML, Lynn RB, et al, "Clinical Value of Esophageal Motility Testing," *Dig Dis*, 1998, 16(4):198-204 (review).

Domenech E and Kelly J, "Swallowing Disorders," *Med Clin North Am*, 1999, 83(1):97-113 (review).

Dray TG, Hillel AD, and Miller RM, "Dysphagia Caused by Neurologic Deficits," *Otolaryngol Clin North Am*, 1998, 31(3):507-24 (review).

Ekberg O and Pokieser P, "Radiologic Evaluation of the Dysphagic Patient," *Eur Radiol*, 1997, 7(8):1285-95 (review).

Ladenheim SE and Marlowe FI, "Dysphagia Secondary to Cervical Osteo-phytes," *Am J Otolaryngol*, 1999, 20(3):184-9.

Mujica VR and Conklin J, "When It's Hard to Swallow. What to Look for in Patients with Dysphagia," *Postgrad Med*, 1999, 105(7):131-4, 141-2, 145.

Palmer JB, Drennan JC, and Baba M, "Evaluation and Treatment of Swal-lowing Impairments," *Am Fam Phys*, 2000, 61(8):2453-62 (review).

Schechter GL, "Systemic Causes of Dysphagia in Adults," *Otolaryngol Clin North Am*, 1998, 31(3):525-35 (review).

Spechler SJ, "AGA Technical Review on Treatment of Patients With Dysphagia Caused by Benign Disorders of the Distal Esophagus," *Gastroenterology*, 1999, 117(1):233-54.

Stoschus B and Allescher HD, "Drug-Induced Dysphagia," *Dysphagia*, 1993, 8(2):154-9 (review).

Tobin RW, "Esophageal Rings, Webs, and Diverticula," *J Clin Gastroenterol*, 1998, 27(4):285-95 (review).

DYSPHAGIA

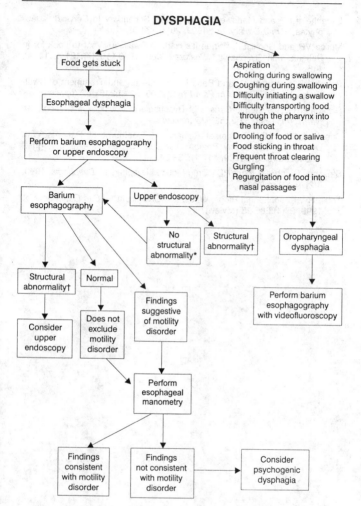

*An unremarkable upper endoscopy should be followed by barium esophagography. Upper endoscopy may miss subtle mucosal rings or webs. In addition, motility disorders cannot be diagnosed by upper endoscopy.

†Structural abnormalities of the esophagus include malignancy, stricture, diverticula, webs, and ring. When a structural abnormality is first identified by barium esophagography, upper endoscopy is often indicated to establish a histologic diagnosis.

DYSURIA (MEN)

STEP 1: *How Common is Dysuria in Men?*

Dysuria refers to pain or burning on urination. Although a more common complaint in women, dysuria does occur in men, increasing significantly as men age. Dysuria is usually the result of inflammation or irritation of the urinary tract.

Proceed to Step 2

STEP 2: *What are the Causes of Dysuria in Men?*

The causes of dysuria in men are listed in the following box.

Causes of Dysuria in Men	
More Common	
Acute pyelonephritis	Prostatitis
Cystitis	Urethritis
Epididymitis	
Less Common	
Behcet's syndrome	Hemorrhagic cystitis
Benign prostatic hyperplasia	Interstitial cystitis
Bladder cancer	Radiation cystitis
Calculi	Reiter's syndrome
Drug-induced cystitis	Urethral cancer
Eosinophilic cystitis	Urethral stricture
Granulomatous cystitis	

While there are noninfectious causes of dysuria in men, most cases are due to infection. This chapter will initially focus on the infectious etiologies of dysuria followed by a discussion of the noninfectious etiologies of dysuria.

Proceed to Step 3

STEP 3: *Are There Any Clues in the Patient's History That Point to the Etiology of the Dysuria?*

Clues in the patient's history that point to the etiology of the dysuria are listed in the following table.

Historical Clue	Condition Suggested
Back pain	Acute pyelonephritis Prostatitis
Fever	Acute prostatitis Acute pyelonephritis Disseminated gonococcal infection Epididymitis Prostatic abscess Reiter's syndrome
Joint pain	Disseminated gonococcal infection Reiter's syndrome
Ocular symptoms	Behcet's syndrome Reiter's syndrome
Rectal pain or perineal aching	Prostatitis
Scrotal pain	Acute prostatitis Epididymitis
Skin rash	Disseminated gonococcal infection Reiter's syndrome
Urethral discharge	Epididymitis Prostatitis Urethritis

Proceed to Step 4

STEP 4: *Are There Any Clues in the Patient's Physical Examination That Point to the Etiology of the Dysuria?*

Physical examination findings that point to the etiology of the dysuria are listed in the following table.

Physical Examination Finding	Condition Suggested
Conjunctivitis	Gonococcal urethritis Reiter's syndrome
Enlargement of prostate	Benign prostatic hyperplasia
Flank tenderness	Acute pyelonephritis
Genital ulceration	HSV urethritis Other sexually transmitted disease
Palpable prostate tenderness*	Acute prostatitis Prostatic abscess
Tender swelling of the epididymis	Epididymitis

*In patients suspected of having prostatitis, a gentle digital rectal exam is recommended to avoid precipitating bacteremia and possible sepsis.

If the history and physical examination provide clues to the diagnosis, the evaluation should be directed accordingly.

If the etiology of the dysuria is unclear after a thorough history and physical examination, *Proceed to Step 5.*

> ## STEP 5: *Does the Patient Have Acute Prostatitis or Epididymitis?*

Acute prostatitis and epididymitis can be readily excluded by performing a thorough physical examination. Digital prostate exam revealing a very tender, boggy prostate is consistent with acute prostatitis. Erythema, edema, and tenderness of the scrotal area should prompt concern for epididymitis.

If the physical examination does not support the diagnosis of either acute prostatitis or epididymitis, *Proceed to Step 6.*

Acute prostatitis and epididymitis will be discussed further in the remainder of this step.

Acute Prostatitis

Acute prostatitis is an acute illness that often begins with nonspecific symptoms of malaise, fever, arthralgias, and myalgias. It is characterized by the presence of irritative and obstructive voiding symptoms such as dysuria, frequency, urgency, and retention. Many patients have pain in the rectum, back, or perineum. At times, this pain may be quite severe.

The clinician should consider performing a digital prostate examination to exclude acute prostatitis in men presenting with dysuria and fever. However, patients suspected of having acute prostatitis should not have a vigorous examination of their prostate since such an examination may precipitate bacteremia. Instead, the clinician should perform a gentle examination. Even with a gentle examination, the great majority of patients with acute prostatitis will "jump off the table" with prostate palpation. The clinician will often be able to palpate a very tender, boggy, and edematous prostate.

When symptoms and signs are consistent with acute prostatitis, the clinician should obtain a urinalysis. In addition, urine and blood cultures are indicated. Urine culture usually reveals the growth of the pathogenic organism. *E. coli* is the major etiologic agent in acute bacterial prostatitis. Less commonly isolated are species of *Proteus*, *Klebsiella*, *Pseudomonas*, *Serratia*, *Enterobacter*, and *Providencia*.

Prostatic abscess, which may occur in patients with acute prostatitis, is also a consideration in men presenting with dysuria and fever. Although a common complication of acute bacterial prostatitis in the past, it is now rare. Nevertheless, it should remain a consideration, especially in diabetic or immunocompromised patients. Digital prostate examination may reveal a localized area of swelling or fluctuance. Transrectal ultrasonography or CT scan can confirm the diagnosis of prostatic abscess.

Epididymitis

Epididymitis is most commonly encountered in men between the ages of 20 and 35. In these men, the cause is usually related to sexually transmitted disease. *Neisseria gonorrhoeae* and *Chlamydia trachomatis* are the main etiologic organisms. Older men may also develop epididymitis. In this age group, there is often an underlying urologic abnormality such as benign prostatic hyperplasia. Other risk factors for epididymitis include vasectomy, prostatectomy, indwelling urinary catheter, and recent urinary tract instrumentation. In older men, the main etiologic organisms include *E. coli*, other enteric bacteria, and staphylococcus species.

Unilateral scrotal swelling and pain are the hallmarks of acute epididymitis. Dysuria occurs in approximately 50% of patients who are sexually active. In these cases, the dysuria may be a manifestation of a preceding urethritis. In older men, dysuria is a less common complaint. Physical examination may reveal a febrile or even toxic appearing patient. The scrotum is noted to be swollen, tender, and erythematous. Tenderness is maximal with palpation of the epididymis.

The clinician should consider obtaining urinalysis and urine culture in patients suspected of having epididymitis. About 25% of patients will have pyuria. The presence of a discharge should prompt testing for sexually transmitted organisms. The causative organism can usually be identified by culture of the urine or urethra.

Epididymitis should be differentiated from testicular torsion, which is a urologic emergency. At times, differentiating between the two can be quite challenging. The reader is referred to the chapter on Scrotal Pain (Acute) *on page 443* for more information.

End of Section.

STEP 6: *Does the Patient Have Acute Pyelonephritis?*

Acute pyelonephritis is a bacterial infection of the kidney. Not uncommonly, one or two days of lower urinary tract symptoms (eg, dysuria, frequency, urgency) precede the onset of the clinical manifestations of acute pyelonephritis. Fever, flank pain, and nausea/vomiting are the symptoms that should prompt the clinician to suspect upper urinary tract infection. Physical examination may reveal costovertebral angle tenderness.

Confirmation of the diagnosis requires urinalysis and culture. The presence of >10 white blood cells per high powered field (centrifuged urine) is considered to represent significant pyuria. Although pyuria is not specific for urinary tract infection, its presence in a male with signs and symptoms of pyelonephritis provides support for the diagnosis. Urine culture should be sent in every male presenting with acute pyelonephritis. Blood cultures should be sent as well.

Clinical features used to distinguish between cystitis and pyelonephritis are listed in the following table.

Comparison Between Cystitis and Pyelonephritis

Signs & Symptoms	Cystitis	Pyelonephritis
Fever	Absent	Usually present
Urgency, frequency	Present	Sometimes present
Flank pain	Absent	Sometimes present
Vomiting	Absent	Often present
Pyuria	Always present*	Always present*
Bacteriuria	Always present	Always present
Positive blood culture	Absent	Often present

*Except in neutropenic patients

Adapted from Nseyo UO, Weinman E, and Lamm DL, *Urology for Primary Care Physicians*, Philadelphia, PA: WB Saunders Co, 1999, 133.

Most urinary tract infections in men are caused by Gram-negative bacilli. *E. coli* causes almost 50% of all infections. Other Gram-negative bacilli including species of *Proteus*, *Providencia*, *Klebsiella*, *Enterobacter*, *Pseudomonas*, and *Citrobacter* are less commonly isolated. Gram-positive cocci, particularly *Enterococcus* species, are causative in 20% of all urinary tract infections in men.

The clinician should consider urologic investigation in men presenting with acute pyelonephritis. Many men have an underlying structural problem that predisposes them to infection of the upper urinary tract.

If the patient has acute pyelonephritis, *Stop Here.*

If the patient has signs and symptoms suggestive of cystitis, *Proceed to Step 7.*

STEP 7: *Does the Patient Have Cystitis or Urethritis?*

Dysuria is a complaint that is common to both cystitis and urethritis. Although frequency, urgency, suprapubic pain, and hematuria are more suggestive of cystitis, the presence of these symptoms is not sufficient to exclude urethritis, particularly in sexually active men.

Urethral discharge in a man presenting with dysuria should prompt consideration of urethritis. It is important to realize, however, that the presence of urethral discharge is not synonymous with urethritis. In fact, urethral discharge may be a manifestation of epididymitis or prostatitis. However, most men with dysuria and urethral discharge are suffering from urethritis. Epididymitis can be readily excluded if physical examination of the scrotum does not reveal tenderness or swelling of the epididymis. In the absence of fever and palpable prostate tenderness, acute prostatitis is unlikely.

Not all men with urethritis will report a urethral discharge. For this reason, it is useful to strip the urethra in an effort to express secretions. Stripping of the urethra can be performed by squeezing the shaft of the penis in a distal direction. Urethral stripping may lead to the appearance of a discharge at the urethral meatus.

If the patient has urethral discharge, *Proceed to Step 8.*

If the patient does not have urethral discharge, *Proceed to Step 15.*

STEP 8: *Is the Clinical Presentation Suggestive of Gonococcal or Nongonococcal Urethritis?*

Urethritis can be divided into gonococcal and nongonococcal infection. A multitude of pathogens have been isolated in patients with nongonococcal urethritis. Between 30% and 50% of nongonococcal urethritis cases, however, are due to *Chlamydia trachomatis*. Although *Ureaplasma urealyticum* has been implicated in most cases of nongonococcal urethritis not due to *C. trachomatis*, there is some controversy regarding the role of this pathogen in nonchlamydial nongonococcal urethritis. Other pathogens are identified in at least 20% of cases.

Although persons of all ages may develop infectious urethritis, it tends to be a disease of young sexually active individuals. Dysuria and urethral discharge are the classic features of infectious urethritis. However, these symptoms may not be present together. Frequency, urgency, and hematuria are not typical of urethritis. The presence of these symptoms should prompt the clinician to consider an alternative diagnosis such as bacterial urinary tract infection.

The patient's clinical presentation may offer clues to the clinician as to the etiologic organism. These classic clues are listed in the following table.

	Gonococcal Urethritis	Nongonococcal Urethritis
Quality of Discharge	Yellow-green	Mucopurulent or mucoid
Amount of Discharge	Profuse	Scant to moderate*
Onset of Symptoms	Acute	Insidious

*The discharge of nongonococcal urethritis tends to be less profuse than gonococcal urethritis. Not uncommonly, the discharge may only be noted after urethral stripping or in the morning before the first void.

It is important to realize that many cases of gonococcal and nongonococcal urethritis do not present classically. Overlap in the clinical presentation of these two causes of infectious urethritis is common. Differentiation between these two forms of urethritis based upon the clinical presentation is only accurate in 75% of cases. Because the clinical presentation does not allow the clinician to accurately differentiate between these two causes, laboratory testing is essential.

Proceed to Step 9

STEP 9: *What are the Results of the Urethral Smear?*

Urethral discharge, either obtained spontaneously or by urethral stripping, should be placed onto a glass slide for Gram staining. If discharge cannot be expressed in a patient suspected of having urethritis, a urethral swab should be inserted into the urethra in order to obtain a specimen. The diagnosis of urethritis is firmly established when more than four PMNs per oil-immersion field are observed.

If >4 PMNs are noted per oil-immersion field, *Proceed to Step 10.*

If ≤4 PMNs are noted per oil-immersion field, *Proceed to Step 13.*

If Gram staining is not available, *Proceed to Step 14.*

STEP 10: *Are Any Intracellular Gram-Negative Diplococci Noted?*

The presence of >4 PMNs per oil-immersion field establishes the diagnosis of urethritis. It does not, however, distinguish between gonococcal and nongonococcal urethritis. To make the distinction, it is necessary to search the Gram-stained slide for any Gram-negative intracellular diplococci. The presence of Gram-negative intracellular diplococci is consistent with gonococcal urethritis. In fact, the sensitivity and specificity of this finding is 95% and 98%, respectively.

If intracellular Gram-negative diplococci are noted, *Proceed to Step 11.*

If intracellular Gram-negative diplococci are not noted, *Proceed to Step 12.*

STEP 11: *Does a Culture for Gonorrhea Need to Be Performed?*

N. gonorrhoeae culture does not need to be performed when the urethral smear reveals Gram-negative intracellular diplococci. In these cases, the clinician should treat the patient for gonococcal urethritis.

Up to 25% of these men, however, will have concomitant nongonococcal urethritis due to *C. trachomatis* or other organisms. As a result, the clinician should perform testing for the detection of *C. trachomatis*, the major cause of nongonococcal urethritis. Because of the expense and complexity involved in culturing *C. trachomatis*, the clinician may wish to perform nonculture tests. It is important to realize that all nonculture tests can detect dead organisms. Therefore, nonculture tests should not be performed within three weeks after treatment for chlamydial infection. The tests that are available in the diagnosis of chlamydial urethritis are listed in the following table.

Test	Sensitivity (%)	Specificity (%)	Comment
EIA*	70-90	95-99	Readily done in high volume
DFA*	70-95	95-99	Depends on skill of microscopist; not amenable to high volume
Culture†	65-80	>99	Requires expert laboratory
DNA Probe†	86-93	98-99.5	Can test for *N. gonorrhoeae* with same swab
DNA Amplification (LCR or PCR)†	94-99	>99	Can use first-voided portion of urine or urethral swab with equal performance, and test for *N. gonorrhoeae* with same specimen

*Compared with culture

†Compared with enhanced reference standard comprising culture and DNA amplification plus culture of DFA test

Adapted from Armstrong D and Cohen J, *Infectious Diseases*, Harcourt Publishing (Mosby), 1999, 2.63.6.

A positive chlamydial test result, irrespective of the type of test performed, warrants treatment for chlamydial infection. Besides testing for *C. trachomatis*, many experts recommend the following in patients diagnosed with gonococcal urethritis:

- Serologic test for syphilis (RPR)
- Referral and treatment of sexual partners

End of Section.

STEP 12: *Does the Patient Have Nongonococcal Urethritis?*

The absence of intracellular Gram-negative diplococci on the Gram-stained urethral smear should prompt consideration of nongonococcal urethritis. These patients should be presumptively treated for nongonococcal urethritis. While the clinician may wish to perform chlamydia testing, treatment should not be delayed until the test results return. In addition, it is important to perform gonococcal testing in these patients since the Gram stain does not always show the typical intracellular Gram-negative diplococci in cases of gonococcal urethritis. Diagnostic tests available for *N. gonorrhoeae* are listed in the following table.

Test	Sensitivity (%)	Specificity (%)	Comment
Gram stain*	95 (symptomatic) 60 (asymptomatic)	98	Results immediately available
Culture	90-97	98-99	Require careful handling and proper facilities
DNA Probe†	93-99	98-99.5	Can test for *C. trachomatis* with same swab
DNA Amplification (LCR or PCR)†	98-99	>99	Can use first-voided portion of urine or urethral swab with equal performance, and *C. trachomatis* with same specimen

*Compared with culture

†Compared with enhanced reference standard comprising DNA amplification or probe competition assay

Adapted from Armstrong D and Cohen J, *Infectious Diseases*, Harcourt Publishing (Mosby), 1999, 2.63.6.

A positive gonococcal test result, irrespective of the type of test performed, should prompt treatment for gonococcal urethritis. Besides gonococcal testing, many experts recommend the following:

- Serologic test for syphilis (RPR)
- Referral and treatment of sexual partners

Persistence or recurrence of the clinical manifestations of nongonococcal urethritis after antimicrobial therapy should prompt the clinician to consider the possibilities listed in the following box.

Possibilities to Consider When Symptoms and Signs of Nongonococcal Urethritis Persist or Recur Following Antimicrobial Treatment
Noncompliance (patient, partner)
Reinfection
Urethritis due to nonchlamydial organisms (HSV, trichomoniasis, *Candida*)

Noncompliance with recommended therapy or recurrence following sexual contact with an untreated partner should prompt the clinician to retreat the patient. The clinician should also consider obtaining a wet mount examination and culture of an intraurethral swab specimen for *Trichomonas vaginalis*.

End of Section.

STEP 13: *Does ≤4 PMNs per Oil-Immersion Field Exclude Gonococcal or Nongonococcal Urethritis?*

Infectious urethritis is not excluded in patients who have <5 PMNs per oil-immersion field for the following reasons:

- Recent urination may result in decreased numbers of PMNs noted on the urethral smear
- Variability in specimen collection and technique
- Intraobserver variability in reading urethral smear

In fact, <5 PMNs per oil-immersion field may be noted in up to 33% of men with chlamydial urethritis. In these cases, further evaluation and treatment is dependent on the presence or absence of discharge.

- Discharge present
  When discharge is present, the clinician should treat presumptively for nongonococcal urethritis. Testing for chlamydia, gonorrhea, and syphilis (RPR) should be performed. Referral and treatment should be offered to sexual contacts.

- Discharge absent
  When discharge is not present, the clinician should try to examine the patient before the first morning void. Alternatively, examination may be performed after a prolonged period of time elapses in which the patient does not urinate. During this examination, the clinician should perform urethral stripping. A repeat urethral smear should be performed on any discharge obtained. Further management should be based on the results of the urethral smear as described in Step 9.

  If no discharge is expressed, the patient should be instructed to provide the first 10 mL of the first void urine to the laboratory for microscopic analysis. When ≥10 white blood cells per high powered field are noted on microscopy, the patient should be managed as having nongonococcal urethritis, as described in Step 12.

  If <10 white blood cells per high powered field are noted, then the clinician should consider alternative diagnoses such as cystitis and prostatitis. In sexually active men, however, the clinician may wish to begin empiric therapy for nongonococcal urethritis, despite the lack of objective evidence for urethritis.

End of Section.

STEP 14: *What Should be Done if Gram Staining is Not Available?*

When Gram staining is not available to confirm the presence of urethritis in patients with urethral complaints, several options are available to the clinician:

- The demonstration of pyuria (>10 to 15 white blood cells per high powered field) in only the first 10 mL of voided urine (rest of urine is unremarkable for significant pyuria) is suggestive of urethritis. Instead of microscopic analysis of the urine for pyuria, the clinician may wish to use the leukocyte esterase test as a surrogate. Equal numbers of white blood cells throughout the urine specimen should prompt the clinician to consider cystitis (see Step 15).

- When microscopic analysis or leukocyte esterase testing of the first 10 mL of voided urine is not available, then the clinician should assume that the urethral discharge is due to infection until proven otherwise.

These patients should be treated for both gonococcal and nongonococcal urethritis while waiting for the results of testing for *N. gonorrhoeae* and *C. trachomatis*. Positive test results mandate referral of sexual partner for treatment.

End of Section.

STEP 15: *Does the Patient Have Bacterial Cystitis?*

When urethral discharge (spontaneous or by urethral stripping) cannot be demonstrated, urethritis becomes less likely. The lack of a discharge does not exclude the diagnosis. It should, however, prompt the clinician to consider other possibilities such as cystitis. If there is any uncertainty, the clinician may wish to perform a urethral smear from a specimen obtained by the insertion of a urethral swab 2 cm into the anterior urethra. The demonstration of >4 PMNs per oil-immersion field establishes the diagnosis of urethritis.

If the urethral smear reveals the presence of >4 PMNs per oil-immersion field, *Proceed to Step 10.*

The presence of ≤4 PMNs per oil-immersion field argues against the diagnosis of urethritis and should prompt the clinician to consider cystitis. When compared to women, urinary tract infection in younger men is fairly uncommon. Risk factors that predispose younger men to the development of a urinary tract infection include HIV infection, sexual contact with infected female partner, and the practice of anal intercourse. Being uncircumcised increases the risk as well. With increasing age, urinary tract infections become more common, reflecting urologic abnormalities such as prostatic enlargement and bladder dysfunction. Many authorities feel that bladder outlet obstruction caused by prostatic enlargement is the most common predisposition in older men.

Symptoms of cystitis include dysuria, frequency, urgency, and suprapubic pressure. Some men may report gross hematuria. A urinalysis should be obtained to determine if significant numbers of white blood cells are present. The presence of >10 white blood cells per high powered field is considered to be significant pyuria. Leukocyte esterase testing can be performed in lieu of the microscopic examination for white blood cells. Significant pyuria or a positive leukocyte esterase test in a male with symptom and signs suggestive of a lower urinary tract infection provides support for the diagnosis of cystitis.

Proceed to Step 16

STEP 16: *Should a Urine Culture be Performed?*

Urine culture should be performed in men with signs and symptoms suggestive of cystitis. In contrast to women, men with suspected cystitis do not have to provide a clean catch midstream urine specimen for culture. The initial void specimen, even without cleansing of the urethral meatus, is suitable for culture. For those who are unable to void, the clinician may wish to perform in and out urethral catheterization or suprapubic aspiration in an effort to obtain a specimen for culture. A urine culture colony count of ≥10^3 cfu/mL of a single or predominant species is considered to be clinically significant.

The results of the culture are usually not available at a time when therapy is instituted. Fortunately, the clinician can select appropriate antibiotic therapy based on knowledge of the urinary pathogens that commonly cause lower urinary tract infections.

Most urinary tract infections in men are caused by Gram-negative bacilli. *E. coli* causes almost 50% of all infections. Other Gram-negative bacilli including species of *Proteus, Providencia, Klebsiella, Enterobacter, Pseudomonas,* and *Citrobacter* are less commonly isolated. Gram-positive cocci, particularly

Enterococcus species, are causative in 20% of all urinary tract infections in men.

If the urine culture reveals the growth of the pathogen, ***Proceed to Step 17.***

If the urine culture does not reveal the growth of the pathogen, ***Proceed to Step 18.***

STEP 17: *Should a Urologic Evaluation be Performed?*

It has traditionally been held that the development of a urinary tract infection in men mandates a urologic investigation since many men have structural abnormalities predisposing them to infection. Thirty percent of younger men with single episodes of bacteriuria have a structural abnormality identified with urologic evaluation. However, it is now known that certain risk factors can predispose men to infection in the absence of structural abnormalities of the urinary tract. In particular, cystitis in homosexual or uncircumcised men may not require urologic evaluation.

There is uncertainty regarding the clinical significance of most genitourinary abnormalities identified in men with urinary tract infection. Since the identification of these abnormalities seldom leads to an alteration in the clinician's treatment plan, many clinicians reserve urologic evaluation for men who present with the following:

- Pyelonephritis

- Recurrent infections

  Chronic bacterial prostatitis should clearly be one consideration in older men who present with relapsing urinary tract infections after appropriate antibiotic therapy. In these cases, persistence of urinary pathogen in the prostate leads to recurrent infection. Many patients with chronic bacterial prostatitis are asymptomatic between episodes of recurrent urinary tract infection. Physical examination is usually unrevealing in these patients. Prostatic localization tests may be performed to establish the diagnosis. A prolonged course of antibiotic therapy is required to eradicate the prostate of the pathogen.

  Other considerations in patients with recurrent infection include iatrogenic infection (after catheterization), structural urologic abnormalities, and upper urinary tract involvement.

- Failure to respond to appropriate antibiotic therapy

  Infection caused by drug-resistant strain, poor renal function (preventing antibiotic from reaching the urine), anatomical abnormality of the urinary tract, and urinary obstruction are all considerations when the patient fails to respond to appropriate antibiotic therapy.

End of Section.

STEP 18: *Does the Patient Have a Noninfectious Cause of Dysuria?*

When the urine culture is negative in the patient suspected of having bacterial cystitis, the clinician should consider other conditions that may present with dysuria. Prior to discussing the noninfectious causes of dysuria, the clinician should realize that the urine culture may be negative in patients with cystitis if antibiotic therapy was started before the specimen was obtained. In addition, atypical pathogens such as mycobacteria and fungi may not be detected on standard culture.

In older men, benign prostatic hyperplasia (BPH) should be considered. Over 50% of men >70 years of age have manifestations of BPH. The clinical manifestations of BPH include both obstructive and irritative symptoms. Although patients with BPH may develop dysuria due to urinary infection because of stasis and obstruction, others present with pain or burning on urination because of inflammation of the distended urethral mucosa (in the absence of infection).

Malignancy is also a consideration in men with dysuria. Both bladder cancer (including carcinoma *in situ*) and urethral cancer may present with dysuria. Dysuria has also been reported in patients with renal cell carcinoma.

Another important cause of dysuria is calculi. Calculi anywhere in the urinary tract may cause inflammation, resulting in dysuria. Other conditions associated with dysuria are listed in the box in Step 2.

REFERENCES

Armstrong D and Cohen J, *Infectious Diseases*, Harcourt Publishing (Mosby), 1999, 2.63.6.

Hooton TM and Stamm WE, "Diagnosis and Treatment of Uncomplicated Urinary Tract Infection," *Infect Dis Clin North Am*, 1997, 11(3):551-81 (review).

Lipsky BA, "Prostatitis and Urinary Tract Infection in Men: What's New; What's True?" *Am J Med*, 1999, 106(3):327-34.

Neu HC, "Urinary Tract Infections," *Am J Med*, 1992, 92(4A):63S-70S (review).

Nseyo UO, Weinman E, and Lamm DL, *Urology for Primary Care Physicians*, Philadelphia, PA: WB Saunders Co, 1999, 133.

Orenstein R and Wong ES, "Urinary Tract Infections in Adults," *Am Fam Phys*, 1999, 59(5):1225-34, 1237.

Roberts RG and Hartlaub PP, "Evaluation of Dysuria in Men," *Am Fam Phys*, 1999, 60(3):865-72.

Schaeffer AJ, "Urinary Tract Infection in Men – State of the Art," *Infection*, 1994, 22(Suppl 1):S19-21 (review).

Teillac P, "Management of Urinary Tract Infection in Elderly Men," *Eur Urol*, 1991, 19(Suppl 1):23-7 (review).

DYSURIA (MEN)

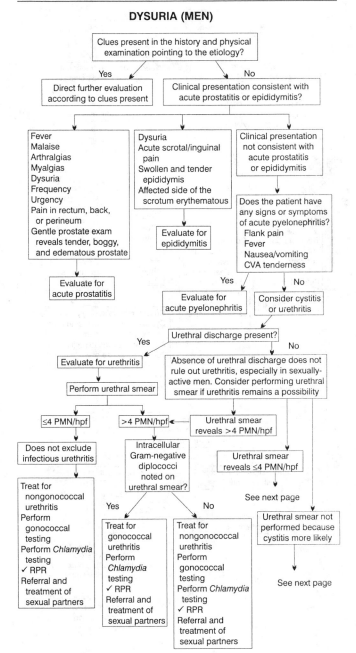

DYSURIA (MEN)
(continued)

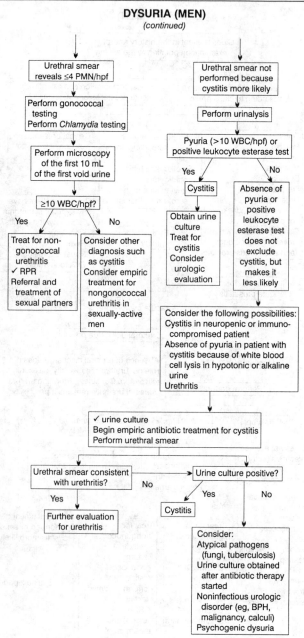

Urethral smear reveals ≤4 PMN/hpf

Perform gonococcal testing
Perform *Chlamydia* testing

Perform microscopy of the first 10 mL of the first void urine

≥10 WBC/hpf?

Yes

Treat for non-gonococcal urethritis
✓ RPR
Referral and treatment of sexual partners

No

Consider other diagnosis such as cystitis
Consider empiric treatment for nongonococcal urethritis in sexually-active men

Urethral smear not performed because cystitis more likely

Perform urinalysis

Pyuria (>10 WBC/hpf) or positive leukocyte esterase test

Yes

Cystitis

Obtain urine culture
Treat for cystitis
Consider urologic evaluation

No

Absence of pyuria or positive leukocyte esterase test does not exclude cystitis, but makes it less likely

Consider the following possibilities:
Cystitis in neuropenic or immuno-compromised patient
Absence of pyuria in patient with cystitis because of white blood cell lysis in hypotonic or alkaline urine
Urethritis

✓ urine culture
Begin empiric antibiotic treatment for cystitis
Perform urethral smear

Urethral smear consistent with urethritis?

No

Yes

Further evaluation for urethritis

Urine culture positive?

Yes

Cystitis

No

Consider:
Atypical pathogens (fungi, tuberculosis)
Urine culture obtained after antibiotic therapy started
Noninfectious urologic disorder (eg, BPH, malignancy, calculi)
Psychogenic dysuria

DYSURIA (WOMEN)

STEP 1: *What is Dysuria?*

Pain or burning on urination is referred to as dysuria. Dysuria is a common problem, accounting for over three million office visits a year. In one study, 20% of women between 20-54 years of age reported at least one episode of dysuria in the past year.

Proceed to Step 2

STEP 2: *What are the Causes of Dysuria in Women?*

The causes of dysuria in women are listed in the following box.

Causes of Dysuria in Women	
Most Common	
Cystitis	Urethritis
Pyelonephritis	Vaginitis
Less Common	
Bladder calculus	Interstitial cystitis
Bladder cancer	Psychogenic dysuria
Drug-induced cystitis	Radiation cystitis
Eosinophilic cystitis	Ureteral calculus
Foreign body	Urethral cancer
Granulomatous cystitis	Urethral diverticulum
Hemorrhagic cystitis	Urethral stricture

The major causes of dysuria in women are principally infectious. Much of this chapter deals with the infectious causes of dysuria. When an infectious etiology is not present, the clinician should consider some of the less common causes of dysuria in women.

Proceed to Step 3

STEP 3: *Are There Any Clues in the Patient's History That Point to the Etiology of the Dysuria?*

Clues in the patient's history that point to the etiology of the dysuria are listed in the following table.

Historical Clue	Condition Suggested
Dysuria accompanied by frequency and urgency	Cystitis*
Dysuria perceived as an internal discomfort	Cystitis*
Dysuria perceived as an external discomfort	Vaginitis
Hematuria	Urinary tract infection (very uncommon in urethritis or vaginitis)
Use of spermicide or diaphragm	Risk factor for urinary tract infection
Suprapubic pain†	Cystitis*
Fever	Acute pyelonephritis Primary genital herpes‡
Vaginal discharge	Vaginitis
Back pain	Acute pyelonephritis
Dyspareunia	Vaginitis
Vaginal pruritus	Vaginitis
Nausea / vomiting	Acute pyelonephritis
History of atrophic vaginitis	Atrophic vaginitis Risk factor for urinary tract infection
History of recurrent urinary tract infection	Risk factor for urinary tract infection

*Some patients with pyelonephritis will have manifestations of cystitis.

†Suprapubic pain is a complaint in only 15% to 20% of cystitis cases.

‡Symptoms that should prompt consideration of primary genital herpes include dysuria, headache, neck pain, photophobia, and fever. Dysuria, which is reported in almost 80% of primary genital herpes cases, is not a feature of recurrent genital herpes.

Proceed to Step 4

STEP 4: *Are There Any Clues in the Patient's Physical Examination That Point to the Etiology of the Dysuria?*

Clues in the physical examination that point to the etiology of the dysuria are listed in the following table.

Physical Examination Finding	Condition Suggested
Suprapubic tenderness*	Cystitis†
Fever (>101.3°F or 38.5°C)	Acute pyelonephritis
Costovertebral angle tenderness	Acute pyelonephritis
Vaginal discharge	Vaginitis Genital herpes‡
Satellite vaginal pustules	Vaginitis (vaginal candidiasis)
Grouped painful vesicles Tender inguinal lymphadenopathy	Genital herpes‡

*Suprapubic tenderness is only appreciated in up to 20% of women with cystitis.

†Some patients with pyelonephritis will also have physical examination findings of cystitis.

‡Physical examination will usually reveal the characteristic lesions of genital herpes along with tender inguinal lymphadenopathy. Nearly 75% of patients will be noted to have vaginal discharge.

If the history and physical examination provide clues to the etiology of the dysuria, the clinician can direct the evaluation accordingly.

If the etiology of the dysuria is unclear after a thorough history and physical examination, **Proceed to Step 5.**

STEP 5: *Does the Patient Have Vaginitis?*

Although it is true that most women with dysuria will be found to have a urinary tract infection, it is important to realize that the symptoms of urinary tract infection are nonspecific. As such, the clinical presentation of vaginitis may mimic that of a urinary tract infection. As a result, it is important to ask the patient with dysuria about the presence of symptoms suggestive of vaginitis. Vaginal symptoms include discharge, itching, irritation, and odor. In one study of women who presented with dysuria and frequency but denied having vaginal symptoms, nearly 80% were found to have a urinary tract infection. Only 1% had vaginitis. Therefore, the absence of vaginal symptoms in a reliable patient provides a strong argument against the diagnosis of vaginitis.

Asking the patient to describe the dysuria further can be helpful in differentiating between vaginitis and urinary tract infection. The dysuria of cystitis is characteristically internal, often described as a deep burning sensation. In contrast, dysuria in patients with vaginitis is typically external, usually appreciated when the urine comes into contact with inflamed perineum.

It is not necessary to perform a pelvic examination in all patients who present with dysuria, especially if there are no clinical features suggestive of vaginitis. The great majority of these patients will be found to have a urinary tract infection. If any uncertainty exists, however, the clinician may elect to perform a pelvic examination to exclude vaginitis.

If the patient has symptoms and signs of vaginitis, proceed to the chapter on Vaginal Discharge *on page 521.*

If the patient does not have signs and symptoms of vaginitis, *Proceed to Step 6.*

STEP 6: *Does the Patient Have Urethritis Secondary to a Sexually Transmitted Disease?*

Some women with acute dysuria will be found to have gonococcal or chlamydial infection. Studies of women have shown that venereal urethritis is a much less common cause of dysuria than urinary tract infection but the proportion of patients with dysuria secondary to urethritis varies in different patient populations.

In women who are not sexually active, urethritis is very unlikely. Urethritis is also rare in patients who have a stable sexual partner, as long as the partner does not have symptoms of urethritis. Gonococcal or chlamydial infection presenting with dysuria should be a concern in women who have the risk factors listed in the following box.

Risk Factors for Gonococcal or Chlamydial Urethritis
History of pelvic inflammatory disease
History of sexually transmitted disease
Multiple sexual partners
New sexual partner
Partner with urethritis symptoms
Urinary symptoms that are "slow and stuttering" (>1 week)

Tenderness in the urethral area may be noted in patients with urethritis. In a minority of cases, the clinician may be able to express urethral discharge. It is important to realize, however, that the signs and symptoms of venereal urethritis are usually overshadowed by the clinical manifestations of coexisting cervicitis. A complete pelvic examination is necessary in these patients. Appropriate diagnostic testing for urethritis and/or cervicitis should be performed.

If the patient has urethritis and/or cervicitis, *Stop Here.*

If the patient does not have urethritis / cervicitis, *Proceed to Step 7.*

STEP 7: *Does the Patient Have Pyuria or a Positive Leukocyte Esterase Dipstick Test Result?*

It is generally agreed that women with acute dysuria should have a urine specimen analyzed for the presence of significant numbers of white blood cells or pyuria. Most women who are found to have pyuria have a bacterial urinary tract infection. A smaller proportion have venereal urethritis. Many clinicians rely on the urine dipstick leukocyte esterase test as a surrogate. Both tests are described in the remainder of this step.

Pyuria

The counting chamber method is the gold standard for the detection of pyuria. In this method, the number of white blood cells per mm^3 is counted in uncentrifuged urine. Although the counting chamber method is widely used in research circles, its use is impractical in the clinical setting. More reasonable in clinical practice is an estimation of the number of white blood cells per high power field using the centrifuged urine sediment. Normal urine should have less than 10 white blood cells per high power field. Greater than 10 white blood cells per high power field signifies the presence of pyuria.

Infection of the urinary tract is the most common cause of pyuria. However, it is important to realize that pyuria is a nonspecific finding. Pyuria has been noted in many noninfectious conditions, as shown in the following box.

Noninfectious Causes of Pyuria	
Contamination during collection	Malignancy
Prepuce secretions	Stones
Vaginal secretions	Transplant rejection
Cyclophosphamide treatment	Trauma
Foreign bodies	Tubulointerstitial disease
Glomerulonephritis	
Infections adjacent to urinary tract	
Appendicitis	
Diverticulitis	

Over 96% of symptomatic adult women with urinary tract infection will have >10 white blood cells per high powered field.

Leukocyte Esterase Dipstick Test

In women with acute dysuria, the leukocyte esterase test can be used as a surrogate to microscopic analysis of the urine for white blood cells. The leukocyte esterase test is a dipstick test that, if positive, indicates the presence of at least 8 white blood cells per high power field. The test has a sensitivity of 88% to 95% and specificity of 94% to 98%. False-negative test results may be due to rifampin, ascorbic acid, nitrofurantoin, blood, or bilirubin. False-positive test results may be seen in patients taking imipenem or amoxicillin/clavulanate.

Also available to the clinician is dipstick testing for nitrite. Nitrite testing is based on the concept that most bacterial pathogens of the urinary tract convert nitrate to nitrite. However, nitrite testing has a sensitivity of only 30%. Nitrite testing on first void urine specimens increases the sensitivity to 60%. Urinary tract infection is present more than 90% of the time if both nitrite and leukocyte esterase dipstick tests are positive.

Since the great majority of women with urinary tract infection will have pyuria, the absence of pyuria (or a negative leukocyte esterase test) should prompt the clinician to consider vaginal or pelvic disorders mimicking the presentation of a urinary tract infection. In these cases, the clinician should perform a pelvic exam, even if the patient denies symptoms suggestive of a vaginal or venereal condition. Also worth considering is whether the negative leukocyte esterase test is falsely negative. The clinician may wish to examine the urine for the presence of white blood cells if there is suspicion for a false-negative test result.

If the patient has pyuria (or positive leukocyte esterase test), ***Proceed to Step 8.***

If the patient does not have pyuria, ***Proceed to Step 18.***

STEP 8: *Does the Patient Have Cystitis or Acute Pyelonephritis?*

Pyuria or a positive leukocyte esterase dipstick test in a woman with acute dysuria supports the diagnosis of urinary tract infection. Urinary tract infection can be divided into upper and lower. The most common types of upper and lower urinary tract infection are acute pyelonephritis and cystitis, respectively. It is important to differentiate between cystitis and acute pyelonephritis for many reasons, some of which include length of treatment and need for hospitalization.

Although there are sensitive procedures available that can differentiate between upper and lower urinary tract infection, these procedures are invasive and impractical to use in the clinical setting. As a result, clinicians must rely on the clinical presentation to make the distinction. The signs and symptoms of lower urinary tract infection are listed in the following box.

Signs & Symptoms of Lower Urinary Tract Infection	
Dysuria	Pelvic discomfort
Fever (low grade, usually <100.4°F)*	Small volume voids
Frequency	Suprapubic tenderness
Hematuria	Urgency

*Most patients with lower urinary tract infection are afebrile.

Up to 30% of patients with acute pyelonephritis have signs and symptoms of lower urinary tract infection. In many cases, these lower urinary tract findings precede the upper urinary tract findings by several days. In addition, classic cases of acute pyelonephritis are characterized by upper urinary tract findings which include progressive flank pain, fever, chills, and nausea/vomiting. Physical examination often reveals a febrile, tachycardic patient. Evidence of volume contraction secondary to nausea and vomiting may be noted. Tenderness to palpation or percussion over the costovertebral angle is considered by many to be pathognomonic for acute pyelonephritis.

The following table offers a comparison between cystitis and acute pyelonephritis.

Signs & Symptoms	Cystitis	Acute Pyelonephritis
Fever	Absent	Usually present
Urgency / Frequency	Present	Sometimes present
Flank Pain	Absent	Sometimes present
Vomiting	Absent	Often present
Pyuria	Always present	Always present
Bacteriuria	Always present	Always present
Positive Blood Cultures	Absent	Often present

Adapted from Nseyo UO, Weinman E, and Lamm DL, *Urology for Primary Care Physicians*, Philadelphia, PA: WB Saunders Co, 1999, 133.

The clinician should realize, however, that many cases of acute pyelonephritis do not present classically. For example, diabetic patients with acute pyelonephritis may not present with flank pain. Confusion may be the sole manifestation of upper urinary tract infection in the elderly. Fever may be absent, especially in the elderly.

The absence of upper urinary tract findings does not exclude acute pyelonephritis. When sophisticated localization studies are performed in patients with suspected cystitis, up to 30% are found to have subclinical pyelonephritis.

If the patient has cystitis, *Proceed to Step 9.*

If the patient has acute pyelonephritis, *Proceed to Step 19.*

STEP 9: *Should a Urine Culture be Performed?*

For years, experts recommended the performance of urine culture and antimicrobial susceptibility testing in all women suspected of having urinary tract infection. Since the etiologic bacterial organisms and their antimicrobial susceptibility profile can easily be predicted in women with acute uncomplicated cystitis, many clinicians decide to manage these patients without urine culture. In addition, there is no data to suggest that pretreatment cultures improve therapeutic outcome.

Although studies investigating the utility of this approach (treatment without urine culture) in the management of acute, uncomplicated cystitis are lacking, there is data to suggest that the empiric treatment is safe and cost-effective. Pretreatment urine cultures and antimicrobial susceptibility testing are recommended, however, in women with complicated cystitis. The term "complicated" refers to the presence of factors (anatomical or functional abnormalities of the urinary tract) that can make eradication of the infection more difficult. It is important to recognize complicated urinary tract infection because resistant organisms are more likely to be encountered. A longer course of antibiotic therapy is often recommended in cases of complicated cystitis.

Complicated Cystitis	
Diabetes mellitus	Known structural or functional
History of frequent infection	urologic abnormalities
History of resistant organisms	Pregnancy
Immunocompromised patient	Recent antibiotic treatment
Indwelling catheter	(prolonged or repeated)
	Recent hospitalization

A urine culture should also be obtained in women who wish proof of infection.

If urine culture is indicated, **Proceed to Step 10.**

If urine culture is not indicated, **Proceed to Step 11.**

STEP 10: *What are the Results of the Urine Culture?*

The most widely used method for obtaining a urine culture is to have the patient collect a clean-voided midstream urine specimen. Contamination will be minimized by discarding the first 10 mL of urine. It is very important to process the specimen expeditiously. If the urine specimen cannot be processed within one hour, the clinician should refrigerate the specimen in an effort to avoid the proliferation of bacteria at room temperature. By doing so, the clinician can avoid high colony counts (of nonpathogenic bacteria) that can be potentially misleading.

Because voided urine specimens can easily become contaminated by perineal flora, it is essential to distinguish culture contamination from true infection. Factors that suggest culture contamination include the following:

- Low bacterial counts
- Growth of nonpathogenic organism (several species may be present)

In contrast, true infection is characterized by higher colony counts of one or more well recognized urinary pathogens. Traditionally, experts have considered $\geq 10^5$ colony forming units (cfu)/mL to be consistent with infection. While this cutoff is very specific in the diagnosis of urinary tract infection, it is now known that acute cystitis may present with colony counts between 10^2 and 10^4 cfu/mL. Investigators now agree that counts $\geq 10^2$ cfu/mL are significant in patients who are symptomatic.

There are several other techniques available in obtaining a urine specimen for culture. Some patients are unable to provide an uncontaminated midstream urine specimen. In these patients, the clinician may elect to obtain a catheterized specimen under sterile conditions. Contamination is less frequently noted in catheterized specimens when compared to voided midstream urine specimens. Suprapubic aspiration is another technique that can be performed when the patient is unable to provide a voided midstream urine specimen.

Because culture results are not usually available at a time when the clinician has to make treatment decisions, many clinicians turn to urine microscopy to provide information to guide therapy. Bacteriuria of $>10^5$ cfu/mL is likely when at least one organism is seen per oil immersion field (unspun urine) of a properly prepared Gram stain. Using the same criterion, the sensitivity of the Gram stain increases from 93% to 98% if centrifuged rather than uncentrifuged urine is examined. It is important to realize, however, that microscopic examination of urine for bacteria does not readily detect bacteria when the infection is characterized by lower bacterial colony counts (10^2 to 10^4 cfu/mL). Therefore the absence of bacteria on microscopic analysis does not exclude the possibility of urinary tract infection.

Proceed to Step 11

STEP 11: *What are the Results of Treatment?*

Once cystitis has been diagnosed, the clinician should treat the patient with an appropriate course of antibiotic therapy. Since therapy is usually instituted without performing a culture in uncomplicated cystitis (or before culture results return in patients with complicated cystitis), knowledge of the incidence of bacterial pathogens in lower urinary tract infections is important in the selection of appropriate antibiotic therapy. The following table lists the common bacterial pathogens in both uncomplicated and complicated lower urinary tract infections.

Pathogen	Incidence (%)
Uncomplicated infection	
Escherichia coli	80
Staphylococcus saprophyticus	10
Proteus mirabilis	5
Klebsiella pneumoniae	4
Enterobacter species	1
Beta-hemolytic streptococci	<1
Complicated infection	
Escherichia coli	35
Enterococcus faecalis	16
Proteus mirabilis	13
Staphylococcus epidermidis	12
Klebsiella pneumoniae	7
Pseudomonas aeruginosa	5
Staphylococcus aureus	4
Enterobacter species	3
Others*	5

*Includes *Serratia*, *Streptococcus*, *Acinetobacter*, and *Citrobacter* species

Adapted from Sweet RL and Gibbs RS, *Infectious Diseases of the Female Genital Tract*, 3rd ed, Baltimore, MD: Williams & Wilkins, 1995; and also adapted from "The Woman with Dysuria," *Am Fam Phys*, 1998, 57(9):2158.

Prior to instituting therapy, the clinician should also consider the possibility of subclinical pyelonephritis. Recall that up to 30% of patients suspected of having cystitis are actually found to have subclinical pyelonephritis when sophisticated localization studies are performed. Investigators have identified risk factors for subclinical pyelonephritis in women presenting with signs and symptoms of cystitis. The presence of these risk factors, which are listed in the following box, should prompt the clinician to treat the patient for subclinical pyelonephritis rather than cystitis (eg, longer course of antibiotic therapy).

Risk Factors for Subclinical Pyelonephritis in Women
Anatomic anomaly of the urinary tract
Diabetes mellitus
History of acute pyelonephritis within past year
Hospital-acquired infection
Immunocompromised
More than 3 UTIs in past year
Pregnancy
Recent antibiotic use
Recent urinary tract instrumentation
Relapse of symptoms within three days of treatment for acute cystitis
Symptoms present for more than one week before seeking treatment
Ureteral obstruction
Vesicoureteral reflux

Adapted from Johnson CC, "Definitions, Classification, and Clinical Presentation of Urinary Tract Infections," *Med Clin North Am*, 1991, 75(2):241-52 (review); also adapted from "The Woman With Dysuria," *Am Fam Physician*, 1998, 57(9):2159.

One of four outcomes is possible with treatment of cystitis:

- Complete response with resolution of symptoms

- Initial response with recurrence of symptoms after two weeks (reinfection)

- Initial response with recurrence of symptoms within two weeks or partial response (relapse)

- No response whatsoever (nonresponder)

If the patient has a complete response with resolution of symptoms and no recurrence, ***Proceed to Step 12.***

If the patient has reinfection (initial response with recurrence of symptoms after two weeks), ***Proceed to Step 13.***

If the patient has relapsing infection (initial response with recurrence within two weeks or partial response), ***Proceed to Step 14.***

If the patient does not respond to therapy (nonresponder), ***Proceed to Step 15.***

STEP 12: *What Further Evaluation is Necessary?*

No further evaluation is necessary in women who have complete resolution of their symptoms with treatment (and no recurrence). It is reasonable to obtain a repeat urinalysis after treatment to demonstrate the resolution of the abnormalities noted on the urinalysis (eg, pyuria, hematuria). In particular, it is important to document resolution of the hematuria, especially in older women or women with risk factors for genitourinary malignancy. Hematuria that is the result of a urinary tract infection will resolve with appropriate treatment of the infection. Persistence of hematuria warrants consideration of other causes of blood in the urine.

End of Section.

STEP 13: *Why is the Patient Prone to Reinfection?*

When treatment of a urinary tract infection results in complete resolution of the symptoms but urinary tract infection recurs after at least two weeks, reinfection is said to be present. Reinfection is usually characterized by infection due to different organisms or a different serotype of the same species of organism.

In these cases, repeated colonization of the periurethral area occurs with enteric organisms. At some point, this colonization may extend into the urethra and bladder with the subsequent development of active infection. Studies have shown that anatomic or functional abnormalities of the genitourinary tract are present in only a small percentage of cases. Of key importance in women with reinfection is prevention. In some women, adherence to the points in the following list may be sufficient in preventing reinfection.

- Avoid a full bladder
- High fluid intake
- Voiding after intercourse
- Consider change in contraceptive method if currently using diaphragm
- Consider change in contraceptive method if currently using spermicide
- Wiping from anterior to posterior following voiding

When more than 2 reinfections are experienced per year in a woman who has followed the previously listed points, the clinician should consider starting prophylactic or suppressive antibiotic therapy. In patients with reinfection, urologic investigation should be considered if prophylactic or suppressive therapy is unsuccessful.

End of Section.

STEP 14: *What is the Cause of the Relapse?*

Relapsing infection is said to be present if symptoms recur within two weeks after an initial response. Women who partially respond to the antibiotic treatment are also considered to have relapsing infection. Causes to consider are the emergence of antibiotic resistance in the pathogenic organism and patient noncompliance. Also worth considering is the possibility of upper urinary tract involvement. In other cases, there may be abnormalities or factors that protect the organism from eradication. These factors responsible for relapsing infection are listed in the following table.

Cause	Pathology
Urinary stasis	Poor emptying Vesicoureteral reflux Hydronephrosis Bladder or urethral diverticula
Sequestered organisms	Necrotic tissue (bladder cancer, papillary necrosis) Foreign body (stones, stents, catheters) Vesicoenteric fistula
Altered immune system	Diabetes mellitus Chemotherapy Corticosteroid use
Altered antibiotic secretion	Azotemia Patient compliance

Adapted from Nseyo UO, Weinman E, and Lamm DL, *Urology for Primary Care Physicians*, Philadelphia, PA: WB Saunders Co, 1999, 157.

These patients often require a prolonged course of antibiotic therapy. Referral to urology is quite reasonable in this group of patients.

End of Section.

STEP 15: *Why Has the Patient Not Responded to Antibiotic Therapy?*

The great majority of women with uncomplicated cystitis should have symptomatic improvement within a few days of appropriate therapy. Failure to improve (nonresponder) warrants further investigation. In particular, the clinician should obtain a urine culture.

If the urine culture is positive, *Proceed to Step 16.*

If the urine culture is negative, *Proceed to Step 17.*

STEP 16: *What is the Significance of the Positive Urine Culture?*

A positive urine culture that is obtained in a woman who is not responding to antibiotic therapy should prompt the clinician to consider the possibilities listed in the following box.

Possibilities to Consider when Positive Urine Cultures are Obtained in Women Not Responding to Antibiotic Therapy for "Urinary Tract Infection"

Organism is resistant to antibiotic chosen*

Patient is noncompliant

Significant renal failure is impairing the effectiveness of the antibiotic chosen

Patient has upper urinary tract involvement†

Patient has urologic disease‡

---

*If a urine culture was obtained prior to the onset of therapy, it may reveal the growth of an organism that is resistant to the antibiotic chosen. In these cases, the antibiotic should be changed depending upon the antimicrobial susceptibility profile of the organism. If a urine culture was not obtained at the onset of therapy, it should be obtained at this point since the patient is not responding to the therapy selected. Further treatment decisions should await results of the culture.

†As mentioned earlier in this chapter, the clinical presentation does not always allow the clinician to differentiate cystitis from pyelonephritis. In fact, up to 30% of patients with suspected cystitis are actually found to have subclinical pyelonephritis if sophisticated localization studies are performed. Also worth considering is the possibility that the infection which was originally consistent with cystitis has progressed to pyelonephritis. Recall that it is not uncommon for pyelonephritis to begin within one or two days of lower urinary tract symptoms and signs.

‡Urologic abnormalities may prevent symptomatic cure in patients with urinary tract infection. In most cases, however, the presence of a urologic abnormality is not known at the time of the patient's presentation. In these cases, it is preferable to delay urologic investigation until the patient has been treated with a prolonged course of antibiotic therapy. Exceptions to this rule are in patients with signs and symptoms of nephrolithiasis, etc, that should prompt the clinician to obtain an urgent urologic consultation.

End of Section.

STEP 17: *What is the Significance of a Negative Urine Culture?*

A negative urine culture that is obtained in a woman who is not responding to antibiotic therapy should prompt the clinician to consider the possibilities listed in the following box.

Possibilities to Consider when Negative Urine Cultures are Obtained in Women Not Responding to Antibiotic Therapy for "Urinary Tract Infection"

Atypical pathogens (tuberculosis, fungal)

Psychogenic dysuria

Urethritis (gonococcal, chlamydial, noninfectious)

Vaginitis (infectious or noninfectious)

Urologic disease

Bladder calculus	Interstitial cystitis
Bladder cancer	Radiation cystitis
Drug-induced cystitis	Ureteral calculus
Eosinophilic cystitis	Urethral cancer
Foreign body	Urethral diverticulum
Granulomatous cystitis	Urethral stricture
Hemorrhagic cystitis	

Also recall that pyuria is not specific for urinary tract infection. In these cases, dysuria and pyuria may be a reflection of a noninfectious disease process in the genitourinary tract.

Of the causes listed in the preceding box, the clinician should especially consider the possibility of venereal urethritis or vaginitis. Pelvic examination is absolutely necessary in these cases as is appropriate diagnostic testing for these conditions.

If the etiology of the dysuria remains unclear, it is reasonable to obtain a urologic consultation.

End of Section.

STEP 18: *Does the Absence of Pyuria Exclude a Urinary Tract Infection?*

The absence of pyuria does not exclude the presence of a urinary tract infection. Since the great majority of women with urinary tract infection have pyuria, its absence, however, does make urinary tract infection less likely. On occasion, pyuria may be absent in lower or upper urinary tract infection, particularly in neutropenic or immunocompromised patients. Patients who have a renal or perinephric abscess may also not present with pyuria. For these reasons, then, it is worthwhile to send a urine culture when pyuria is not present in a woman suspected of having a urinary tract infection.

The absence of pyuria should also prompt the clinician to consider other causes of dysuria. In particular, vaginal or pelvic conditions warrant consideration. As such, these patients deserve a thorough pelvic examination. In the absence of a pelvic or vaginal condition, the clinician may choose to begin empiric treatment for a urinary tract infection while awaiting culture results. A positive urine culture should prompt continued treatment with an adequate course of antibiotics. A negative urine culture should prompt consideration of the conditions listed in the box in Step 17.

End of Section.

STEP 19: *What Tests Should be Performed in Patients With Acute Pyelonephritis?*

Prior to discussing the tests that should be obtained in patients with acute pyelonephritis, brief mention will be made here regarding the differential diagnosis of acute pyelonephritis. These conditions, some of which have the potential to be life-threatening, are listed in the following box.

Differential Diagnosis of Acute Pyelonephritis	
Acute cholecystitis	Herpes zoster (prior to vesicular eruption)
Acute hepatitis	Intra-abdominal abscess
Appendicitis	Myocardial infarction
Bacterial pneumonia	Other intra-abdominal conditions
Diverticulitis	Pelvic inflammatory disease

The preceding box is included in this section to remind the clinician that acute pyelonephritis may be confused with other illnesses. Other considerations in the patient presenting with acute pyelonephritis include the need for hospitalization which should be individualized.

Besides obtaining a urine specimen for pyuria and/or leukocyte esterase testing, the clinician should also perform the following tests in the patient with acute pyelonephritis:

- Urine culture (discussed in Step 10)

    Although the growth of a single uropathogen is typical, in some cases, multiple organisms may be cultured, particularly in immunocompromised hosts.

- Gram stain of the urine

    A properly prepared Gram stain may help the clinician select the appropriate antibiotic therapy, especially since the culture results are usually not available at a time when the clinician wishes to start therapy.

- Blood cultures

    Approximately 25% of patients with acute pyelonephritis will have positive blood cultures.

Imaging studies are not indicated in most patients with acute pyelonephritis. In those who are particularly ill, the clinician may wish to obtain a standard abdominal film. The radiograph may reveal findings consistent with calculi, obstruction, or other urologic abnormalities. If the diagnosis of acute pyelonephritis is not clear, the clinician may wish to obtain a CT scan. Contrast-enhanced CT is the imaging test of choice in patients with acute pyelonephritis. Streaky or wedge-shaped hypodense areas in the kidney reflect the inflammatory changes that characterize acute pyelonephritis. These areas of inflammation fail to concentrate contrast material when compared to normal kidney parenchyma. Diffuse swelling is also typical. In some cases, focal bulges or inflammatory stranding in the perinephric fat may be noted. If pyelonephritis develops in the setting of nephrolithiasis, nonenhanced spiral CT is the imaging test of choice in the detection of calculi.

Proceed to Step 20

STEP 20: *What is the Expected Time Course for Symptomatic Improvement?*

Most women with acute pyelonephritis notice symptomatic improvement within the first few days following the start of appropriate antibiotic therapy. Failure to improve should prompt the clinician to consider the possibilities listed in the following box.

Possibilities to Consider When Symptoms of Acute Pyelonephritis Do Not Improve After 48-72 Hours of Antibiotic Therapy
Patient does not have acute pyelonephritis (consider alternative diagnoses)
Organism is resistant to antibiotic
Noncompliance
Abscess
Obstruction

In these cases, the clinician should ensure that the pathogenic organism is susceptible to the antibiotic chosen. A review of the patient's chart should be done to ensure that the patient has been receiving antibiotic therapy (appropriate dose, interval, etc). If treatment was started as an outpatient, the clinician should seriously consider hospitalization for intravenous antibiotics and further evaluation.

When acute pyelonephritis is complicated by the development of an abscess, the clinician may be able to palpate a flank mass. The absence of a flank mass, however, does not exclude an abscess. Therefore, the clinician should consider performing imaging tests (ultrasound or CT). Contrast-enhanced CT scan will help determine whether the infection has been complicated by abscess development. Although smaller abscesses may resolve with a prolonged course of antibiotic therapy, larger abscesses may require drainage along with medical therapy.

An obstruction to urine flow (calculi or malignancy) can also be diagnosed with imaging tests. In these patients, symptomatic improvement often does not occur until either the obstruction is relieved or alternative urinary drainage is established. Urology consultation is recommended in these complicated cases.

Proceed to Step 21

STEP 21: *Does the Patient Need Urologic Referral After Resolution of the Acute Pyelonephritis?*

Urologic referral is indicated when the likelihood of finding a correctable genitourinary abnormality is high. In most women, the yield of extensive testing is low. However, in women who develop relapsing infection (same organism), it may be worthwhile to perform urologic investigation. This is especially true if relapse occurs after a prolonged course of antibiotic therapy for the first relapse. There is much uncertainty regarding whether women who have recurrent pyelonephritis due to different organisms should have urologic studies.

End of Section.

REFERENCES

Hooton TM and Stamm WE, "Diagnosis and Treatment of Uncomplicated Urinary Tract Infection," *Infect Dis Clin North Am*, 1997, 11(3):551-81.

Johnson CC, "Definitions, Classification, and Clinical Presentation of Urinary Tract Infections," *Med Clin North Am*, 1991, 75(2):241-52 (review).

Kurowski K, "The Women With Dysuria," *Am Fam Phys*, 1998, 57(9):2155-64, 2169-70.

Neu HC, "Urinary Tract Infections," *Am J Med*, 1992, 92(4A):63S-70S (review).

Nseyo UO, Weinman E, and Lamm DL, *Urology for Primary Care Physicians*, Philadelphia, PA: WB Saunders Co, 1999, 133, 157.

Orenstein R and Wong ES, "Urinary Tract Infections in Adults," *Am Fam Phys*, 1999, 59(5):1225-34, 1237.

Sweet RL and Gibbs RS, *Infectious Diseases of the Female Genital Tract*, 3rd ed, Baltimore, MD: Williams & Wilkins, 1995.

"The Woman with Dysuria," *Am Fam Phys*, 1998, 57(9):2158-9.

DYSURIA (WOMEN)

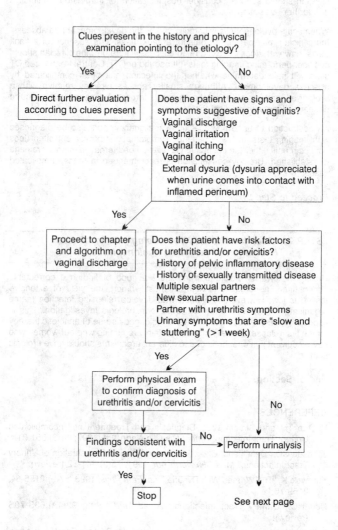

Clues present in the history and physical examination pointing to the etiology?

Yes → Direct further evaluation according to clues present

No → Does the patient have signs and symptoms suggestive of vaginitis?
- Vaginal discharge
- Vaginal irritation
- Vaginal itching
- Vaginal odor
- External dysuria (dysuria appreciated when urine comes into contact with inflamed perineum)

Yes → Proceed to chapter and algorithm on vaginal discharge

No → Does the patient have risk factors for urethritis and/or cervicitis?
- History of pelvic inflammatory disease
- History of sexually transmitted disease
- Multiple sexual partners
- New sexual partner
- Partner with urethritis symptoms
- Urinary symptoms that are "slow and stuttering" (>1 week)

Yes → Perform physical exam to confirm diagnosis of urethritis and/or cervicitis

Findings consistent with urethritis and/or cervicitis

No → Perform urinalysis

Yes → Stop

No (risk factors) → Perform urinalysis

See next page

DYSURIA (WOMEN)
(continued)

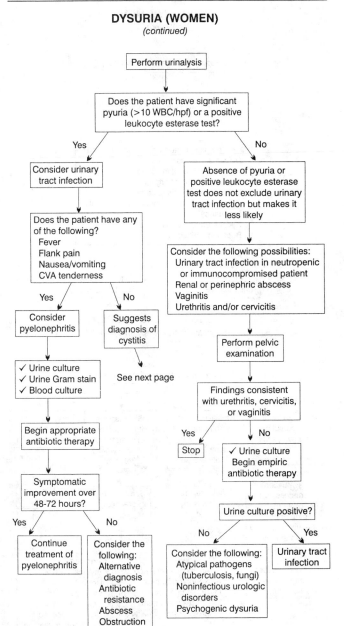

Perform urinalysis

Does the patient have significant pyuria (>10 WBC/hpf) or a positive leukocyte esterase test?

Yes

Consider urinary tract infection

Does the patient have any of the following?
Fever
Flank pain
Nausea/vomiting
CVA tenderness

Yes

Consider pyelonephritis

✓ Urine culture
✓ Urine Gram stain
✓ Blood culture

Begin appropriate antibiotic therapy

Symptomatic improvement over 48-72 hours?

Yes

Continue treatment of pyelonephritis

No

Consider the following:
Alternative diagnosis
Antibiotic resistance
Abscess
Obstruction

No

Suggests diagnosis of cystitis

See next page

No

Absence of pyuria or positive leukocyte esterase test does not exclude urinary tract infection but makes it less likely

Consider the following possibilities:
Urinary tract infection in neutropenic or immunocompromised patient
Renal or perinephric abscess
Vaginitis
Urethritis and/or cervicitis

Perform pelvic examination

Findings consistent with urethritis, cervicitis, or vaginitis

Yes

Stop

No

✓ Urine culture
Begin empiric antibiotic therapy

Urine culture positive?

No

Consider the following:
Atypical pathogens (tuberculosis, fungi)
Noninfectious urologic disorders
Psychogenic dysuria

Yes

Urinary tract infection

DYSURIA (WOMEN)
(continued)

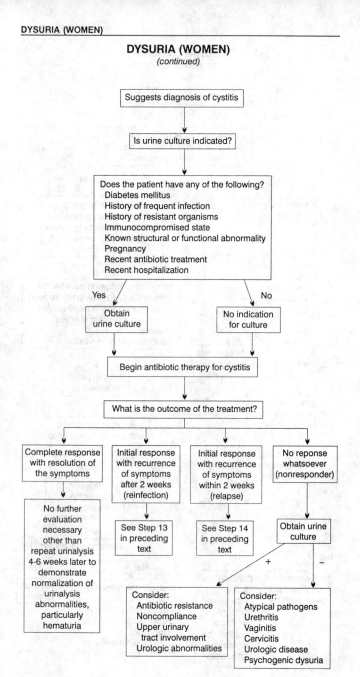

Suggests diagnosis of cystitis

Is urine culture indicated?

Does the patient have any of the following?
Diabetes mellitus
History of frequent infection
History of resistant organisms
Immunocompromised state
Known structural or functional abnormality
Pregnancy
Recent antibiotic treatment
Recent hospitalization

Yes → Obtain urine culture

No → No indication for culture

Begin antibiotic therapy for cystitis

What is the outcome of the treatment?

Complete response with resolution of the symptoms → No further evaluation necessary other than repeat urinalysis 4-6 weeks later to demonstrate normalization of urinalysis abnormalities, particularly hematuria

Initial response with recurrence of symptoms after 2 weeks (reinfection) → See Step 13 in preceding text

Initial response with recurrence of symptoms within 2 weeks (relapse) → See Step 14 in preceding text

No reponse whatsoever (nonresponder) → Obtain urine culture

+ → Consider:
Antibiotic resistance
Noncompliance
Upper urinary tract involvement
Urologic abnormalities

− → Consider:
Atypical pathogens
Urethritis
Vaginitis
Cervicitis
Urologic disease
Psychogenic dysuria

EPISTAXIS

STEP 1: *How Common is Epistaxis?*

Epistaxis is a common complaint that prompts patients to visit emergency rooms. In fact, 10% of adults have sought medical attention for epistaxis. Between 60% and 70% of adults have experienced at least one episode. In most cases, the epistaxis is mild, easily controlled by conservative therapy. On occasion, however, the bleeding may be profuse. Although deaths due to epistaxis are rare, they have occurred. It is important to realize, then, that epistaxis has the potential to be life-threatening.

Proceed to Step 2

STEP 2: *How Serious is the Nosebleed?*

When a patient presents with epistaxis, the initial focus should center on the basics of airway, breathing, and circulation. In particular, the clinician should assess the following:

- **Vital Signs**

  In the hypotensive patient, the clinician should be particularly concerned about significant blood loss. Most patients, however, will be noted to have reactive hypertension secondary to the apprehension that accompanies the nosebleed. Since epistaxis is anxiety provoking, tachycardia is not uncommon in these patients. However, tachycardia, like hypotension, may also be a sign of significant blood loss.

- **Airway**

  The presence of any signs suggestive of airway compromise should prompt the clinician to consider airway intervention.

- **General Appearance**

- **Mental Status**

  A change in mental status is suggestive of significant blood loss. Cool skin temperature and pallor of the conjunctiva may also be noted with massive epistaxis.

The goals, then, during the initial evaluation are stabilization of the patient. To that end, fluid resuscitation and airway intervention take precedence over performing a thorough history and physical examination. Only after the patient with epistaxis has been stabilized should the clinician consider the causes and management of the nosebleed.

Proceed to Step 3

STEP 3: *What are the Causes of Epistaxis?*

The causes of epistaxis are listed in the following box.

Causes of Epistaxis	
Environmental factors	Medications
Cold, dry air	Aspirin
Local factors	Coumadin
Trauma	Dipyridamole
Nose picking	Heparin
Facial trauma	NSAIDs
Nasal septal deviation	Steroid nasal inhalers
Surgery	Thioridazine
Inflammation	Ticlid
Acute respiratory infection	Topical hyperosmolar sodium chloride
Chronic sinusitis	Systemic conditions
Allergic rhinosinusitis	Hypertension
Foreign body	Coagulation disorders
Cocaine inhalation	Thrombocytopenia
Malignancy	Hemophilia
Chemicals	von Willebrand's disease
	Disseminated intravascular coagulation
	Liver disease
	Chronic renal failure
	Alcoholism
	Hereditary hemorrhagic telangiectasia

These conditions will be discussed in further detail below.

Environmental Factors

When hospital admissions for epistaxis are examined with regards to time of the year, there is clearly an increase noted during the winter months. It is thought that this seasonal predilection is secondary to exposure to cold, dry air.

Trauma

The most common cause of epistaxis is self-inflicted trauma through nose picking. Facial trauma that occurs with motor vehicle accidents is commonly associated with epistaxis, which, in severe cases, can be life-threatening. A nosebleed that develops days to weeks after trauma sustained to the base of the skull should prompt the clinician to consider a post-traumatic pseudoaneurysm of the internal carotid artery. This potentially life-threatening condition is characterized by the triad of massive epistaxis, unilateral blindness, and orbital fracture.

Nasal Septal Deviation

In several studies, nasal septal deviation was more commonly found in epistaxis patients when compared to a control group. That this association exists is well recognized but, unfortunately, how nasal septal deviation predisposes to nosebleeds is not clearly understood.

Surgery

Epistaxis occurring within the first several weeks after certain types of facial surgery is not uncommon. It tends to occur more often in patients who have undergone septal, turbinate, orbital, or sinus surgery.

Inflammation

Common causes of epistaxis include acute respiratory infection, chronic sinusitis, and allergic rhinosinusitis. Mucosal hyperemia is common in patients with viral or allergic rhinitis. In these patients, forceful nose blowing or nose picking can easily lead to epistaxis. When epistaxis is accompanied by a unilateral purulent discharge, the clinician should consider the possibility of a foreign body impaction. Foreign body impaction should be more of a consideration in children and mentally-impaired individuals.

Malignancy

Both benign and malignant tumors can present with epistaxis. In some patients, nosebleeding may be the only symptom. In other cases, symptoms such as foul discharge, change in smell, and nasal obstruction may accompany the epistaxis. When other symptoms are present, typically they are unilateral. Common malignancies that may present with epistaxis include the following:

- Squamous cell carcinoma
- Melanoma
- Inverted papilloma
- Adenoid cystic carcinoma

Juvenile angiofibroma is a consideration in male adolescents, often presenting with recurrent episodes of severe epistaxis.

Chemicals

The clinician should determine if there has been any exposure to any airborne irritants or toxic chemicals. Some toxic chemicals that can damage the nasal mucosa include ammonia, gasoline, sulfuric acid, and chromates. Cigarette smoke is a well recognized irritant.

Hypertension

In studies performed examining the relationship between hypertension and epistaxis, investigators have not found a higher incidence of hypertension among individuals with epistaxis when compared to a control group. While it is true that most patients with epistaxis present with an elevated blood pressure, the elevation is likely to be related to the anxiety that accompanies epistaxis. All patients with epistaxis who present with hypertension should have their blood pressure rechecked to ensure normalization of the blood pressure. In many cases, the blood pressure returns to normal after the epistaxis is controlled. In a minority, follow up of the patient's blood pressure may reveal that the patient had previously undiagnosed hypertension.

Chronic Renal Failure

There seems to be a relationship between chronic renal failure and epistaxis, the etiology of which is thought to be multifactorial. Some factors that may predispose these individuals to nosebleeding include platelet dysfunction and the use of heparin during hemodialysis.

Coagulation Disorders

In hereditary conditions such as hemophilia and von Willebrand's disease, epistaxis is commonly encountered. Epistaxis may occur in other hematologic conditions such as leukemia, thrombocytopenia, and multiple myeloma.

Hereditary Hemorrhagic Telangiectasia

Hereditary hemorrhagic telangiectasia, also known as the Osler-Weber-Rendu syndrome, is characterized by telangiectatic blood vessels throughout the body including the nasal cavity. Because of their fragility, these vessels can rupture quite easily, often leading to recurrent epistaxis. Almost all patients with hereditary hemorrhagic telangiectasia are symptomatic by the age of 40. Epistaxis is quite common. In fact, it is the presenting symptom in approximately 90% of cases.

Alcoholism

The risk of epistaxis is increased in patients who consume large amounts of alcohol. One factor thought to play a role in the increased risk is the elevation in the bleeding time that accompanies heavy alcohol use. In addition, alcoholic patients are often malnourished. In these patients, vitamin deficiencies (eg, vitamin K) can lead to an impairment in the production of coagulation factors. With prolonged use of large amounts of alcohol, chronic liver disease or cirrhosis may ensue, leading to coagulation disturbances.

Medications

A thorough medication history is essential in the patient presenting with epistaxis since many different medications can affect the normal clotting process. NSAIDs and aspirin, for example, impair platelet aggregation. Patients anticoagulated with heparin or coumadin are at higher risk for the development of epistaxis. Thioridazine does not interfere with normal clotting. The epistaxis that has been noted with this medication is thought to be due to excessive drying which is an anticholinergic side effect.

Proceed to Step 4

STEP 4: *Are There Any Clues in the Patient's History That Point to the Etiology of the Epistaxis?*

Clues in the patient's history that may point to the etiology of the patient's epistaxis are listed in the following table.

Historical Clue	Condition Suggested
History of hypertension	Relationship between hypertension and epistaxis (controversial)
Cocaine use (intranasal)	Cocaine use (causing mucosal inflammation)
Recent nose picking, scratching, or vigorous nose blowing	Trauma

(continued)

Historical Clue	Condition Suggested
Recent motor vehicle accident	Facial trauma
	Post-traumatic pseudoaneurysm of the internal carotid artery
History of liver disease	Liver disease (coagulation disturbances)
Family history of epistaxis	Hereditary hemorrhagic telangiectasia
	Hemophilia
	von Willebrand's disease
Recurrent, spontaneous epistaxis	Consider bleeding or coagulation disorder
Recent facial surgery	Surgery
Recent chemotherapy	Thrombocytopenia
Purulent nasal discharge	Foreign body
	Sinusitis
Recent or current upper respiratory tract infection	Upper respiratory tract infection
Medication use	Medication predisposing to epistaxis
Triad of unilateral blindness, orbital fracture, and massive epistaxis	Post-traumatic pseudoaneurysm of the internal carotid artery

Proceed to Step 5

STEP 5: *Are There Any Clues in the Patient's Physical Examination That Point to the Etiology of the Epistaxis?*

Before performing the physical examination, it is essential to ensure that the proper equipment is available. The necessary equipment includes the following:

- Headlight
- Nasal speculum
- Suction tips
- Emesis basin
- Bayonet forceps
- Gown / gloves / face mask / eyeglasses

As preparations are being made for the physical examination, the patient should be instructed to apply direct pressure to the nose. This can be done by having the patient compress the nose between two fingers. In many cases, direct pressure is all that is needed to stop the bleeding. Prior to the nasal examination, the clinician should anesthetize the nasopharynx by using an anesthetic and vasoconstrictive agent. This may also be helpful in temporarily ceasing the bleeding when direct pressure is unsuccessful. Some choices available to the clinician include the following:

- Phenylephrine with lidocaine
- Oxymetazoline with lidocaine
- Epinephrine with lidocaine

Once the topical medication has been applied, the examination of the nose begins with attempts to clear the nose of all clots and debris by asking the patient to blow the nose. Alternatively, the clinician may elect to use the suction. The key to a proper physical examination of the nose is visualization of as much of the nasal vestibule as possible. To ensure that this occurs, the clinician should ask the patient to keep the head upright. Patients have a tendency to tilt their head backwards but this will only allow the clinician to visualize the roof of the nasal cavity.

Proceed to Step 6

STEP 6: *Does the Patient Have Anterior or Posterior Epistaxis?*

Epistaxis may be anterior or posterior. This classification refers to the source of the nasal bleeding. Although posterior epistaxis (5% of epistaxis cases) is much less common than anterior epistaxis, it is important for the clinician to recognize features in the patient's presentation that help differentiate posterior from anterior epistaxis. Making a distinction between anterior and posterior epistaxis is important because the type of epistaxis present dictates the treatment. Clues in the history and physical examination that may help to make this distinction are listed in the following table.

	Anterior Epistaxis	Posterior Epistaxis
Is the epistaxis unilateral or bilateral?	More commonly unilateral	More commonly bilateral
Is the epistaxis mild or profuse?	More commonly mild	More commonly profuse
Is blood flowing down the posterior oropharynx?	Usually not	Usually
How difficult is it to control the epistaxis?	Less difficult	More difficult

Most cases of epistaxis are due to an anterior source. In these cases, the clinician can often visualize the area of bleeding. Examination of the nose may reveal bleeding, ulceration, or erosion. If the source of the bleeding is easily visualized, the management of choice is chemical or electrical cautery. Cautery should not, however, be performed in thrombocytopenic or anticoagulated patients. In the event that cautery is unsuccessful in ceasing the bleeding, the clinician may elect to perform anterior nasal packing. In approximately 25% of cases, anterior nasal packing does not halt the bleeding. In these cases, the clinician should ascertain whether or not the patient feels any blood trickling down the posterior pharynx. If the patient describes this sensation or blood is noted flowing down the posterior pharynx, then posterior epistaxis is likely. Regardless of how the patient answers this question, however, the clinician should obtain an emergent ENT consultation when anterior nasal packing fails to control the bleeding.

With posterior epistaxis, it may be difficult to visualize the area that is bleeding. In these cases, it may be necessary to perform fiberoptic nasopharyngoscopy to identify the source of the bleeding. All patients with posterior epistaxis require an emergent consultation with ENT. The reader is referred to a specialty text for further information regarding the management of posterior epistaxis.

Proceed to Step 7

STEP 7: What Laboratory Tests Need to be Obtained in the Patient With Epistaxis?

The clinician may forego laboratory testing in minor nosebleeds that do not recur. With more severe bleeds or with those that recur, the following laboratory tests are recommended:

- PT / PTT
- CBC with platelet count

In addition, type and crossmatch may be needed in patients with serious or massive epistaxis in whom significant blood has been lost. Coagulation studies are likely to be normal unless the patient has any of the following features:

- Recurrent epistaxis
- Prolonged episode
- Failure to respond to conservative management
- History of liver disease
- History of bleeding disorder (hemophilia, von Willebrand's disease)
- Anticoagulation with heparin or coumadin

Serum BUN and creatinine should be obtained in the patient suspected of having chronic renal failure. Liver function tests may be necessary if epistaxis is thought to be secondary to the coagulation disturbances that accompany chronic liver disease or cirrhosis. A DIC panel should only be obtained in those who have signs and symptoms of DIC.

Proceed to Step 8

STEP 8: What Issues Need to be Followed-Up Once the Epistaxis is Controlled?

A thorough history, physical examination, and laboratory studies (when indicated) will reveal the etiology in most cases of epistaxis. Regardless of whether the cause is identified at the time of the nosebleed, the patient should be instructed to follow up with a primary care or ENT physician two to three days after control of the nosebleed. At this visit, the clinician should examine the nose carefully again in an attempt to identify the cause of the epistaxis. In these cases, the cause may be more evident during examination when the patient is not actively bleeding. In some patients, however, the cause remains elusive despite a thorough evaluation.

In the event that the history and physical examination are concerning for malignancy (eg, mass visualized on endoscopic nasal exam), the clinician may elect to perform CT or MRI. All such patients should be referred to the ENT physician for consideration of biopsy.

REFERENCES

Alvi A and Joyner-Triplett N, "Acute Epistaxis. How to Spot the Source and Stop the Flow," *Postgrad Med,* 1996, 99(5):83-90, 94-6 (review).

Okafor BC, "Epistaxis: A Clinical Study of 540 Cases," *Ear Nose Throat J*, 1984, 63(3):153-9.

Pfaff JA and Moore GP, "Eye, Ear, Nose, and Throat," *Emerg Med Clin North Am*, 1997, 15(2)327-40 (review).

Tan LK and Calhoun KH, "Epistaxis," *Med Clin North Am*, 1999, 83(1):43-56 (review).

ERECTILE DYSFUNCTION

STEP 1: *How Common is Erectile Dysfunction?*

Erectile dysfunction refers to the inability to develop or maintain an erection of sufficient degree necessary for sexual activity. Based upon a 1992 NIH consensus statement, the term "erectile dysfunction" is favored over impotence because the latter was considered to be too pejorative. Nonetheless, it is a common problem, one that increases with age. In fact, up to 33% of men over the age of 65 have erectile dysfunction. Erectile dysfunction accounts for over 500,000 ambulatory visits a year.

Proceed to Step 2

STEP 2: *Does the Patient Truly Have Erectile Dysfunction?*

Because many patients are reluctant to discuss erectile dysfunction, it is important for the clinician to take a thorough sexual history in every patient. Not uncommonly, patients with erectile dysfunction will wait several years before seeking medical attention. There are many reasons accounting for this delay in presentation. Some of these reasons include the following:

- Reluctance to seek medical help because of the belief that the erectile dysfunction may improve or resolve spontaneously
- Difficulty believing that the clinician can help in such a matter
- Shame and embarrassment

In addition, healthcare professionals also play a role in the delay in presentation. Many clinicians are uncomfortable discussing sexual function with their patients. But not doing so prevents the identification of a common problem that often has a significant impact on the patient's quality of life. With new treatments now available, it behooves the clinician to discuss these issues with every patient.

One approach used by many clinicians in eliciting a history of erectile dysfunction is to begin the sexual history with the question "Are you sexually active?" If the answer to this question is "no", the clinician should determine why the patient is not sexually active. There are a number of reasons why a patient may refrain from sexual activity. While some patients choose to abstain from sexual activity, it is best not to assume so. In fact, a major reason why patients refrain from sex is erectile dysfunction.

In those who are sexually active, it is useful to ask the patient, "Are you satisfied with your sex life?" An affirmative response argues against the presence of erectile dysfunction. A "no" response should be followed by asking how the sex life could be better. In many cases, this series of questions will elicit a history of difficulty in initiating or maintaining an erection.

The general public also has many misconceptions as to what constitutes normal sexual function. It is not uncommon for otherwise healthy individuals to experience erectile dysfunction from time to time. In many cases, the difficulty in initiating or maintaining the erection is due to fatigue, boredom, anxiety, lack of sleep, depression, or relationship troubles.

If erectile dysfunction is not present, ***Stop Here.***

If erectile dysfunction is present, ***Proceed to Step 3.***

STEP 3: *What are the Causes of Erectile Dysfunction?*

The causes of erectile dysfunction are listed in the following box.

Causes of Erectile Dysfunction	
Anatomic	Recreational drugs
Penile trauma	Cocaine
Peyronie's disease	Heroin
Priapism	Marijuana
Endocrine / metabolic	Psychogenic
Estrogen-producing neoplasms	Systemic conditions
(adrenal, testis)	Diabetes mellitus
Hyperprolactinemia	Hyperlipidemia
Hyperthyroidism	Hypertension
Hypogonadism	Liver disease
Hypopituitarism	Renal failure
Hypothyroidism	Vasculogenic
Medications / toxins	Major artery
Neurogenic	Aortoiliac disease
Autonomic neuropathy	(Leriche syndrome)
Diabetic neuropathy	Atheroma of the pudendal vessels
Multiple sclerosis	Internal iliac atheroma
Peripheral neuropathy	Microvascular
Spinal cord trauma / damage	Venous leak
Surgery	
Abdominoperineal resection	
Cystectomy	
Perineal prostatectomy	
Rectal pull-through procedures	
Sympathectomy	
Transurethral resection of the prostate	
Urethrectomy	
Vascular surgery	

Proceed to Step 4

STEP 4: *Are There Any Clues in the Patient's History That Point to the Etiology of the Erectile Dysfunction?*

Clues in the patient's history that point to the etiology of the patient's erectile dysfunction are listed in the following table.

Historical Clue	Condition Suggested
History of priapism	Cavernosal fibrosis
Preservation of morning erection	Suggests psychogenic cause of erectile dysfunction
Absence of morning erections	Suggests organic cause of erectile dysfunction
Circumstantial erectile dysfunction: Intact erectile function with masturbation but not with interactive sex Intact erectile function with one partner but not another Intact erectile function upon awakening but not with interactive sex	Suggests psychogenic cause of erectile dysfunction
Decreased libido	Testosterone deficiency Psychogenic cause of erectile dysfunction
Rectal / bladder / prostate surgery	Surgery (neurogenic cause of erectile dysfunction)
Intact libido	Testosterone deficiency unlikely
New medication recently started	Medication-induced erectile dysfunction
Improvement in erectile function after discontinuation of suspect medication	Medication-induced erectile dysfunction
Alcohol use	Alcoholism
History of diabetes mellitus	Diabetes mellitus (vascular and/or neurogenic mechanism)
History of neurologic condition	Neurogenic cause of erectile dysfunction
Smoker	Cigarette smoke is an independent risk factor for erectile dysfunction
Marijuana, heroin, or cocaine use	Erectile dysfunction secondary to recreational drug use
Recent change in stress, marriage, loss of job, bereavement	Psychogenic cause of erectile dysfunction
Pain in calves when walking	Claudication (major vascular disease)
Polyuria Polydipsia	Diabetes mellitus
History of one of more of the following conditions: Hypertension Diabetes mellitus Hyperlipidemia Cigarette smoking	Risk factors for major vascular disease (atherosclerosis)
Decreased frequency of shaving	Hypogonadism
History of pelvic or perineal trauma	Erectile dysfunction secondary to trauma (vasculogenic or neurogenic)
Headache	Pituitary tumor

Proceed to Step 5

STEP 5: *Are There Any Clues in the Patient's Physical Examination That Point to the Etiology of the Erectile Dysfunction?*

Clues in the patient's physical examination that point to the etiology of the erectile dysfunction are listed in the following table.

Physical Examination Finding	Condition Suggested
Testicle size <4 cm in diameter	Testicular atrophy (suggests hypogonadism)
Decreased distal muscle strength Diminished reflexes in lower extremities Impaired vibration, position, and tactile sensation	Peripheral neuropathy
Diminished or absent pulses in lower extremities Cool skin temperature Loss of hair Bruits	Major vascular disease
Fibrotic penile plaques	Peyronie's disease
Absence of bulbocavernous reflex*	Suggests neurogenic cause of erectile dysfunction

One or more of the following:
  Palmar erythema
  Spider angioma
  Parotid / lacrimal gland enlargement
  Testicular atrophy
	Chronic liver disease or cirrhosis

Reduced or absent secondary sex characteristics	Hypogonadism
Gynecomastia	Hypogonadism
Tremor Warm, moist skin Tachycardia	Hyperthyroidism
Nodularity of testis	Suggests Leydig cell estrogen-secreting tumor
Dry, scaly skin Puffy face Sparse eyebrows Low-pitched and rough voice Delay in relaxation phase of deep tendon reflexes (hung-up reflex)	Hypothyroidism

*When gentle pinching of the glans penis results in contraction of the external anal sphincter, the bulbocavernous reflex is present.

If there are clues in the history and physical examination that point to the etiology of the erectile dysfunction, the clinician should tailor the work-up accordingly.

If the cause of the erectile dysfunction is not clear after a thorough history and physical examination, *Proceed to Step 6.*

STEP 6: *Does the Patient Have Medication-Induced Erectile Dysfunction?*

A thorough medication history is essential in the patient presenting with erectile dysfunction. In fact, medications are probably the most common cause of erectile dysfunction, accounting for up to 25% of cases. In addition to prescribed medications, the clinician should determine if the patient is taking any over-the-counter or herbal preparations. Medications considered to be common offenders are listed in the following box.

Medications That Commonly Cause Erectile Dysfunction	
Alcohol	Antihypertensives
α-adrenergic antagonists	Diuretics
Analgesics	Thiazide
Narcotics	Spironolactone
NSAIDs	β-blockers
Antiandrogens	Sympatholytics
5-α-reductase inhibitors	Reserpine
LH-releasing hormone agonists	Guanethidine
Cyproterone acetate	α-methyldopa
Flutamide	Clonidine
Casodex	Calcium channel blockers
Estrogens	ACE inhibitors
Anticholinergics	Hydralazine
Anticonvulsants	Antipsychotics
Phenytoin	Phenothiazines
Phenobarbital	Thioxanthines
Antidepressants	Butyrophenones
Tricyclic	Anxiolytics
Monoamine oxidase inhibitors	Benzodiazepines
Selective serotonin reuptake inhibitors	H_2-receptor blockers
Antihistamines	Cimetidine
Recreational drugs	Ranitidine
Marijuana	Lipid-lowering therapy
Nicotine	Clofibrate
Others	Niacin
	Miscellaneous
	Baclofen
	Digoxin
	Metoclopramide

Particularly useful in establishing the diagnosis is eliciting a history of erectile dysfunction that began shortly after the institution of a new medication. It is important to realize, however, that not all medication-induced erectile dysfunction begins shortly after a new medication is started. With thiazide diuretics and antidepressants, for example, the onset of the erectile dysfunction may be delayed. Resolution of the erectile dysfunction after the suspect medication is discontinued confirms the diagnosis.

If the patient's erectile dysfunction is medication-related, **Stop Here.**

If the patient's erectile dysfunction is not medication-related, **Proceed to Step 7.**

> **STEP 7:** *What Laboratory Tests Need to Be Performed in the Evaluation of Erectile Dysfunction?*

Laboratory tests useful in the evaluation of the patient with erectile dysfunction may be divided into basic and endocrinologic tests. Basic tests that should be obtained in all patients include the following:

- CBC
- Urinalysis
- BUN, creatinine
- Liver function tests
- Glucose

Abnormal glucose intolerance is identified in nearly 15% of previously healthy men who complain of erectile dysfunction. Over 40% of individuals with diabetes report erectile dysfunction.

The purpose of these basic tests is to screen for systemic disease that may be causing or contributing to the erectile dysfunction.

There is some debate as to whether all patients presenting with erectile dysfunction should have endocrinologic testing. Some argue that testing should be reserved for patients who present with signs and symptoms of an underlying endocrinopathy. There is merit to this argument because the incidence of an endocrinopathy in patients presenting with erectile dysfunction alone is low. Others, however, feel that testing is warranted in all patients in an effort to identify the minority of patients who may have a serious underlying condition such as a prolactinoma.

Although there is no universal agreement on the degree of endocrinologic testing that should be performed, most authorities agree that, at a minimum, clinicians should obtain the following tests:

- Testosterone Level

  A low testosterone level supports the diagnosis of hypogonadism. Once the presence of hypogonadism has been established, it is necessary to determine FSH and LH levels to differentiate primary from secondary hypogonadism. Elevated FSH and LH levels indicate the presence of primary hypogonadism (testicular abnormality). Low to normal FSH and LH levels, however, suggest hypothalamic-pituitary dysfunction or secondary hypogonadism.

- Prolactin Level

  An elevated prolactin level should prompt consideration of the causes of hyperprolactinemia. In particular, the clinician should perform imaging of the hypothalamic-pituitary region to exclude a mass lesion.

Erectile dysfunction can occur in both hypothyroidism and hyperthyroidism. In general, signs and symptoms of thyroid hormone deficiency or excess are present. Erectile dysfunction alone would be an unusual presentation of thyroid disease. As such, many do not routinely obtain thyroid function tests unless the clinical presentation is suggestive of hyperthyroidism or hypothyroidism. Some, however, obtain these tests routinely, irrespective of the clinical presentation.

If the laboratory testing establishes the etiology of the erectile dysfunction, *Stop Here.*

If the laboratory testing does not establish the etiology of the erectile dysfunction, *Proceed to Step 8.*

STEP 8: *Does the Patient Have a Psychogenic Cause of the Erectile Dysfunction?*

Psychogenic erectile dysfunction should be considered in any of the following situations:

- The history, physical examination, and laboratory data do not elucidate an organic etiology of the erectile dysfunction

- An organic etiology is identified but treatment or correction of the etiology does not improve erectile function

  Some individuals have considerable anxiety about their sexual performance. This may be a primary problem or alternatively, may stem from the stress and frustration that accompanies organic erectile dysfunction.

  In patients with both organic and psychogenic erectile dysfunction, successful treatment of the organic cause may not lead to an improvement of the sexual function if the clinician fails to recognize that psychogenic factors are also contributing. In these cases, there is often intense preoccupation about performing successfully. These patients are so concerned about their performance that they lose the ability to focus on the sexual stimuli that is so integral to maintaining their arousal. Erectile dysfunction then ensues.

  The most common cause of psychogenic erectile dysfunction is excessive life stressors. Some examples include loss of a family member or job.

Features in the patient's clinical presentation that suggest a psychogenic cause of the erectile dysfunction are listed in the following box.

Clinical Features Suggestive of Psychogenic Cause of Erectile Dysfunction
Sudden, complete loss of function
Onset at young age
Intact erectile function with one partner but not another
Maintenance of erections upon awakening or with masturbation
Circumstantial (erectile dysfunction in some settings while normal erectile function in other settings)
Previous history of erectile dysfunction with spontaneous improvement
Excessive life stressors
Mental status findings consistent with depression, anxiety disorder, or psychosis

Psychogenic erectile dysfunction is often apparent from the patient's clinical presentation. When identified, in some cases, brief counseling is all that is needed to restore erectile function. When brief counseling is not effective or there is uncertainty regarding the presence of psychogenic erectile dysfunction, the clinician may consider performing nocturnal penile tumescence studies to verify the presence of psychogenic erectile dysfunction. During sleep, the psychological factors that weigh so heavily on individuals with psychogenic erectile dysfunction are not operative, allowing the patient to have the nocturnal erections that normally accompany REM sleep. In contrast, organic erectile dysfunction is characterized by the persistence of erectile dysfunction throughout sleep. Findings consistent with an organic etiology should prompt the clinician to search for the underlying cause.

In patients who have psychogenic erectile dysfunction, brief counseling may be all that is necessary. When brief counseling fails to improve erectile function, the clinician should send the patient to a sex therapist for further treatment.

REFERENCES

Dinsmore W and Evans C, "ABC of Sexual Health: Erectile Dysfunction," *BMJ*, 1999, 318(7180):387-90.

Jordan GH, "Erectile Function and Dysfunction," *Postgrad Med*, 1999, 105(2):131-4, 137-8, 143-4.

Kaiser FE, "Erectile Dysfunction in the Aging Man," *Med Clin North Am*, 1999, 83(5):1267-78.

Keene LC and Davies PH, "Drug-Related Erectile Dysfunction," *Adverse Drug React Toxicol Rev*, 1999, 18(1):5-24.

Korenman SG, "New Insights into Erectile Dysfunction: A Practical Approach," *Am J Med*, 1998, 105(2):135-44.

Lue TF, "Erectile Dysfunction," *N Engl J Med*, 2000, 342(24):1802-13.

Miller TA, "Diagnostic Evaluation of Erectile Dysfunction," *Am Fam Phys*, 2000, 61(1):95-104, 109-10.

Morgentaler A, "Male Impotence," *Lancet*, 1999, 354(9191):1713-8.

Wierman ME, "Advances in the Diagnosis and Management of Impotence," *Dis Mon*, 1999, 45(1):1-20 (review).

Wierman ME, "Advances in the Diagnosis and Management of Impotence," *Adv Intern Med*, 1999, 44:1-17 (review).

ERECTILE DYSFUNCTION

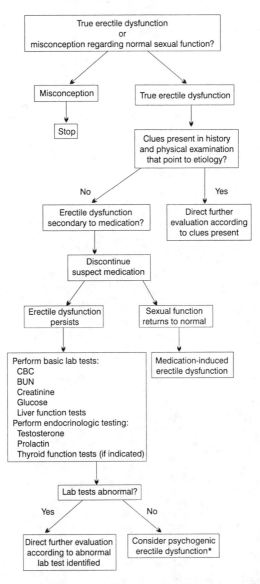

True erectile dysfunction
or
misconception regarding normal sexual function?

Misconception → Stop

True erectile dysfunction

Clues present in history and physical examination that point to etiology?

No → Erectile dysfunction secondary to medication?

Yes → Direct further evaluation according to clues present

Discontinue suspect medication

Erectile dysfunction persists

Sexual function returns to normal → Medication-induced erectile dysfunction

Perform basic lab tests:
  CBC
  BUN
  Creatinine
  Glucose
  Liver function tests
Perform endocrinologic testing:
  Testosterone
  Prolactin
  Thyroid function tests (if indicated)

Lab tests abnormal?

Yes → Direct further evaluation according to abnormal lab test identified

No → Consider psychogenic erectile dysfunction*

*Psychogenic causes of erectile dysfunction should also be considered when an organic etiology is identified but treatment or correction of the etiology does not restore sexual function.

FATIGUE

STEP 1: *How Common is Fatigue?*

Fatigue is a commonly encountered complaint in the primary care setting. In fact, in the United States alone, fatigue accounts for approximately 10 million visits a year. In community-based surveys, nearly 50% of the population, if asked, report fatigue.

Not all patients with fatigue present for medical attention. Many of these patients do not seek medical care because the fatigue is transient, perhaps caused by a recent viral illness, inadequate sleep, or overwork. In these cases, then, the affected individual is able to recognize the cause of the fatigue and steps taken to correct the cause lead to the resolution of the symptom.

Patients do, however, get concerned when fatigue is persistent or not easily explained. In these situations, there is worry that the fatigue may be due to a serious underlying condition.

Proceed to Step 2

STEP 2: *What Does the Patient Mean by the Term "Fatigue"?*

Prior to embarking on an evaluation for fatigue, the clinician should ascertain just what the patient means by the term "fatigue." Fatigue means different things to different people. Fatigue is not easily defined. There is no universally accepted definition of this commonly encountered complaint. Popular definitions include the following:

- Sensation of exhaustion during or after normal activities
- Not enough energy to initiate an activity

The clinician should encourage the patient to describe the sensation. When asked to describe the sensation, patients may offer any of the terms listed in the following box.

What the Patient Might Mean By "Fatigue"	
Boredom	Reduced output or performance
Distaste for work	Sleepiness
Dyspnea with exertion	Tiredness
Exhaustion	Unwillingness to work
Lack of energy	Weakness
Lassitude	Weariness
Listlessness	

Adapted from Greene WL, *Clinical Medicine*, 2nd ed, Fincher RM, Johnson WP, Kaufmann L, et al (eds), St Louis, MO: Mosby, 1995, 183.

In particular, it is important to separate patients with fatigue from those who are having weakness, dyspnea on exertion, and sleepiness.

Sleepiness

Sometimes patients use the word "fatigue" to refer to excessive daytime sleepiness. In fact, nearly 5% of the population has difficulty with excessive daytime sleepiness. In some of these cases, patients do not volunteer that they are sleepy during the day because they may not realize that their symptoms are sleep-related. Excessive daytime sleepiness may manifest with fatigue, sleepiness, decreased motivation, poor concentration, forgetfulness, irritability, or depression. If a history of excessive daytime sleepiness is elicited in the patient complaining of fatigue, the clinician should determine if the patient has a primary sleep disorder. Primary sleep disorders include sleep apnea, narcolepsy, nocturnal myoclonus, and cataplexy.

Weakness

Weakness refers to a reduction in muscle strength. True weakness is said to be present when a reduction in muscle strength is demonstrated by physical examination. This is to be contrasted with the complaint of weakness that often accompanies many medical conditions such as congestive heart failure, renal insufficiency, and anemia. In these conditions, objective assessment of muscle strength will usually reveal that the patient has normal strength. In these cases, weakness can be considered synonymous with fatigue. It is important to differentiate true weakness from fatigue because the demonstration of true weakness warrants a thorough evaluation searching for a neurologic or muscular cause of the patient's complaint.

Dyspnea With Exertion

Some patients will describe fatigue with exertion. While fatigue is often exertional, it is important to ensure that the patient is not referring to shortness of breath with exertion. It is important to differentiate between the two because the approach to the patient with dyspnea with exertion differs from that of fatigue.

If the fatigue that the patient reports really refers to sleepiness, dyspnea with exertion, or true weakness, **Stop Here.**

If the patient truly has fatigue, **Proceed to Step 3.**

STEP 3: *Does the Patient Have Physiologic Fatigue?*

Normal individuals may develop fatigue. Most often, fatigue develops in these individuals because of one or more of the following factors:

- Inadequate sleep
- Not enough rest
- Overactivity
- Poor physical conditioning
- Stress
- Change in diet

When one or more of the above factors are the cause of the patient's fatigue, the patient is said to have physiologic fatigue. Physiologic fatigue is easily recognized if the clinician takes time to explore the above factors. In many cases, patients are aware of the habits that are predisposing them to the fatigue. Some groups that are prone to developing physiologic fatigue include the following:

- Pregnant women
- New parents
- Individuals working evening or night hours
- Shift work that rotates
- Students
- Healthcare professionals

Correction of the cause leads to a rapid improvement in the patient's fatigue. Further evaluation is warranted, however, when the fatigue is persistent despite attempts to correct the suspected cause or if the fatigue is of sufficient severity to impair the patient's ability to perform normal activities.

If the patient's physiologic fatigue resolves with correction of the etiology, *Stop Here.*

If the patient's fatigue does not resolve with correction of the cause or if it is of sufficient severity to impair the patient's ability to perform normal activities, *Proceed to Step 4.*

STEP 4: *What are the Causes of Fatigue?*

Physiologic causes of fatigue are considered in the preceding step. In this step, other causes of fatigue will be considered, particularly those that should be considered when the fatigue is persistent or of sufficient severity that it impacts upon the patient's abilities to perform normal activities. The causes of fatigue are listed in the following box.

Causes of Fatigue	
Anemia	Infection
Chronic fatigue syndrome	Brucellosis
Chronic liver disease / cirrhosis	Endocarditis
Chronic obstructive pulmonary disease	Hepatitis
Chronic renal failure	HIV / AIDS
Congestive heart failure	Mononucleosis
Connective tissue diseases	Osteomyelitis
Rheumatoid arthritis	Pharyngitis
SLE	Toxoplasmosis
Endocrine / Metabolic disorders	Tuberculosis
Adrenal insufficiency	Urinary tract infection
Diabetes mellitus	Viral illness
Electrolyte disorders	Malignancy
Hyperthyroidism	Medications / Toxins
Hypoglycemia	Alcohol
Hypothyroidism	Drug abuse
Obesity	Poisons
Starvation or dieting	Side effect of medication
	Psychosocial conditions
	Adjustment reaction
	Anxiety disorders
	Depression
	Occupational stress / professional burnout
	Situational life stresses

Proceed to Step 5

> ## STEP 5: Which Causes of Fatigue Previously Listed are More Common?

Studies have been performed examining the frequencies of the various causes of fatigue. The results of two such studies are shown in the following table.

Cause	280 Patients	54 Patients
Psychogenic disorder	142	10
Organic disorder	109	25
Endocrine	24	12
Cardiovascular	23	0
Respiratory	21	2
Hematologic	19	1
Cancer	7	0
Gastrointestinal (usually hepatic)	6	2
Renal	5	0
Obesity	3	0
Arthritic	2	3
Malnutrition	1	0
Medication side effect	0	4
Miscellaneous	0	5
Undetermined	27	18

Adapted from Greene WL, *Clinical Medicine*, 2nd ed, Fincher RM, Johnson WP, Kaufmann L, et al (eds), St Louis, MO: Mosby, 1995, 183.

Proceed to Step 6

> ## STEP 6: Are There Any Clues in the Patient's Clinical Presentation That Point to the Etiology of the Fatigue?

Although psychogenic causes account for 50% to 60% of fatigue cases, it is important to exclude organic etiologies. Fatigue that is due to a systemic illness often has the features listed in the following box.

Clinical Features of "Fatigue" Due to Systemic Illness
Absent on arising in the morning
Develops as the day progresses
Worsens with activities
Relieved by resting
Progressively worsens if underlying disease is not treated

The key to identifying the cause of the fatigue is a thorough history and physical examination. In most cases, other symptoms and signs are present when the fatigue is due to a systemic illness. For example, fatigue is not uncommon in patients with congestive heart failure. When present, however, it is usually accompanied by shortness of breath or leg swelling. A thorough review of systems is necessary, then, to identify localizing symptoms and signs that would guide further evaluation.

If the history and physical examination provide clues to the etiology of the fatigue, the approach should be tailored to the signs and symptoms present, **Stop Here.**

If the history and physical examination do not provide clues to the etiology of the fatigue, **Proceed to Step 7.**

STEP 7: What Laboratory Tests are Helpful in the Evaluation of the Patient With Fatigue?

If there are any historical or physical examination features pointing to a particular etiology, the clinician should perform appropriate testing to confirm the diagnosis. In the absence of clues in the history and physical examination, it is reasonable to obtain the following tests:

- BUN, creatinine
- CBC
- Electrolytes
- ESR
- Glucose
- Liver function tests
- TSH
- Urinalysis

Note: An elevated TSH but normal free T_4 is consistent with subclinical hypothyroidism. Thyroid hormone replacement has not consistently improved fatigue in these patients.

Other tests including CXR, EKG, and PPD may be indicated depending upon the patient's clinical presentation. A HIV test should be considered if risk factors can be identified in the patient's history.

When there are no clues in the patient's clinical presentation pointing to the etiology of the fatigue, the clinician should realize that the yield of the above laboratory tests is low. In a minority of cases, however, the lab test results may uncover the etiology of the fatigue.

If the etiology of the fatigue has been identified, **Stop Here.**

If the etiology of the fatigue has not been identified, **Proceed to Step 8.**

STEP 8: Is the Fatigue Medication-Induced?

Medications are a common cause of fatigue. In some cases, the fatigue is due directly to the medication. In other cases, the medication may interfere with normal sleep patterns. Common offending medications are listed in the following box.

Medications Commonly Causing Fatigue
Analgesics
Narcotics
NSAIDs
Antibiotics
Tetracycline
Antihistamines
Antihypertensive agents
β-blockers
Centrally-acting
Colchicine
Corticosteroids
Oral contraceptives
Psychotropic
Antidepressants
Sedatives and hypnotics
Tranquilizers

It is important to realize, however, that any medication could potentially be the cause of the fatigue. When fatigue develops shortly after the introduction of a new medication, the clinician should suspect medication-induced fatigue. This is irrespective of whether the medication is a common offender. Withdrawal of the medication followed by resolution of the fatigue supports the diagnosis.

It is important to realize that medications that do not commonly cause fatigue may do so if drug levels rise above therapeutic levels. Digoxin toxicity is an example. When patients are on medications that are monitored periodically by drug levels, it is reasonable to obtain these levels when a patient presents with fatigue.

Illicit drug use is also a cause of fatigue. Herein lies the importance of a thorough substance abuse history. In addition, both alcohol use and withdrawal may be associated with fatigue.

If the patient has medication-induced fatigue, *Stop Here.*

If the patient does not have medication-induced fatigue, *Proceed to Step 9.*

STEP 9: *Does the Patient Have Malignancy?*

When the cause of the fatigue is not apparent, of concern to both patients and clinicians alike is the possibility of malignancy. While it is true that fatigue is common in patients with malignancy, it is usually present with advanced cancer. In these cases, fatigue is usually accompanied by signs and symptoms of the underlying neoplasm. Isolated fatigue is a very uncommon initial presentation of an occult malignancy. Therefore, an extensive evaluation searching for malignancy is not warranted. Rather the clinician should take this opportunity to perform age-specific screening tests for cancer.

If the patient has a malignancy, *Stop Here.*

If the patient does not have malignancy, *Proceed to Step 10.*

STEP 10: *Does the Patient Have Psychogenic Fatigue?*

Psychogenic causes of fatigue are quite common, accounting for over 50% of cases. Features in the patient's clinical presentation that suggest the presence of psychogenic fatigue are listed in the following box.

Features that Suggest the Fatigue is Psychogenic
Present all the time
Present on awakening
Often improves later in the day
Fluctuates with changes in mood or stress
Symptoms of depression, anxiety, or somatization disorder may be present

Of the psychogenic causes of fatigue, depression is the most common. Psychologic screening tests are available to help the clinician in the diagnosis of these psychogenic causes of fatigue.

The clinician should also consider chronic fatigue syndrome as the cause of the patient's fatigue. This is a syndrome that has predilection for young women. It is characterized by debilitating fatigue often in conjunction with other symptoms, some of which may include sore throat, muscle aches, joint pain, headaches, and memory loss. There is an increased prevalence of psychiatric illness in patients with chronic fatigue syndrome.

Criteria for the diagnosis of the chronic fatigue syndrome have been proposed by the Centers for Disease Control and Prevention. These criteria are listed in the following box.

Revised CDC Criteria for Chronic Fatigue Syndrome
A case of chronic fatigue syndrome is defined by the presence of:
1. Clinically evaluated, unexplained, persistent or relapsing fatigue that is of new or definite onset; is not the result of ongoing exertion; is not alleviated by rest; and results in substantial reduction of previous levels of occupational, educational, social, or personal activities; and
2. Four or more of the following symptoms that persist or recur during six or more consecutive months of illness and that do not predate the fatigue:
A. Self-reported impairment in short-term memory or concentration
B. Sore throat
C. Tender cervical or axillary nodes
D. Muscle pain
E. Multijoint pain without redness or swelling
F. Headaches of a new pattern or severity
G. Unrefreshing sleep
H. Postexertional malaise lasting ≥ 24 hours

Adapted from *Harrison's Principles of Internal Medicine*, 14th ed, Fauci AS, Braunwald E, Isselbacher KJ, et al (eds), New York, NY: McGraw-Hill: 1998, 2484; also adapted from Fukuda K, Straus SE, Hickie I, et al, "The Chronic Fatigue Syndrome: A Comprehensive Approach to its Definition and Study," International Chronic Fatigue Syndrome Study Group, *Ann Intern Med*, 1994, 121(12):953-9.

If the patient has a psychogenic cause of the fatigue, *Stop Here.*

If the patient does not have a psychogenic cause of the fatigue, *Proceed to Step 11.*

> STEP 11: *What are Considerations in the Fatigued Patient Who Has No Identifiable Organic or Psychogenic Cause?*

Despite a thorough evaluation, no diagnosis can be established in up to 30% of patients with fatigue. It is important to follow these patients over time because some may develop signs and symptoms of an organic disorder. In others, a psychogenic cause may become more apparent with the passage of time. When no medical or psychiatric cause can be identified, the patient should be considered to have idiopathic chronic fatigue.

REFERENCES

Ang DC and Calabrese LH, "A Common-Sense Approach to Chronic Fatigue in Primary Care," *Cleve Clin J Med*, 1999, 66(6):343-50, 352 (review).

Chew WM and Birnbaumer DM, "Evaluation of the Elderly Patient With Weakness: An Evidence Based Approach," *Emerg Med Clin North Am*, 1999, 17(1):265-78 (review).

Epstein KR, "The Chronically Fatigued Patient," *Med Clin North Am*, 1995, 79(2):315-27 (review).

Fukuda K, Straus SE, Hickie I, et al, "The Chronic Fatigue Syndrome: A Comprehensive Approach to its Definition and Study," International Chronic Fatigue Syndrome Study Group, *Ann Intern Med*, 1994, 121(12):953-9.

Greene HL, *Clinical Medicine*, 2nd ed, Fincher RM, Johnson WP, Kaufmann L, et al (eds), St Louis, MO: Mosby, 1995, 183.

Harrison's Principles of Internal Medicine, 14th ed, Fauci AS, Braunwald E, Isselbacher KJ, et al (eds), New York, NY: McGraw-Hill: 1998, 2484.

Katon WJ and Walker EA, "Medically Unexplained Symptoms in Primary Care," *J Clin Psychiatry*, 1998, 59(Suppl 20):15-21 (review).

Llewelyn MB, "Assessing the Fatigued Patient," *Br J Hosp Med*, 1996, 55(3):125-9 (review).

Portenoy RK and Itri LM, "Cancer-Related Fatigue: Guidelines for Evaluation and Management," *Oncologist*, 1999, 4(1):1-10 (review).

Ruffin MT and Cohen M, "Evaluation and Management of Fatigue," *Am Fam Phys*, 1994, 50(3):625-34 (review).

FATIGUE

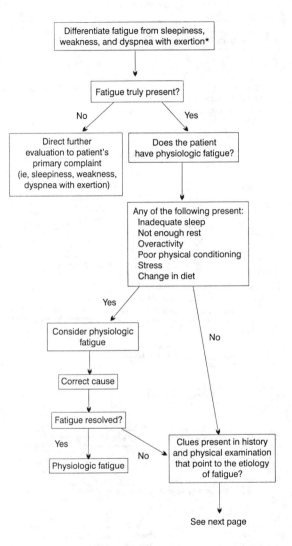

*Weakness differs from fatigue in that the former is characterized by a reduction in muscle strength as demonstrated by the physical exam.

FATIGUE
(continued)

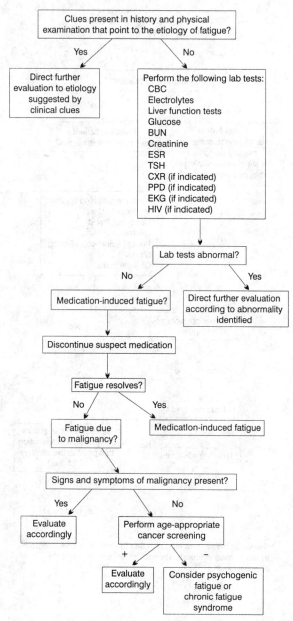

GENITAL ULCER

STEP 1: *What are the Causes of Genital Ulcer?*

While infection is a major consideration in the patient presenting with genital ulcer, the clinician should realize that there are noninfectious conditions that may give rise to this complaint. The causes of genital ulcer are listed in the following box.

Causes of Genital Ulcer	
Infectious	**Noninfectious**
Amebiasis	Aphthous ulcers
Candidiasis	Behcet's syndrome
Chancroid	Fixed drug eruption
Donovanosis	Inflammatory bowel disease
Herpes simplex virus	Malignancy
Histoplasmosis	Reiter's syndrome
Lymphogranuloma venereum	Trauma
Mycobacterial	
Syphilis	
Tularemia	

Proceed to Step 2

STEP 2: *Are There Any Clues in the Patient's History That Point to the Etiology of the Genital Ulcer?*

The history can offer clues that point to the etiology of the patient's genital ulcer.

Historical Clue	Condition Suggested
Exposure to multiple sexual partners	Sexually transmitted disease
Sexual partner having genital symptoms	Sexually transmitted disease
Recent treatment of sexually transmitted disease in sexual partner	Sexually transmitted disease
Vigorous coitus or masturbation Biting during sex	Trauma
Recent travel	Consider less common infectious conditions such as LGV and donovanosis (in addition to common causes)*
Recent immigrant	Consider less common infectious conditions such as LGV and donovanosis (in addition to common causes)*

(Continued)

(continued)

Historical Clue	Condition Suggested
Recent use of tetracycline or other drug	Fixed drug eruption
Prodrome of local paresthesia prior to ulcer	Recurrent genital herpes (not in primary infection)
History of "zipper accident"	Trauma
History of mental disorder	Self-induced ulcer
Recent application of topical agents such as cosmetics, lubricants, aphrodisiacs, and chemicals used in contraceptives	Contact dermatitis
In association with urethritis, conjunctivitis, and arthritis	Reiter's syndrome

*Common infectious causes of genital ulcer include genital herpes, syphilis, and chancroid.

Proceed to Step 3

STEP 3: *Does the Patient Have a Sexually Transmitted Disease?*

Although Step 1 described both the infectious and noninfectious causes of genital ulcer, this approach will begin with consideration of the infectious causes. It is essential to identify the patient with genital ulcer disease due to a sexually transmitted disease. By establishing the appropriate diagnosis, treatment can then be offered not only to the patient but also to sexual partners (if infected), thus impacting upon the spread of the disease.

Studies have shown that genital ulcer patients who have HIV transmit HIV more readily when a genital ulcer is present. Also, the presence of a genital ulcer places an individual at higher risk of acquiring HIV during sexual contact.

Between 5% and 10% of visits to STD clinics involve genital ulceration. The cause of genital ulceration is clearly dependent on geographic location. In the United States, the most common infectious causes of genital ulceration, in descending order of frequency, are herpes simplex virus, syphilis, and chancroid.

Lymphogranuloma venereum and donovanosis should be more of a consideration outside of the United States, particularly in developing countries. LGV is common in Africa and the Far East. Endemic areas for donovanosis include India, West Indes, Africa, South America, and Papua New Guinea. In the patient presenting in the United States, a history of foreign travel should prompt consideration of these two possibilities. Genital ulceration in the immigrant from an area endemic for LGV and donovanosis also warrants consideration of these infections.

Proceed to Step 4

> **STEP 4:** *What is the Clinical Presentation of the Common Infectious Causes of Genital Ulcer?*

In this step, the clinical presentation of the common infectious causes of genital ulcer will be considered.

Genital Herpes

Although both herpes simplex virus type I and II can cause genital ulceration, type II is more commonly encountered. The presentation of genital herpes differs to some extent depending on whether the infection is primary or recurrent. Primary infection is characterized by the presence of systemic symptoms including fever, headache, dysuria, anorexia, myalgias, and malaise. Extragenital manifestations of primary HSV infection include aseptic meningitis and urinary bladder retention, occurring in 8% and 2% of patients, respectively. Manifestations of genital herpes typically develop 2-20 days after exposure with a mean of six days.

At the time of presentation, the lesions of genital herpes may be present in various stages. Vesicles, pustules, and erythematous ulcers may be appreciated. Particularly suggestive of herpes simplex viral infection is the finding of multiple vesicular lesions on an erythematous base. Spontaneous rupture of these vesicles result in the formation of painful ulcerations. Tender inguinal lymphadenopathy often accompanies the lesions of genital herpes (only in primary infection). The lesions usually resolve within two weeks.

Recurrent genital herpes simplex virus infection occurs in 50% and 75% of HSV type 1 and II infection, respectively. Many report a prodrome of burning, itching, or tingling prior to the development of the genital lesions. Recurrent infection is generally less severe, often healing in a shorter period of time. Recurrent infection also tends to be more localized. Systemic manifestations are not a feature of recurrent genital herpes infection.

Syphilis

Although multiple ulcers (as many as 50% of cases) may occur in primary syphilis, most often, a single lesion is present. After an incubation period ranging from 9-90 days (mean: 21 days), the lesion usually starts as a painless papule, eroding to form an ulcer soon thereafter. The base is typically smooth, clean, and indurated. The borders of the lesion are raised and firm (well-defined). This lesion, known as a chancre, heals in 3-6 weeks. Occasionally, the lesion may take up to 12 weeks to resolve. Nontender inguinal lymphadenopathy, that is often bilateral, frequently accompanies the chancre.

Three to eight weeks later, untreated patients may develop signs and symptoms of secondary syphilis. In rare cases, the patient may present with the manifestations of secondary syphilis while the chancre is still present. The classic manifestations of secondary syphilis include rash which may be macular, maculopapular, papular, or pustular. Approximately 75% of patients develop constitutional symptoms such as anorexia, low-grade fever, malaise, sore throat, weight loss, and arthralgia. In some, generalized lymphadenopathy may be noted.

Chancroid

Genital infection due to *H. ducreyi*, also known as chancroid, is less common in the United States than syphilis and genital herpes. Nonetheless, major outbreaks of chancroid have been reported, usually occurring in nonwhite, uncircumcised men. Many authorities feel that chancroid is an under-reported disease, mainly because diagnostic tests are not widely available.

After an incubation period of 4-7 days, the infection begins with a tender papule surrounded by erythema. Several days later, a pustule forms only to rupture soon thereafter, resulting in the formation of an ulcer. In some cases, multiple ulcers are present. The lesion is typically described as nonindurated, ragged, painful, and undermined. Often covered by a gray or yellow purulent exudate, the base of the ulcer bleeds readily if manipulated. The size of the ulcers vary from 1-20 mm.

Tender lymphadenopathy, usually unilateral, often accompanies the genital ulcer (50%). The overlying skin is often erythematous. If left untreated, suppuration may result in abscess (bubo) formation. Rupture of the abscess may occur spontaneously, resulting in the development of draining sinuses. Without treatment, the genital ulcers and inguinal abscesses may persist for months or even years.

Lymphogranuloma Venereum

The etiologic agent of lymphogranuloma venereum is *Chlamydia trachomatis*. Infection is caused by the L1, L2, and L3 serovars of the organism. The illness can be considered to occur in three stages. It is in the first stage of the illness that a genital ulcer may be noted.

Some 3-30 days after exposure, a small papule or ulcer may develop, usually in the genital area. In many cases, the lesion goes unnoticed. Days to weeks later, infected patients develop inguinal lymphadenopathy (second stage), the major manifestation of the illness. The lymphadenopathy is typically unilateral, discrete, and tender. Overlying erythema is not uncommon. Both superficial and deep inguinal nodes are involved, sometimes giving rise to the characteristic "groove sign."

The matted and enlarged lymph nodes may coalesce and suppurate, resulting in the formation of buboes. The lymphadenopathy is often accompanied by systemic manifestations including fever, headache, and myalgias.

Donovanosis

Donovanosis, also known as granuloma inguinale, is caused by *Calymmatobacterium granulomatis*. Less than 100 cases of donovanosis are described yearly in the United States. After an incubation period of 8-80 days, a small painless papule or indurated nodule develops. Soon thereafter, ulcers may be noted which give way to heaped-up areas of beefy red granulation tissue. Lymphadenopathy is unusual. However, extension of the granulomatous process into the inguinal area may result in pseudobubo formation.

Proceed to Step 5

> **STEP 5:** *Are There Any Clues in the Patient's Physical Examination That Point to the Etiology of the Genital Ulcer?*

The morphologic appearance of the genital ulcer can provide clues to the etiology. In the following table, only the three most common infectious causes of genital ulceration are compared.

	Syphilis	Genital Herpes	Chancroid
Agent	*Treponema pallidum*	Herpes simplex virus type II	*H. ducreyi*
Incubation Period	10-90 days	Up to 1 week	Up to 21 days
Initial Lesion	Papule	Vesicle	Papule
Number of Ulcers	Single (60%) or multiple	Single or multiple (usually)	Single or multiple (usually 1-3)
Base	Clean (red and smooth)	Clean (red and smooth)	Yellow-gray exudate (rough and uneven)
Pain	No	Yes	Yes
Induration	Yes	No	No
Adenopathy	Yes Nontender Unilateral or bilateral	Yes (but only in primary infection) Usually bilateral Tender	Yes Tender, fluctuant Unilateral (rarely bilateral) Overlying erythema
Duration	Up to 6 weeks	2-3 weeks (often recurrent)	Up to 6 weeks

Unfortunately, none of the features in the above table allows the clinician to definitively identify the etiologic organism. In many cases of genital ulcer disease, the lesion does not present as described classically in textbooks. There are many factors which may play a role in altering the appearance of the genital ulcer. These factors include the following:

- Delay in seeking care

- Self-treatment with topical and oral agents (including antibiotics)

- HIV infection

- Mixed infection

- Secondary bacterial infection

Even in the absence of these factors, the clinical presentation of genital ulcerations often does not fit into what is considered "classic." In studies that have examined the utility of the clinical examination, the sensitivity has not been found to exceed 50%. A recent study assessed the sensitivity and specificity of the so-called "classic" physical examination findings in the diagnosis of syphilis, genital herpes, and chancroid. The findings of this study are listed in the following table.

	Classic Physical Examination Findings	Sensitivity (%)	Specificity (%)
Syphilis	Painless, indurated clean-based ulcer	31	98
Genital Herpes	Multiple, shallow, tender ulcers	35	94
Chancroid	Deep, undermined, purulent ulcer	34	94

As a result, the key to establishing the etiology is laboratory confirmation.

Proceed to Step 6

STEP 6: *What Laboratory Tests are Available to Establish the Diagnosis?*

Laboratory testing can establish the etiology of genital ulcer in patients with a sexually transmitted disease. Appropriate laboratory testing, however, is not always available. Quite often, the clinician must offer the patient what is termed "syndromic management." With syndromic management, the clinician may prescribe therapy for more than one type of infection. This is often necessary because either the laboratory test results have not returned at the time of the visit or the appropriate testing is not available.

Which tests to obtain is largely a reflection of the geographic location and the clinician's suspicion for the various infectious causes of genital ulceration. In industrialized countries, major causes of genital ulcers are genital herpes and syphilis. In these patients, the clinician should obtain the following tests:

- Serologic test for syphilis
- Darkfield microscopy or direct immunofluorescence staining of genital ulcer material for *T. pallidum*
- Culture for herpes simplex virus or detection of HSV antigen with ELISA or direct immunofluorescence tests

These, of course, are not rigid rules and should be modified on the basis of the patient's presentation and the availability of laboratory tests. Chancroid deserves consideration in some cases as do LGV and donovanosis, especially if a history of recent travel is elicited.

In developing countries, the less common causes of ulceration in industrialized countries are more commonly encountered. As such, testing for *H. ducreyi*, LGV, and donovanosis should be considered, if available. Of course, testing for syphilis and genital herpes are also important considerations in these parts of the world.

The laboratory tests available in the diagnosis of these sexually transmitted diseases are discussed below.

Genital Herpes

Viral isolation remains a widely used method in establishing the definitive diagnosis of genital herpes infection. However, viral culture may be negative in up to 50% of recurrent infection. Reasons for a negative culture include the following:

- Absence of viral shedding (average duration of viral shedding is 4 days)
- Type of genital lesion present (yield higher from vesicles than erosions or crusts)
- Errors in preparation/processing

Other tests available to establish the diagnosis include the following:

- HSV DNA detection by PCR
- HSV antigen detection by immunoperoxidase or immunofluorescence techniques
- Tzanck preparation revealing the characteristic multinucleated giant cells

    A Tzanck smear is prepared by staining a smear from a fresh vesicle with either Wright's or Giemsa stain. Microscopy is then performed looking for multinucleated giant cells. Of note, a positive Tzanck smear does not allow the clinician to differentiate HSV from VZV. Since VZV typically does not cause genital ulceration, this is usually not clinically significant. The utility of the Tzanck smear is dependent on the presence or absence of intact vesicles. In the absence of vesicles, the sensitivity is lower. Identification of multinucleated giant cells also requires considerable experience.

- HSV serology

    In general, a rise in antibody titer is only found in patients with primary genital herpes infection.

Syphilis

Testing available in the diagnosis of syphilis includes the following:

- Darkfield microscopy or direct immunofluorescence staining of the genital ulcer material for *T. pallidum*

    The spirochetal organisms causing syphilis may be directly visualized using darkfield microscopy. Because serologic tests are not always positive in early syphilis, darkfield microscopy is essential. The utility of the microscopy depends not only on the skill of the examiner but also the adequacy of specimen preparation. The sensitivity varies between 70% and 95% depending on the skill of the examiner. Because darkfield microscopy has some limitations in the diagnosis of syphilis, the clinician may elect to perform direct immunofluorescence staining of ulcer material.

- Serological testing for syphilis

    The diagnosis of primary syphilis can be verified serologically. Serologic tests used in the diagnosis of syphilis can be divided into nontreponemal and treponemal tests. Nontreponemal tests include VDRL and RPR while FTA-ABS and MHA-TP are treponemal tests. One of the nontreponemal tests should be obtained initially. It is important to realize that these tests have a sensitivity of about 80% in the patient with primary syphilis. A positive test result should be followed by one of the treponemal tests to ensure that the result is not a false-positive. The clinician may elect to repeat the nontreponemal test after a few weeks in those having a negative result to detect the patient who initially presents before a serologic response can be detected. Quantitative RPR or VDRL levels should also be obtained. This will serve as a baseline to assess the response to therapy, should the patient have syphilis.

Chancroid

Microscopic examination has poor sensitivity and specificity in the diagnosis of chancroid because genital ulcers not due to *H. ducreyi* are often colonized with gram-negative rods that closely resemble *H. ducreyi*. Definitive diagnosis requires culture. Material obtained from the base of the ulceration may be sent for *H. ducreyi* culture which has a sensitivity of approximately 80%. Culture of a bubo aspirate has a sensitivity of about 50%.

The diagnosis of chancroid can be a difficult one, however, since most STD clinics in the United States do not have the capability of performing culture for *H. ducreyi*. In those that do, experience in culturing the organism is lacking, impacting upon the usefulness of the culture. Because of these limitations, treatment for chancroid is often administered when a patient presents with genital ulcer disease compatible with chancroid. The CDC has proposed criteria for the diagnosis of chancroid. The diagnosis is probable if the following criteria are met:

- Clinical findings compatible with chancroid
- Negative darkfield microscopy
- Negative serologic test for syphilis
- Negative culture for herpes simplex virus or clinical presentation not typical of genital herpes

LGV

Culture may be performed to confirm the diagnosis of LGV. Cultures of the ulcer may be revealing. However, rarely is the ulcer cultured because, in most cases, the lesion goes unnoticed. False-positive results may occur if non-LGV strains of *C. trachomatis* contaminate the ulceration. This may occur in patients who have concomitant cervical infection or nongonococcal urethritis. Bubo aspiration for culture has low yield in establishing the diagnosis.

The most widely used serologic test in the diagnosis of LGV is the complement fixation test. A single titer equal to or exceeding 1:64 is considered diagnostic. Rising titers are also supportive of infection.

Donovanosis

The etiologic agent of donovanosis, *C. granulomatis*, cannot be cultured. As a result, establishing the diagnosis requires direct visualization of the organism within biopsy specimens. Specimens should be examined for the characteristic "Donovan bodies" which represent the bacillary organisms within histiocytes. The demonstration of intracytoplasmic encapsulated Donovan bodies within mononuclear cells in Giemsa- or Wright-stained specimens establishes the diagnosis of donovanosis.

The following table summarizes the laboratory tests available in the diagnosis of the infectious causes of genital ulcer.

	Syphilis	Genital Herpes	Chancroid	LGV	Donovanosis
Microscopy	Darkfield or indirect immuno-fluorescence	Antigen detection	Gram-staining has low sensitivity and specificity	Not available	Giemsa- or Wright-stained tissue smears and sections
Culture	Not available except by rabbit testicular inoculation	Cell culture	Sensitive, selective media available	Cell culture	Not available
Serology	RPR/VDRL, FTA-ABS, TPHA, MHA-TP	Rarely useful (primary herpes)	Experimental	Complement fixation and immuno-fluorescent antibody test	Experimental
Molecular Techniques	PCR (experimental)	PCR (experimental)	PCR (experimental)	PCR	Not available

Adapted from *Sexually Transmitted Diseases*, Holmes KK, Mardh P, Sparling PF (eds), New York, NY: McGraw-Hill, 1999, 890.

Despite our best efforts, in 25% of patients with genital ulcer disease, the etiology will remain unclear. Often this is due to the lack of sensitivity of the laboratory tests previously described. Therefore, it is reasonable to treat patients suspected of having a sexually transmitted disease even if laboratory data corroborating the diagnosis is lacking. In those who do not respond to treatment, noninfectious etiologies of genital ulceration should be considered. These are described below.

If the patient has a sexually transmitted disease, *Stop Here.*

If the patient does not have a sexually transmitted disease, *Proceed to Step 7.*

STEP 7: *What are the Noninfectious Causes of Genital Ulcer?*

Noninfectious causes of genital ulcer are described below.

Aphthous Ulcers

Also known as canker sores, aphthous ulcers are ulcerations of the mucous membranes. Aphthous ulcers are quite common on the oral mucosa. Less commonly, such ulcerations may occur over the genitalia. When they do affect the genital area, often a history of oral canker sores can be elicited. Oral and genital lesions are not always present together, however. Aphthous ulcerations of the genital area are often large and irregular with a white base. With deeper ulcerations, the base may be red. The lesions are typically painful.

Aphthous ulcerations of the genital region may occur in Behcet's disease, an illness characterized by systemic manifestations which include arthritis, skin rash, and inflammatory eye disease. Inflammatory bowel disease is also associated with aphthous ulcers, usually of the oral mucosa. Genital lesions may also occur. When genital lesions are present, the lesions characteristically wax and wane with the activity of the bowel disease.

Fixed Drug Eruptions

Although uncommon, fixed drug eruptions have been reported with a number of medications. The most common offending medications are listed in the following box.

Common Offending Drugs Causing Fixed Drug Eruption	
Acetaminophen	Penicillins
Barbiturates	Phenolphthalein
NSAIDs	Sulfonamides
Oral contraceptives	Tetracycline

In the typical case, one or several erosions or ulcers develop 1-2 days following the institution of a new medication. The lesions may be large, even reaching 3 cm. With subsequent exposure to the same medication, the lesions recur in the same location. Lesions may also be present outside the genital area.

Trauma

Trauma is a common cause of genital ulcer, especially among men. Men may have "zipper accidents." Men may also develop traumatic genital ulceration after sexual intercourse, particularly if the activity was vigorous. In these cases, however, every effort must be made to exclude infectious causes of genital ulceration.

Reiter's Syndrome

Reiter's syndrome is one type of HLA B27 spondyloarthropathy. It is characterized by the following triad:

- Inflammatory arthropathy
- Conjunctival inflammation
- Clinical manifestations usually follow urethritis or diarrhea

One of the extra-articular manifestations of Reiter's syndrome is circinate balanitis which may manifest with shallow, painless ulcerations of the penis.

The other uncommon causes of genital ulceration are listed in the box in Step 1. The reader is encouraged to consult appropriate sources for information regarding these uncommon causes of genital ulceration should the etiology of the ulcer remain unexplained.

REFERENCES

Augenbraun MH and McCormack WM, "Sexually Transmitted Diseases in HIV-Infected Persons," *Infect Dis Clin North Am*, 1994, 8(2):439-48. (review).

Birnbaum NR, Goldschmidt RH, and Buffett WO, "Resolving the Common Clinical Dilemmas of Syphilis," *Am Fam Phys*, 1999, 59(8):2233-40, 2245-6 (review).

Brown TJ, Yen-Moore A, and Tyring SK, "An Overview of Sexually Transmitted Diseases. Part I," *J Am Acad Dermatol*, 1999, 41(4):511-32 (review).

Clyne B and Jerrard DA, "Syphilis Testing," *J Emerg Med*, 2000, 18(3):361-7 (review).

Goldman BD, "Herpes Serology for Dermatologists," *Arch Dermatol*, 2000, 136(9):1158-61 (review).

Hart G, "Donovanosis," *Clin Infect Dis*, 1997, 25(1):24-30 (review).

Lewis DA, "Diagnostic Tests for Chancroid," *Sex Transm Infect*, 2000, 76(2):137-41 (review).

Miller KE and Graves JC, "Update on the Prevention and Treatment of Sexually Transmitted Diseases," *Am Fam Phys*, 2000, 61(2):379-86 (review).

Mroczkowski TF and Martin DH, "Genital Ulcer Disease," *Dermatol Clin*, 1994, 12(4):753-64 (review).

Rosen T and Brown TJ, "Genital Ulcers. Evaluation and Treatment," *Dermatol Clin*, 1998, 16(4):673-85 (review).

Sexually Transmitted Diseases, Holmes KK, Mardh P, Sparling PF (eds), New York, NY: McGraw-Hill, 1999, 890.

Singh AE and Romanowski B, "Syphilis: Review With Emphasis on Clinical, Epidemiologic, and Some Biologic Features," *Clin Microbiol Rev*, 1999, 12(2):187-209 (review).

Wicher K, Horowitz HW, and Wicher V, "Laboratory Methods of Diagnosis of Syphilis for the Beginning of the Third Millennium," *Microbes Infect*, 1999, 1(12):1035-49 (review).

GYNECOMASTIA

STEP 1: *What is Gynecomastia?*

Gynecomastia is the proliferation of the glandular component of the male breast. Clinically, this manifests as palpable breast tissue in men. There are times, however, when the presence of palpable breast tissue is normal. These times include the following:

- Newborn

- Puberty

- Elderly

Many authorities maintain that palpable breast tissue is abnormal outside these age ranges. In recent years, however, investigators have challenged this traditional thinking. In fact, several studies have shown that 35% of normal men between 17-80 years of age have palpable breast tissue.

It is also necessary to differentiate gynecomastia from lipomastia, which refers to breast enlargement secondary to the deposition of adipose tissue. Lipomastia, also known as pseudogynecomastia, can be differentiated from gynecomastia by the following:

- Breast palpation

  Gentle squeezing of the tissue between the index finger and thumb may allow the clinician to differentiate gynecomastia from lipomastia. In patients with gynecomastia, slight resistance is often appreciated when the tissue is pinched. In addition, true breast tissue feels ropy and coiled.

- Mammography / ultrasonography

  If the physical examination does not allow the clinician to distinguish gynecomastia from lipomastia, imaging with either mammography or ultrasonography can help to make the distinction.

If the patient has lipomastia, *Stop Here*.

If the patient has gynecomastia, *Proceed to Step 2.*

STEP 2: *What are the Causes of Gynecomastia?*

The causes of gynecomastia are listed in the following box.

Causes of Gynecomastia
Physiologic
Newborn
Pubertal
Aging
Pathologic
Congenital
Klinefelter's syndrome
Congenital anorchia
Androgen resistance (testicular feminization)
Defects in testosterone synthesis
Primary hypogonadism
Orchitis
Trauma
Castration
Neurologic diseases
Granulomatous diseases
Chemotherapy
Radiation therapy
Secondary hypogonadism
Chronic disease
Liver disease
Renal disease
Malnutrition
Hyperthyroidism
Malignancy
Testicular tumors
Bronchogenic carcinoma
Adrenal carcinoma
Other tumors producing hCG
Medications
Idiopathic

Although most cases of gynecomastia are benign, on occasion, a serious underlying cause may be present. The challenge for the clinician is to recognize features in the patient's clinical presentation that are suggestive of a serious underlying condition.

Proceed to Step 3

STEP 3: *Does the Patient Have Physiologic Gynecomastia?*

During a man's life, there are three time periods in which gynecomastia is considered physiologic. These time periods include the following:

- Newborn

    The physiologic gynecomastia that is appreciated in newborns usually disappears within the first few weeks of life.

- Pubertal

  Enlargement of the breasts in adolescent boys is common. In most cases, the gynecomastia is bilateral. Even when there is bilateral involvement, it is important for the clinician to realize that asymmetry of breast size is common. Many patients with pubertal gynecomastia complain of breast tenderness. With the passage of time, the gynecomastia resolves. In 90% of cases, it resolves within three years of onset. It is not difficult to recognize pubertal gynecomastia as it usually occurs in conjunction with sexual development.

- Aging

  For years, it has been known that healthy elderly men may develop gynecomastia. Because advancing age is associated with an increased incidence of many of the pathologic conditions listed in Step 2, the clinician should consider the gynecomastia of aging to be a diagnosis of exclusion.

If the gynecomastia is physiologic, **Stop Here**.

If the gynecomastia is pathologic, **Proceed to Step 4.**

STEP 4: *What are the Common Causes of the Gynecomastia?*

The percentage of cases of gynecomastia due to the causes listed in Step 2 are shown in the following table.

Condition	Percentage of Cases (%)
Idiopathic (related to aging)	25
Persistent pubertal gynecomastia	25
Medication-related	10-20
Cirrhosis and/or malnutrition	8
Primary hypogonadism	8
Testicular tumor	3
Secondary hypogonadism	2
Hyperthyroidism	1.5
Renal disease	1

Proceed to Step 5

STEP 5: *Are There Any Clues in the Patient's History That Point to the Etiology of the Gynecomastia?*

Clues in the patient's history that may point to the etiology of the gynecomastia are listed in the following table.

Historical Clue	Condition Suggested
Tall, thin body habitus	Klinefelter's syndrome
History of testicular torsion	Primary hypogonadism
History of mumps	Mumps orchitis leading to primary hypogonadism
History of testicular trauma	Trauma leading to primary hypogonadism
Neurologic diseases, especially those involving the spinal cord	Testicular atrophy (primary hypogonadism)
History of leprosy	Primary hypogonadism
History of renal failure	Renal disease or failure
History of liver disease or cirrhosis	Liver disease or cirrhosis
Nervousness Increased sweating Palpitations Fatigue Weight loss Increased appetite Heat intolerance	Hyperthyroidism
History of radiation exposure	Primary hypogonadism
History of uncorrected cryptorchidism	Primary hypogonadism Testicular cancer
Loss of libido / impotence	Hypogonadism
Headache	Secondary hypogonadism
History of chemotherapy	Primary hypogonadism
Starvation or malnutrition	Starvation or malnutrition
Body builder, weight lifter, or athlete	Medication-induced (androgens)
Administration of testosterone/ androgens	Medication-induced

Proceed to Step 6

STEP 6: *Are There Any Clues in the Patient's Physical Examination That Point to the Etiology of the Gynecomastia?*

Clues in the patient's physical examination that point to the etiology of the gynecomastia are listed in the following table.

Physical Examination Finding	Condition Suggested
Palmar erythema Spider angioma Parotid gland enlargement	Chronic liver disease or cirrhosis
Visual field deficits demonstrated by confrontation testing	Pituitary mass (secondary hypogonadism)

(Continued)

(continued)

Physical Examination Finding	Condition Suggested
Small or atrophic testis	Primary or secondary hypogonadism
Tachycardia Weight loss Tremor Thin, soft, and velvety hair Sweating Brisk reflexes	Hyperthyroidism
Testicular mass or nodule Nontender enlarged testes	Testicular tumors
Clubbing	Bronchogenic carcinoma

Also important to note on physical examination is the presence of asymmetric gynecomastia. Although asymmetric gynecomastia is quite common and usually benign, the clinician should ensure that the unilateral breast enlargement does not represent male breast cancer. Male breast cancer classically presents as a unilateral, eccentric mass that is often fixed to the underlying tissue. Findings such as nipple discharge, dimpling of the skin, and axillary lymphadenopathy are also concerning for breast cancer. Unilateral and eccentric breast enlargement may also be seen in other disorders such as mastitis, abscess, hematoma, lipoma, dermoid cyst, neurofibroma, and lymphangioma.

If breast cancer is a possibility, the evaluation should be tailored appropriately.

If there are clues in the patient's history and physical examination that point to the etiology of the gynecomastia, the evaluation should be tailored accordingly.

If there are no clues in the patient's history and physical examination that point to the etiology of the gynecomastia, *Proceed to Step 7*.

STEP 7: *What are the Results of the Laboratory Tests?*

When the history and physical examination do not provide clues to the etiology of the gynecomastia, the clinician should obtain the following laboratory tests:

- Liver function tests

    Chronic liver disease or cirrhosis is a common cause of gynecomastia. The history may not always reveal risk factors for liver disease. In addition, the signs and symptoms of chronic liver disease and cirrhosis are often nonspecific. The stigmata of chronic liver disease are not always present. For these reasons, then, liver function tests are reasonable tests to obtain so as not to miss the patient with gynecomastia secondary to liver disease.

- BUN and creatinine

    Although a less common cause of gynecomastia than liver disease, renal disease or failure can readily be excluded by obtaining a serum BUN and creatinine.

- TSH and free T$_4$ or free thyroxine index

  Not all patients with gynecomastia secondary to hyperthyroidism have signs and symptoms of thyroid hormone excess. Therefore, measurement of the TSH and free T$_4$ or free thyroxine index can help exclude hyperthyroidism.

If the results of the above laboratory testing reveal the etiology of the gynecomastia, *Stop Here*.

If the results of the above laboratory testing do not reveal the etiology of the gynecomastia, *Proceed to Step 8*.

STEP 8: *Does the Patient Have Medication-Induced Gynecomastia?*

The medications that may cause gynecomastia are listed in the following box.

Medications that Can Cause Gynecomastia	
Antiandrogen or inhibitors of	Drugs of abuse
androgen synthesis	Alcohol
Bicalutamide	Amphetamine
Cyproterone	Heroin
Flutamide	Marijuana
Zanoterone	Hormones
Antibiotics	Androgens and anabolic steroids*
Isoniazid	Chorionic gonadotropin
Ketoconazole	Estrogens and estrogenic agonists
Metronidazole	Diethylstilbestrol
Antiulcer agents	Exposure to dermal ointments
Cimetidine	containing estrogen
Omeprazole	Industrial exposure
Ranitidine	Sexual intercourse with partners
Cancer chemotherapeutic agents	who use vaginal creams
Cardiovascular agents	containing estrogen
Amiodarone	Psychoactive
Captopril	Diazepam
Digoxin	Haloperidol
Enalapril	Phenothiazines
Methyldopa	Tricyclic antidepressants
Reserpine	Other
Spironolactone	Penicillamine
Verapamil	Phenytoin

*When given in conventional doses, testosterone replacement therapy does not usually lead to gynecomastia. Weight lifters, body builders, and athletes often take supraphysiologic amounts of androgens, which leads to the increased production of estradiol by extraglandular aromatization. Gynecomastia is commonly noted in these groups. Not all androgens lead to gynecomastia, however. The clinician should not ascribe gynecomastia to androgen use unless the androgen being used has been clearly linked to the development of gynecomastia.

Adapted from Braunstein GD, "Gynecomastia," *N Engl J Med*, 1993, 328(7):490-5 (review).

Withdrawal of the suspect medication followed by resolution of the gynecomastia supports the diagnosis of medication-induced gynecomastia. However, gynecomastia that has been present for more than one year, irrespective of the cause, is not likely to be reversible even with cessation of the offending medication.

If the patient has medication-induced gynecomastia, **Stop Here**.

If the patient does not have medication-induced gynecomastia, **Proceed to Step 9**.

STEP 9: *What are the Results of Endocrinologic Testing?*

Endocrinologic testing should be considered in patients with unexplained gynecomastia. The clinician should obtain the following tests:

- Testosterone
- hCG
- Luteinizing hormone (LH)
- Estradiol

The results of the above endocrinologic tests may elucidate the etiology of the gynecomastia, as shown in the following table.

Laboratory Test Result	Condition Suggested	Proceed to Step ?
Elevated hCG	Testicular germ cell tumor Extragonadal germ cell tumor hCG-secreting nontrophoblastic neoplasm	Step 10
Decreased testosterone Elevated LH	Primary hypogonadism	Step 11
Decreased testosterone Decreased or normal LH	Secondary hypogonadism	Step 12
Increased testosterone Increased LH	Androgen resistance	Stop Here
Increased estradiol Decreased or normal LH	Leydig or Sertoli cell tumor Adrenal neoplasm Increased extraglandular aromatase activity	Step 13
All normal	Idiopathic gynecomastia	Step 14

STEP 10: *What are the Causes of an Elevated hCG?*

Gynecomastia has been appreciated in patients with trophoblastic or germ cell tumors. In these tumors, the production of hCG or hCG fragments is responsible for the development of gynecomastia. Human chorionic gonadotropin may also be produced by nontrophoblastic malignancies, including cancers of the lung, kidney, adrenal gland, and liver.

A mass noted on testicular ultrasound supports the diagnosis of a testicular germ cell tumor. When a mass is not apparent on ultrasonography, the clinician should consider one of the following possibilities:

- Extragonadal germ cell tumor

- hCG-secreting nontrophoblastic tumor

Chest radiography and abdominal / pelvic CT scan are reasonable imaging tests to obtain in an effort to identify the malignancy.

End of Section.

STEP 11: *What is the Etiology of the Primary Hypogonadism?*

A high LH level in the setting of testosterone deficiency establishes the diagnosis of primary hypogonadism. The causes of primary hypogonadism are listed in the following box.

Causes of Primary Hypogonadism	
Congenital	Trauma†
Viral orchitis*	Radiation exposure
Mumps	Medications
Echovirus	Autoimmune
Lymphocytic choriomeningitis virus	Granulomatous disease‡
Group B arboviruses	Neurologic disease#

* Viral orchitis is a common cause of testicular failure. Although many different viruses may cause testicular failure, mumps is the most important cause. Orchitis occurs in 25% of patients with mumps infection. Typically occurring several days after the onset of parotitis, mumps orchitis may be unilateral or bilateral. Unilateral involvement is more common, occurring in 66% of patients. Not all patients with mumps orchitis will develop testicular atrophy. It develops in approximately 33% of the cases.

† Trauma is also a common cause of testicular atrophy, second only to viral orchitis.

‡ Granulomatous involvement of the testis in patients with leprosy may lead to the development of testicular atrophy.

Testicular atrophy is commonly noted in patients with spinal cord disease. Other neurologic conditions may be associated with testicular atrophy as well.

End of Section.

STEP 12: *What is the Etiology of the Secondary Hypogonadism?*

Low or normal LH levels in the patient with testosterone deficiency should prompt consideration of secondary hypogonadism. Secondary hypogonadism refers to hypothalamic or pituitary conditions that may result in hypogonadism. These conditions are listed in the following box.

Causes of Secondary Hypogonadism		
Congenital	Inflammatory disease	Infiltration
Malignancy	Granulomatous disease	Hemochromatosis
Pituitary adenoma	Tuberculosis	Amyloidosis
Hypothalamic tumors	Sarcoidosis	Vascular event
Craniopharyngioma	Syphilis	Head trauma
Germinoma	Lymphocytic hypophysitis	Surgery
Meningioma	Histiocytosis X/	Radiation
Glioma	eosinophilic granuloma	
Metastatic cancer		

It is reasonable to obtain prolactin levels in these patients since some of the conditions listed in the above box are associated with hyperprolactinemia. In particular, an elevated prolactin level should prompt consideration of a prolactin-secreting pituitary adenoma. It is important to realize that prolactin is not a growth hormone for the breast. As a result, the gynecomastia that may be seen with prolactin-secreting pituitary adenomas is not a reflection of hyperprolactinemia. Rather, the tumor mass may impair the ability of the pituitary gland to secrete LH and FSH, leading to secondary hypogonadism.

Alternatively, the high prolactin level may directly inhibit secretion of LH and FSH in the pituitary gland. CT or MRI of the sella is usually performed in patients with secondary hypogonadism, irrespective of the prolactin level.

End of Section.

STEP 13: *What are the Results of the Testicular Ultrasound?*

Increased estradiol levels in the setting of a decreased or normal LH level should prompt consideration of the following conditions:

- Leydig or Sertoli cell tumor
- Adrenal cancer
- Increased extraglandular aromatase activity

A mass noted on the testicular ultrasound should prompt consideration of a Leydig or Sertoli cell tumor. Because these tumors are often small, physical examination may not reveal the presence of a palpable mass. When the testicular ultrasound is unremarkable, the clinician should consider the following possibilities:

- Adrenal cancer
- Increased extraglandular aromatase activity

To differentiate between these two possibilities, the clinician should obtain an abdominal/pelvic CT scan. The presence of an adrenal mass warrants consideration of an adrenal cancer.

End of Section.

STEP 14: *Does the Patient Have Idiopathic Gynecomastia?*

When the results of endocrinologic testing are unremarkable, idiopathic gynecomastia is the likely diagnosis. In these cases, it is important to reassure the patient that the gynecomastia will not have any serious impact upon the patient's health.

REFERENCES

Braunstein GD, "Gynecomastia," *N Engl J Med*, 1993, 328(7):490-5 (review).

Glass AR, "Gynecomastia," *Endocrinol Metab Clin North Am*, 1994, 23(4):825-37.

Lemack GE, Poppas DP, and Vaughan ED, "Urologic Causes of Gynecomastia: Approach to Diagnosis and Management," *Urology*, 1995, 45(2):313-9.

Neuman JF, "Evaluation and Treatment of Gynecomastia," *Am Fam Phys*, 1997, 55(5):1835-44, 1849-50.

Thompson DF and Carter JR, "Drug-Induced Gynecomastia," *Pharmacotherapy*, 1993, 13(1):37-45.

GYNECOMASTIA

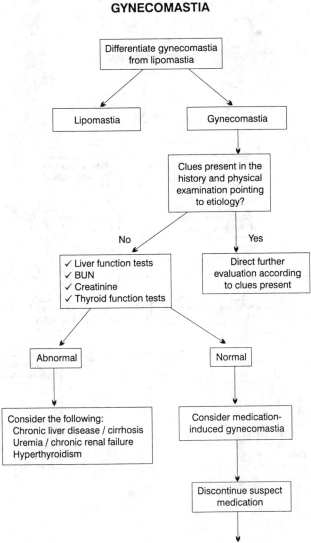

Differentiate gynecomastia from lipomastia

Lipomastia

Gynecomastia

Clues present in the history and physical examination pointing to etiology?

No

Yes

✓ Liver function tests
✓ BUN
✓ Creatinine
✓ Thyroid function tests

Direct further evaluation according to clues present

Abnormal

Normal

Consider the following:
  Chronic liver disease / cirrhosis
  Uremia / chronic renal failure
  Hyperthyroidism

Consider medication-induced gynecomastia

Discontinue suspect medication

See next page

GYNECOMASTIA
(continued)

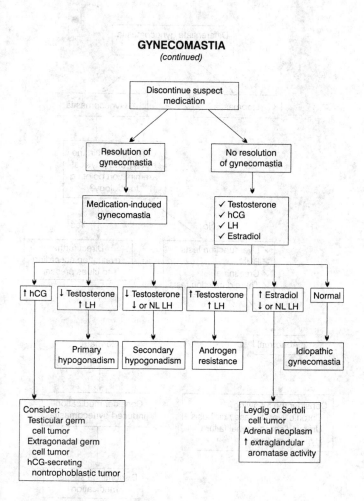

HEMATEMESIS AND / OR MELENA

STEP 1: *Does the Patient Have Hematemesis, Melena, or Both?*

Hematemesis refers to the vomiting of fresh blood or clots. An upper gastrointestinal source of bleeding (source proximal to the ligament of Treitz) is invariably present in patients with hematemesis. Melena refers to black, tarry stools. It is important to realize that there are other causes of black stool. Since licorice, bismuth, and iron supplements are just a few of the substances that may darken stool, it is important to do a guaiac test on all black stool to ensure that melena is present.

Although melena is most commonly appreciated in patients with upper gastrointestinal bleeding, it may also be noted in the patient having a process affecting the small intestine or ascending colon.

Clinical Presentation of Upper Gastrointestinal Bleeding	
Hematemesis	50%
Hematemesis and melena	20%
Melena	30%

On occasion, a patient with upper gastrointestinal bleeding may present with neither hematemesis or melena. In these cases, unexplained syncope may be the only manifestation of the bleed, particularly when a large amount of blood is lost into the gastrointestinal tract. Shortly thereafter, hematemesis or the passage of blood per rectum may be noted.

Proceed to Step 2

STEP 2: *How Concerning is the Patient's Clinical Presentation?*

Stabilization of the patient's hemodynamic status takes precedence in the patient presenting with melena and/or hematemesis. To do so, it is important to make a rapid assessment of the urgency of the patient's presentation. The following should be assessed or performed:

- Vital signs (including orthostatic measurements of blood pressure and pulse)
- Examination of the skin and mucous membranes for pallor
- Examination for findings consistent with shock
- Sending blood for CBC, routine chemistry, and clotting studies (PT/PTT)
- Sending blood for type and cross
- Two large bore intravenous catheters should be placed; a central line should be inserted if the patient is presenting with shock

When orthostatic changes are present (fall in SBP of >10 mm Hg and/or a heart rate increase of >10 bpm), approximately 20% of the circulating volume has been lost. When the volume loss exceeds 40%, shock is invariably present. Acute volume replacement is required in either case as part of the resuscitation process. Further information regarding the stabilization and resuscitation of the patient presenting with melena and/or hematemesis will not be discussed here.

If the patient has melena but no hematemesis, *Proceed to Step 3.*

If the patient has hematemesis but no melena, *Proceed to Step 4.*

If the patient has hematemesis and melena, *Proceed to Step 4.*

STEP 3: *Is the Source of the Melena From the Upper Gastrointestinal Tract?*

Less than 50% of patients with melena have accompanying hematemesis. In the absence of hematemesis, it can be difficult to ascertain if the melena is secondary to a process in the upper gastrointestinal tract, small intestine, or ascending colon. The presence of melena, however, usually implies an upper gastrointestinal source of bleeding. Uncommonly, melena is the manifestation of bleeding in the small intestine or ascending colon. Nasogastric lavage and the BUN to creatinine ratio may be used to help localize the source of the gastrointestinal bleed.

- Nasogastric lavage

   When the location of the bleeding is uncertain, the clinician should place a nasogastric tube. An upper gastrointestinal source of bleeding is present if the aspirate is bloody. While a nonbloody nasogastric aspirate argues against an upper gastrointestinal source of bleeding, it is important to realize that the aspirate may be nonbloody in up to 15% of patients with an upper gastrointestinal bleed. Many of these patients have a duodenal source of bleeding.

   In summary, a clear aspirate does not exclude upper gastrointestinal bleeding because episodic bleeding can occur. Also, a competent pylorus may prevent duodenogastric reflux of blood in patients with lesions located distal to the stomach.

   The presence of bile in the aspirate argues against an upper gastrointestinal source of bleeding. However, it has been shown that clinicians have difficulty discriminating between the presence or absence of bile based upon visual inspection alone.

- BUN / Creatinine ratio

   An elevation of the BUN that is disproportionate to the serum creatinine (ratio >25) suggests an upper gastrointestinal source of bleeding. The presence of such a ratio should be considered a soft clue pointing towards the presence of upper gastrointestinal bleeding.

Nasogastric lavage and the BUN to creatinine ratio may not always permit the clinician to differentiate an upper from a lower gastrointestinal source of bleeding.

If the bleeding clearly originates from the upper gastrointestinal tract, *Proceed to Step 4.*

If it is not clear where the bleeding originates from, it is best to consider the patient as having an upper gastrointestinal source. *Proceed to Step 4.*

STEP 4: *What are the Causes of Upper Gastrointestinal Bleeding?*

The causes of upper gastrointestinal bleeding are listed in the following box.

Causes of Upper Gastrointestinal Bleeding
Duodenum
Aortoenteric fistula
Peptic ulcer disease
Vascular malformations
Esophageal
Erosive esophagitis
Esophageal carcinoma
Mallory-Weiss tear
Varices
Stomach
Benign tumors
Adenoma
Fibroma
Hemangioma
Leiomyoma
Lipoma
Neurofibroma
Dieulafoy's lesion
Erosive gastritis
Malignant tumor
Carcinoid
Gastric carcinoma
Kaposi's sarcoma
Leiomyosarcoma
Lymphoma
Metastatic
Peptic ulcer disease
Portal hypertensive gastropathy
Recurrent marginal ulcer
Rupture of splenic artery aneurysm
Stress erosions
Vascular malformations
Varices
Other
Amyloidosis
Blood dyscrasia
DIC
Leukemia
Thrombocytopenia
von Willebrand's disease
Connective tissue disease
Hemobilia
Hemosuccus pancreaticus
Vasculitis

Proceed to Step 5

STEP 5: *What are the Major Causes of Upper Gastrointestinal Bleeding?*

While the differential diagnosis of upper gastrointestinal bleeding is extensive, the major causes are listed in the following table.

Causes of Upper Gastrointestinal Bleeding
Among 948 Patients

Diagnosis	Percentage of Patients (%)
Peptic ulcer disease	55
Esophageal varices	14
Vascular malformations	6
Mallory-Weiss tear	5
Tumor	4
Erosions	4
Dieulafoy's lesion	1
Other	11

Data obtained from the Center for Ulcer Research and Education
(CURE) Hemostasis Research Group, UCLA School of Medicine and
the West Los Angeles VA Medical Center.

Proceed to Step 6

STEP 6: *Are There Any Clues in the Patient's History That Point to the Etiology of the Upper Gastrointestinal Bleed?*

Ascertaining the cause of the gastrointestinal bleeding requires a thorough history and physical examination. Unfortunately, even after a thorough history and physical examination performed by gastroenterologists, the etiology of the bleeding is uncertain in 50% of cases. Clues in the patient's history that may point to the etiology of the upper gastrointestinal bleed are listed in the following table.

Historical Clue	Disease Suggested
History of peptic ulcer disease or dyspepsia	Peptic ulcer disease
NSAID use	Gastritis Peptic ulcer disease
Alcohol use	Gastritis Esophageal varices
History of cirrhosis	Esophageal varices*
Prior aortic graft surgery	Aortoenteric fistula
Right upper quadrant abdominal pain Jaundice	Hemobilia
Trauma Burns Sepsis	Risk factors for stress erosions
Chronic renal failure Aortic stenosis Prior radiation therapy	Conditions associated with vascular ectasia and angiodysplasia
History of peptic ulcer disease surgery	Recurrent ulcer
History of cancer	Upper gastrointestinal bleed secondary to malignancy
Recent retching followed by hematemesis	Mallory-Weiss tear
Personal or family history of nosebleeds	Osler-Weber-Rendu syndrome

*Many patients with cirrhosis presenting with an upper gastrointestinal bleed have a nonvariceal source of bleeding.

Some of the causes of upper gastrointestinal bleeding are considered in more depth below.

Peptic Ulcer Disease

Peptic ulcer disease is the most common cause of upper gastrointestinal bleeding, accounting for about 50% of cases. While a prior history of peptic ulcer disease is helpful in supporting the diagnosis, 33% of patients with peptic ulcer disease present with bleeding as their initial manifestation. A history of NSAID use is important to elicit as this is the most important risk factor for the development of bleeding in patients with peptic ulcer disease.

Esophageal Varices

Variceal bleeding characteristically occurs in patients with portal hypertension secondary to cirrhosis. In the United States, alcoholic cirrhosis is the leading cause of portal hypertension. Nonetheless, it is important to realize that any disease associated with portal hypertension may manifest with upper gastrointestinal bleeding at some point in the disease course. A history of chronic liver disease or cirrhosis may not be apparent in the patient with a variceal bleed. Herein lies the importance of performing a thorough history and physical examination. In particular, the clinician should search for stigmata of chronic liver disease which include spider angioma, palmar erythema, testicular atrophy, gynecomastia, splenomegaly, ascites, and encephalopathy. Abnormal liver function tests (hypoalbuminemia, elevated PT, elevated aminotransferases) lend further support to esophageal varices as the cause of the upper gastrointestinal bleed.

Even though a variceal bleed must be a major consideration in the cirrhotic patient presenting with upper gastrointestinal bleeding, approximately 25% of cirrhotic patients will be bleeding secondary to a nonvariceal etiology.

Mallory-Weiss Tear

Hematemesis that follows repeated retching or vomiting is a classic history for upper gastrointestinal bleeding from a Mallory-Weiss tear, a mucosal tear in the region of the esophagogastric junction. Retching, however, may not be present in nearly 50% of cases. Recent alcohol use is quite common.

Gastritis

Inflammation of the gastric mucosa is referred to as gastritis. As such, it is a histologic diagnosis. There is no data to support gastritis (as defined by histology) as a cause of upper gastrointestinal bleeding. The so called "gastritis" that is often invoked as a cause of upper gastrointestinal bleeding really refers to subepithelial hemorrhages and erosions that may be appreciated during endoscopy. These endoscopically visualized lesions may develop secondary to drug ingestion (NSAIDs), stress, or alcohol use.

Stress Ulceration

Stress ulcers and erosions may develop in critically ill patients. Risk factors for the development of these lesions include the following:

Risk Factors for the Development of Stress Ulceration	
CNS injury	Multiple organ failure
Coagulopathy	Renal failure
Hepatic failure	Sepsis
Hypotension / shock	Severe burns
Major surgery	Trauma
Mechanical ventilation	

The most common manifestation of stress ulceration is painless gastrointestinal hemorrhage. Although the bleeding is characteristically mild, on occasion, it may be life-threatening. Of note, ulcers that develop after severe burns are known as Curling's ulcers while those that develop in association with intracranial injury are referred to as Cushing's ulcers.

Esophagitis

Esophagitis is an uncommon cause of overt upper gastrointestinal hemorrhage. Several studies have shown that esophagitis is the cause of bleeding in 2% to 8% of cases. Among the different types of esophagitis, clinically-significant bleeding is most often due to that associated with gastroesophageal reflux disease. Less common causes include pill-induced injury, infection, nasogastric tube injury, and corrosive ingestion.

Tumors

There are many different types of upper gastrointestinal neoplasms. Taken together, they are responsible for 1% to 5% of all cases of upper gastrointestinal bleeding. Many of these malignancies tend to present with occult rather than overt gastrointestinal bleeding. Overt hemorrhage may occur in 10% to 20% of patients with gastric cancer. While lymphoma and leiomyosarcoma are not common tumors, the clinician should realize that these tumors have a predilection to bleed. In the AIDS patient, Kaposi's sarcoma is clearly a consideration. In rare cases, metastatic tumors may present with upper gastrointestinal bleeding.

Vascular Malformations

Under the term, vascular malformations, one may place angioma, vascular ectasia, angiodysplasia, telangiectasia, and hemangioma. Although these are not synonyms, endoscopic visualization of the lesion does not allow the clinician to discriminate between these different types of vascular malformations.

The mean age at which angiodysplasia typically presents is 60 years. These lesions may develop in any part of the gastrointestinal tract. Conditions associated with angiodysplasia include aortic stenosis, renal failure, CREST syndrome, and von Willebrand's disease.

Gastric antral vascular ectasia, also known as watermelon stomach, is another type of vascular malformation. The diagnosis is established by identifying its characteristic endoscopic appearance. Watermelon stomach has a predilection for women and tends to present later in life (mean age of 70).

Osler-Weber-Rendu syndrome, or hereditary hemorrhagic telangiectasia, is an uncommon, autosomal-dominant condition characterized by the presence of vascular malformations. Both visceral and mucocutaneous malformations are usually present. A history of recurrent epistaxis in childhood or young adulthood should prompt the clinician to suspect the diagnosis. Another common presentation is gastrointestinal bleeding which typically does not occur until the fourth or fifth decade of life.

Gastric Varices

Gastric varices develop in 20% of patients with portal hypertension. These varices may also be appreciated in up to 10% of patients following esophageal variceal obliteration. The presence of isolated gastric varices should raise concern for the possibility of splenic vein thrombosis.

Portal Hypertensive Gastropathy

Portal hypertensive gastropathy, also known as congestive gastropathy, is a major cause of upper gastrointestinal bleeding in patients with portal hypertension. It tends to be more frequently appreciated in portal hypertension that is secondary to cirrhosis. In noncirrhotic causes of portal hypertension, upper gastrointestinal bleeding secondary to portal hypertensive gastropathy is rare.

Hemobilia

Hemobilia may result when there is communication between the biliary tree and a blood vessel, resulting in biliary tract hemorrhage. The classic triad of right upper quadrant pain, jaundice, and upper gastrointestinal bleeding is only appreciated in 40% of cases. It is important to realize that the upper gastrointestinal bleed may be delayed weeks to months after the initial bile duct injury. The causes of hemobilia are listed in the following box.

Causes of Hemobilia	
Trauma	Nontraumatic
Blunt abdominal	Gallstones
Iatrogenic	Tropical infection
Endobiliary prosthesis	Ascariasis
Hepatic artery catheter infusion	Clonorchiasis
Liver biopsy	Tumor
Operative	Biliary
Percutaneous transhepatic	Gallbladder
cholangiography	Vascular aneurysms
Penetrating abdominal	

Liver function tests may reveal findings consistent with cholestasis.

Hemosuccus Pancreaticus

Hemosuccus pancreaticus is characterized by bleeding from the pancreatic duct. The major causes of hemosuccus pancreaticus include pancreatic pseudocyst and malignancy. It typically occurs when a pseudocyst or tumor erodes into a blood vessel.

Aortoenteric Fistula

Aortoenteric fistula is a rare cause of upper gastrointestinal bleeding. It may be classified as primary or secondary. Primary aortoenteric fistula is exceedingly rare. Secondary aortoenteric fistula may develop after aortic aneurysm repair when a communication develops between bowel and graft prosthesis. Although any part of the intestinal tract may be the site of the communication, in about 75% of cases, the duodenum is involved. Most cases present 3-5 years after the surgery although cases have been reported as early as the postoperative period or as late as 14 years. Over 90% of patients have a "herald or sentinel" bleed that resolves spontaneously. This initial bleed may be followed hours to days later by a massive bleed.

Dieulafoy's Lesion

Dieulafoy's lesion is a rare cause of upper gastrointestinal hemorrhage but one that certainly may be life-threatening. It presents at a mean age of 50 years and tends to have a predilection for men. The lesion refers to a large, tortuous, submucosal artery that is prone to thrombosis and perforation, manifesting as an upper gastrointestinal bleed. While the most common location of this lesion is the stomach, it has been described elsewhere in the gastrointestinal tract as well.

Proceed to Step 7

STEP 7: Are There Any Clues in the Patient's Physical Examination That May Point to the Etiology of the Upper Gastrointestinal Bleed?

Findings in the physical examination that may point to the etiology of the upper gastrointestinal bleed are listed in the following table.

Physical Examination Finding	Disease Suggested
Stigmata of cirrhosis	Esophageal varices
Lymphadenopathy or abdominal mass	Malignancy
Epigastric tenderness	Peptic ulcer disease
Telangiectasias	Osler-Weber-Rendu syndrome
Hepatosplenomegaly	Liver disease or malignancy
Distended abdominal veins	Portal hypertension (esophageal varices)

Physical examination of the skin may provide important clues to the etiology of the upper gastrointestinal bleed, as shown in the following table.

Skin Finding	Condition Suggested
Café-au-lait spots	Neurofibromatosis
Telangiectasias Calcinosis	Scleroderma
Skin hyperextensibility Severe bruising	Ehlers-Danlos syndrome
Raised, waxy papules or plaques Purpura	Amyloidosis
Erythematous macules Purpura Urticarial lesions	Henoch-Schönlein purpura

(Continued)

(continued)

Skin Finding	Condition Suggested
Purpura Nodules Livedo reticularis Cutaneous infarcts	Polyarteritis nodosa Other vasculitides
Tylosis palmaris et plantaris	Esophageal cancer
Flushing Telangiectasias	Carcinoid syndrome
Acanthosis nigracans Cutaneous and subcutaneous nodules (eg, Sister Mary Joseph nodule)	Gastric adenocarcinoma
Nodules and plaques of varying colors	Kaposi's sarcoma
Acquired ichthyosis	Gastrointestinal lymphoma
Epidermoid cysts	Gardner's syndrome
Bluish nevi with rubbery texture	Blue rubber bleb nevus syndrome
Hemangiomas on arms, legs, trunk	Klippel-Trenaunay-Weber syndrome
Telangiectasias	Osler-Weber-Rendu syndrome
Melanotic freckles	Peutz-Jeghers syndrome

Proceed to Step 8

STEP 8: *What Laboratory Tests are Useful in the Evaluation of the Patient Presenting With an Upper Gastrointestinal Bleed?*

Essential laboratory tests to obtain in the patient presenting with an upper gastrointestinal bleed include the following:

- Hemoglobin / hematocrit
- Platelet count
- Liver function tests (ie, albumin, AST, ALT, alkaline phosphatase)
- PT / PTT
- BUN
- Creatinine

The initial hemoglobin / hematocrit obtained usually does not reflect the degree of blood loss. With acute hemorrhage, both red blood cells and plasma volume are lost. As a result, the ratio between the two does not change. With time, there is a shift of body fluid into the intravascular space. This coupled with the administration of intravenous fluids results in a decrease in the hemoglobin, which will become more apparent after a few days. The finding of a low hemoglobin or hematocrit at the time of presentation suggests acute bleeding in the setting of chronic blood loss. The CBC may also reveal thrombocytopenia.

Azotemia (increased BUN) is the result of the absorption of nitrogenous breakdown products of blood present in the intestinal lumen. Another contributing factor to the azotemia is the volume depletion that accompanies gastrointestinal bleeding. Abnormal liver function tests (eg, hypoalbuminemia, etc) may suggest liver disease complicated by portal hypertension.

Proceed to Step 9

STEP 9: *What are the Results of the Upper Endoscopy?*

The upper endoscopy is the initial test of choice in the patient presenting with an upper gastrointestinal bleed. The source of the bleeding can be identified in over 90% of patients. Upper endoscopy allows risk stratification of patients into high-and low-risk groups for rebleeding. For example, stigmata of recent ulcer hemorrhage such as active bleeding, adherent clot, or visible vessel are lesions that are at higher risk of rebleeding.

Endoscopic Appearance of an Ulcer and the Risk of Rebleeding

Endoscopic Appearance	Risk of Bleeding (%)
Actively bleeding or oozing ulcer	55
Nonbleeding, visible vessel	43
Ulcer with adherent clot	14-36

Indications for urgent endoscopy are listed in the following box.

Indications for Urgent Endoscopy in Upper Gastrointestinal Bleeding

- Bleeding does not stop spontaneously (ie, bright-red aspirate that does not clear with nasogastric lavage)
- Known or suspected cirrhosis
- Suspicion for aortoenteric fistula
- Clinical presentation consistent with shock
- Presence of orthostatic hypotension
- Decrease in hematocrit of at least 6%
- Transfusion requirement >2 U PRBC

In patients who do not have the above features and in whom bleeding has ceased, upper endoscopy may be postponed for 24 hours without impairing the diagnostic accuracy. Nor is the clinical outcome affected by delaying the upper endoscopy in these patients. Upper endoscopy is relatively contraindicated in patients with tenuous cardiopulmonary status and in those with a decreased level of consciousness. It is preferable to perform the upper endoscopy after endotracheal intubation in such patients.

There is no role for upper GI barium radiography in the patient presenting with upper gastrointestinal bleeding. When compared to upper endoscopy, disadvantages of barium studies in the evaluation of the patient with upper gastrointestinal bleeding include:

- Barium studies are successful in identifying the etiology in only 30% to 50% of cases.

- Barium studies may interfere with the ability to perform an angiogram or upper endoscopy.

- Barium studies have difficulty in detecting superficial mucosal sources of bleeding.

On occasion, angiography may be required in the patient with upper gastrointestinal bleeding. Angiography should be a consideration, particularly in the patient presenting with massive gastrointestinal hemorrhage. In these cases, angiography may localize the source of bleeding in 75% of cases. Furthermore, angiographic therapy may be successful in halting the bleeding.

If the upper endoscopy reveals the etiology of the upper gastrointestinal bleed, *Stop Here*.

If the upper endoscopy does not reveal the etiology of the upper gastrointestinal bleed, *Proceed to Step 10*.

STEP 10: *What are Some Possibilities in the Patient With an Upper Gastrointestinal Bleed Who Has a Negative Upper Endoscopy?*

It is important to realize that upper endoscopy fails to identify the source of the upper gastrointestinal bleeding in up to 10% of patients with hematemesis. This percentage is even higher in patients presenting with melena alone.

A considerable number of these patients may have had a Mallory-Weiss tear. These tears, which are often small, heal rapidly. As a result, an upper endoscopy performed ≥24 hours after the patient's presentation may be unrevealing. In these cases, it is reasonable to assume that the etiology of the upper gastrointestinal bleed is a Mallory-Weiss tear, particularly if the history reveals retching/vomiting that preceded the upper gastrointestinal bleed. A history of recent alcohol consumption can be elicited in many patients with a Mallory-Weiss tear.

Other reasons why the upper endoscopy may fail to establish the diagnosis include the following:

- On occasion, hematemesis and/or melena may result from a process outside the gastrointestinal tract. These cases involve the swallowing of blood from the nose (epistaxis) or lung (hemoptysis). Fabrication of an upper gastrointestinal bleed has been reported in the Munchausen syndrome.

- Some sources of upper gastrointestinal bleeding may have a subtle appearance. An example of this is Dieulafoy's lesion.

- The source of the bleeding may be small intestinal, in which case the lesion is inaccessible to upper endoscopy.

Angiography is also useful in the identification of the source in patients having a normal upper endoscopy. Findings may be consistent with vascular ectasia, hemobilia, or hemosuccus pancreaticus. Angiography can demonstrate the presence of vascular ectasia but, in the absence of bleeding, it is difficult to ascribe the bleeding to this etiology because ectasia is a common lesion.

If the history is characteristic of a Mallory-Weiss tear, *Stop Here*.

If the history is not characteristic of a Mallory-Weiss tear in the patient having melena alone, *Proceed to Step 11*.

STEP 11: *Is the Melena Secondary to a Process in the Ascending Colon?*

Recall that melena does not invariably indicate an upper gastrointestinal source of bleeding. A minority of these patients will have a lower gastrointestinal source of bleeding (distal to the ligament of Treitz).

In these patients, the right side of the colon should be examined prior to pursuing a small intestinal source of bleeding. The diagnostic test of choice to examine the right colon is colonoscopy.

If the colonoscopy reveals the source of the melena, ***Stop Here***.

If the colonoscopy does not reveal the source of the melena, ***Proceed to Step 12***.

STEP 12: *Does the Patient Have Obscure-Overt Bleeding?*

When a source is not identified after upper endoscopy and colonoscopy, the clinician should determine if the patient satisfies the definition of obscure gastrointestinal bleeding. The American Gastroenterological Association defined obscure gastrointestinal bleeding as "bleeding of unknown origin that persists or recurs after a negative initial or primary endoscopy (colonoscopy and/or upper endoscopy) result."

Tests available in establishing the etiology of obscure-overt bleeding are discussed in further detail below.

Repeat Upper Endoscopy

One study revealed that repeat upper endoscopy established the diagnosis in 30% of patients with obscure-overt bleeding. Upper gastrointestinal tract lesions that have been found during repeat upper endoscopy are listed in the following box.

Upper Gastrointestinal Lesions Found During Repeat Upper Endoscopy in Patients with Obscure-Overt Bleeding	
Blue rubber bleb nevus syndrome	Gastric cancer
Celiac sprue	Gastritis
Dieulafoy's lesion	Osler-Weber-Rendu syndrome
Duodenitis	Peptic ulcer disease
Esophageal cancer	Polyps
Esophagitis	Varices
Gastric antral vascular ectasia	Vascular malformations

Many of the lesions above are rare lesions, the detection of which is dependent upon the skill of the endoscopist.

Repeat Colonoscopy

While it is true that colonoscopy is considered the gold standard for the diagnosis of lesions in the large intestine, the chance of missing a lesion is dependent on the skill and expertise of the endoscopist. Lesions that have been found during repeat colonoscopy include cancer and vascular malformations. There may be a role, then, for repeat colonoscopy in the evaluation of the patient with obscure-overt gastrointestinal bleeding.

Enteroscopy

Visualization of the small intestine is possible with the use of push enteroscopy. Push enteroscopy is diagnostic in up to 57% of patients with obscure gastrointestinal bleeding. Of note, many of the lesions discovered during push enteroscopy are within the reach of upper endoscopy. Only 3% to 5% of obscure gastrointestinal bleeding is due to a small intestinal lesion. Vascular lesions are the most common cause of small intestinal bleeding, accounting for up to 80% of cases.

Vascular Causes of Small Intestinal Bleeding	
Angiodysplasia	Hemangioma
Arteriovenous malformations	Telangiectasia
Dieulafoy's ulcer	Venous ectasia

Small intestinal tumors account for nearly 10% of cases of small intestinal bleeding. Certain conditions increase the risk of developing small intestinal malignancy. These conditions include:

- Celiac disease
- Crohn's disease
- Familial polyposis
- Peutz-Jegher's syndrome
- HIV

Other lesions of the small intestine that may be detected include Crohn's disease, varices, diverticula, Meckel's diverticulum, Zollinger-Ellison syndrome, celiac sprue, vasculitis, and aortoenteric fistula.

Enteroclysis and Small Bowel Follow-Through (SBFT)

Small bowel follow-through and enteroclysis are both radiologic imaging techniques available in the evaluation of small intestinal disease. These imaging techniques are most useful in identifying prominent abnormalities of the small intestinal mucosa such as small intestinal tumors. Vascular malformations, the most common cause of small intestinal bleeding, are rarely identified. Recent studies suggest that it may be preferable to perform one of these studies if a lesion is not discovered during enteroscopy.

Angiography

Bleeding rates as low as 0.5 mL/minute can be detected by angiography. Active arterial bleeding is necessary in order to obtain a positive test. Therefore, angiography should only be performed during active bleeding. Because nuclear scans can detect bleeding at a rate of 0.1 mL/minute, some authorities suggest performing a nuclear scan prior to angiography. Those who have a positive nuclear scan are more likely to have a positive angiographic study. On occasion, angiography may identify a possible lesion when bleeding has stopped.

Nuclear Scan

The source of the obscure-overt bleeding may be localized with the use of a technetium-99m-labeled red blood cell scan. The nuclear scan has the ability to detect lesions with low bleeding rates (about 0.1 mL/minute). Nuclear scans that are immediately positive are often followed by angiographic studies, which are positive in 60% of these cases. Nuclear scans that are not immediately positive may still be considered positive if a delayed "blush" is appreciated. However, angiography has lower yield in this setting, being positive in only 7% of patients.

Meckel's Scan

In young patients, it is important to consider Meckel's diverticulum in the differential diagnosis of obscure-overt bleeding. Meckel's diverticulum, which occurs in 2% of the population, has a predilection for men. It may be diagnosed by nuclear scanning using sodium pertechnetate Tc 99m. In adults, the sensitivity of the scan is approximately 65%. The sensitivity of the test can be increased by administering cimetidine prior to the scan.

REFERENCES

Apel D and Riemann JF, "Emergency Endoscopy," *Can J Gastroenterol*, 2000, 14(3):199-203.

Gupta PK and Fleischer DE, "Nonvariceal Upper Gastrointestinal Bleeding," *Med Clin North Am*, 1993, 77(5):973-92.

Hamlin JA, Petersen B, Keller FS, et al, "Angiographic Evaluation and Management of Nonvariceal Upper Gastrointestinal Bleeding," *Gastrointest Endosc Clin N Am*, 1997, 7(4):703-16.

Katz PO and Salas L, "Less Frequent Causes of Upper Gastrointestinal Bleeding," *Gastroenterol Clin North Am*, 1993, 22(4):875-89.

Lieberman D, "Gastrointestinal Bleeding: Initial Management," *Gastroenterol Clin North Am*, 1993, 22(4):723-36.

Peter DJ and Dougherty JM, "Evaluation of the Patient With Gastrointestinal Bleeding: An Evidence Based Approach," *Emerg Med Clin North Am*, 1999, 17(1):239-61.

HEMATEMESIS

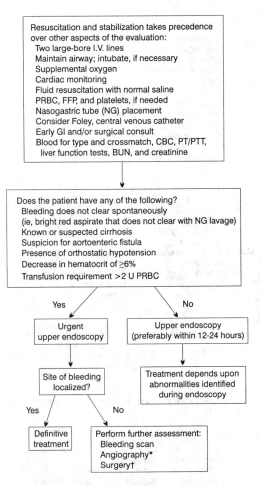

Resuscitation and stabilization takes precedence
over other aspects of the evaluation:
  Two large-bore I.V. lines
  Maintain airway; intubate, if necessary
  Supplemental oxygen
  Cardiac monitoring
  Fluid resuscitation with normal saline
  PRBC, FFP, and platelets, if needed
  Nasogastric tube (NG) placement
  Consider Foley, central venous catheter
  Early GI and/or surgical consult
  Blood for type and crossmatch, CBC, PT/PTT,
    liver function tests, BUN, and creatinine

Does the patient have any of the following?
  Bleeding does not clear spontaneously
  (ie, bright red aspirate that does not clear with NG lavage)
  Known or suspected cirrhosis
  Suspicion for aortoenteric fistula
  Presence of orthostatic hypotension
  Decrease in hematocrit of ≥6%
  Transfusion requirement >2 U PRBC

Yes → Urgent upper endoscopy

No → Upper endoscopy (preferably within 12-24 hours)

Urgent upper endoscopy → Site of bleeding localized?

Upper endoscopy (preferably within 12-24 hours) → Treatment depends upon abnormalities identified during endoscopy

Site of bleeding localized?
  Yes → Definitive treatment
  No → Perform further assessment:
    Bleeding scan
    Angiography*
    Surgery†

*Angiography should be considered if bleeding is severe or persists despite
 endoscopic methods or if endoscopic treatment is not available. It also should
 be considered if surgery is associated with a high risk.
†Criteria for emergency surgery in patients with hematemesis include:
 - Failure to control bleeding by nonoperative methods
 - Prior surgery or anatomic anomaly makes lesion inaccessible to upper
   endoscopy
 - Upper endoscopy is complicated by perforation or lesion with worsening
   bleeding
 - Severe rebleeding despite two attempts to achieve hemostasis by
   endoscopic means
 - To prevent exsanguination in patients with severe shock

MELENA

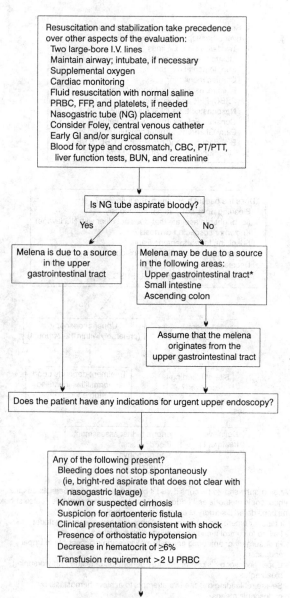

Resuscitation and stabilization take precedence
over other aspects of the evaluation:
  Two large-bore I.V. lines
  Maintain airway; intubate, if necessary
  Supplemental oxygen
  Cardiac monitoring
  Fluid resuscitation with normal saline
  PRBC, FFP, and platelets, if needed
  Nasogastric tube (NG) placement
  Consider Foley, central venous catheter
  Early GI and/or surgical consult
  Blood for type and crossmatch, CBC, PT/PTT,
    liver function tests, BUN, and creatinine

Is NG tube aspirate bloody?

Yes | No

Melena is due to a source
in the upper
gastrointestinal tract

Melena may be due to a source
in the following areas:
  Upper gastrointestinal tract*
  Small intestine
  Ascending colon

Assume that the melena
originates from the
upper gastrointestinal tract

Does the patient have any indications for urgent upper endoscopy?

Any of the following present?
  Bleeding does not stop spontaneously
    (ie, bright-red aspirate that does not clear with
    nasogastric lavage)
  Known or suspected cirrhosis
  Suspicion for aortoenteric fistula
  Clinical presentation consistent with shock
  Presence of orthostatic hypotension
  Decrease in hematocrit of ≥6%
  Transfusion requirement >2 U PRBC

See next page

MELENA
(continued)

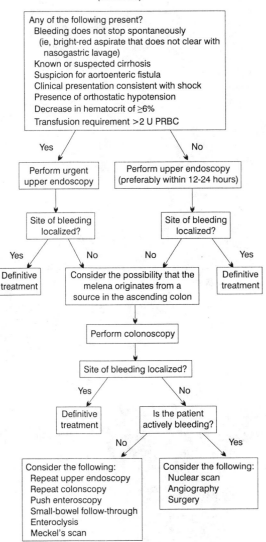

Any of the following present?
- Bleeding does not stop spontaneously (ie, bright-red aspirate that does not clear with nasogastric lavage)
- Known or suspected cirrhosis
- Suspicion for aortoenteric fistula
- Clinical presentation consistent with shock
- Presence of orthostatic hypotension
- Decrease in hematocrit of ≥6%
- Transfusion requirement >2 U PRBC

Yes → Perform urgent upper endoscopy

No → Perform upper endoscopy (preferably within 12-24 hours)

Site of bleeding localized?
- Yes → Definitive treatment
- No → Consider the possibility that the melena originates from a source in the ascending colon

Site of bleeding localized?
- No → Consider the possibility that the melena originates from a source in the ascending colon
- Yes → Definitive treatment

Perform colonoscopy

Site of bleeding localized?
- Yes → Definitive treatment
- No → Is the patient actively bleeding?

No → Consider the following:
- Repeat upper endoscopy
- Repeat colonscopy
- Push enteroscopy
- Small-bowel follow-through
- Enteroclysis
- Meckel's scan

Yes → Consider the following:
- Nuclear scan
- Angiography
- Surgery

*A nonbloody nasogastric aspirate does not rule out an upper gastrointestinal source of bleeding. In fact, up to 15% of patients with upper gastrointestinal tract bleeding have a nonbloody aspirate.

HEMATOCHEZIA

STEP 1: *What is Hematochezia?*

The passage of bright red blood per rectum is known as hematochezia. While hematochezia is the most common presentation of lower gastrointestinal bleeding, bright red blood per rectum may also be appreciated in brisk upper gastrointestinal or small intestinal bleeding.

Site of Bleeding in Patients Presenting with Hematochezia	
Colon	74%
Upper gastrointestinal tract	11%
Small intestine	9%
No site identified	6%

Uncommonly, lower gastrointestinal bleeding may manifest with melena, which refers to black, tarry stools. In these cases, a small intestinal or right colonic source is usually present.

Proceed to Step 2

STEP 2: *How Concerning is the Patient's Presentation?*

Prior to embarking any further in the evaluation of the patient with hematochezia, it is essential to perform a rapid assessment of the degree of blood loss. The following should be assessed or performed:

- Vital signs (including orthostatic measurements of blood pressure and pulse)
- Examination of the skin and mucous membranes for pallor
- Examination for findings consistent with shock
- Sending blood for CBC, routine chemistry, and clotting studies (PT/PTT)
- Sending blood for type and cross
- Two large bore intravenous catheters should be placed; a central line should be inserted if the patient is presenting with shock

Further information regarding the stabilization and resuscitation of the patient presenting with hematochezia will not be discussed here. This step is a reminder that assessment and resuscitation should take precedence over a history and physical examination. In many cases, however, both can be done concurrently.

Proceed to Step 3

STEP 3: *What are the Causes of Lower Gastrointestinal Bleeding?*

The causes of lower gastrointestinal bleeding are listed in the following box.

Causes of Lower Gastrointestinal Bleeding	
Anal fissure	Ischemic colitis
Angiodysplasia	Malignancy
Aortoenteric fistula	Meckel's diverticulum
Dieulafoy's lesion	Polyps
Diverticulosis	Portal colopathy
Hemorrhoids	Postpolypectomy
Ileal or colonic varices	Radiation-induced colitis
Infectious colitis	Solitary rectal ulcer
Inflammatory bowel disease	Upper gastrointestinal bleed
Intussusception	

Proceed to Step 4

STEP 4: *What are the Most Common Causes of Lower Gastrointestinal Bleeding?*

The most common causes of lower gastrointestinal bleeding are listed in the following table.

Cause	Patients (%)
Diverticulosis	30
After polypectomy	7
Ischemia	6
Ulcerations	6
Malignancy	5
Angiodysplasia	4
Radiation proctopathy	2
Inflammatory bowel disease	2
Miscellaneous	12
Undiagnosed*	26

*In this group of patients, the investigators assumed that an unseen vascular lesion was the likely cause of the lower gastrointestinal bleeding. Examples include angiodysplasia and Dieulafoy's lesion.

Adapted from *Clinical Practice of Gastroenterology*, Brandt LJ (ed), Philadelphia, PA: Current Medicine, Inc, 1999, 652.

Proceed to Step 5

STEP 5: *Are There Any Clues in the History That Point to the Etiology of the Hematochezia?*

Clues in the patient's history that may point to the etiology of the hematochezia are listed in the table below.

Historical Clue	Disease Suggested
Abdominal pain/cramping	Inflammatory bowel disease
	Infectious colitis
	Intussusception
	Ischemic colitis
Age <40 years	Meckel's diverticulum
	AIDS
	Inflammatory bowel disease
	Internal hemorrhoids
	Colon cancer (less likely)
Weight loss and anorexia	Malignancy
History of portal hypertension	Portal colopathy
Bright red blood on toilet tissue or around stool (but not mixed with stool)	Hemorrhoid
	Anal fissure
	Rectal polyp
	Rectal cancer
Rectal / anal pain	Anal fissure
	Hemorrhoids
	Radiation proctitis
	Inflammatory bowel disease
History of aortic stenosis	Angiodysplasia
History of atherosclerotic vascular disease	Ischemic colitis
Chronic renal failure	Angiodysplasia
On anticoagulants	Coagulopathy
Current NSAID use	Cecal or intestinal ulcer
History of radiation therapy	Radiation-induced colitis
Ostomy	Ileal or colonic varices
"Currant jelly" appearance of the stools	Meckel's diverticulum
History of abdominal aortic aneurysm repair	Aortoenteric fistula

Proceed to Step 6

STEP 6: *Are There Any Physical Examination Findings that Point to the Etiology of the Hematochezia?*

Clues in the physical examination that point to the etiology of the hematochezia are listed in the following table.

Physical Examination Finding	Disease Suggested
Abdominal tenderness	Infectious colitis Inflammatory bowel disease Intussusception Ischemic colitis
Palpable mass	Inflammatory bowel disease (Crohn's disease) Malignancy
Mass on rectal examination	Rectal cancer
Large, protruding hemorrhoids on rectal examination	Hemorrhoids
Ostomy	Ileal or colonic varices
Sausage-shaped mass	Intussusception
Systolic murmur radiating from base of heart to carotid area Pulsus parvus et tardus	Aortic stenosis (associated with angiodysplasia)

Proceed to Step 7

STEP 7: *What are the Results of the Laboratory Tests?*

Laboratory tests recommended in the evaluation of the patient presenting with hematochezia include the following:

- Hemoglobin/hematocrit
- Platelet count
- PT/PTT
- BUN
- Creatinine

A baseline EKG should be obtained in older patients. An EKG is also recommended in any patient who has a history of cardiopulmonary disease, irrespective of age.

Proceed to Step 8

STEP 8: *What is the Severity of the Bleeding?*

The clinician should strive to differentiate mild from severe bleeding. Severe bleeding is much less common than mild bleeding (15% versus 85%, respectively). Features consistent with severe bleeding include the following:

- Orthostatic change in blood pressure (systolic drop ≥20 mm Hg)
- Orthostatic change in heart rate (increase >20 bpm)
- Hypotension (systolic blood pressure <100 mm Hg)
- Tachycardia (heart rate >100 bpm)
- Decrease in hematocrit of ≥8%
- Hematocrit <30%
- Transfusion requirement >2 units PRBC

The features consistent with mild bleeding include the following:

- Hemodynamic stability
- Hematocrit stable
- Intermittent passage of small amounts of blood

If the patient has mild bleeding, **Proceed to Step 9**.

If the patient has severe bleeding, **Proceed to Step 10**.

STEP 9: *What is the Approach to the Patient With Mild Bleeding?*

Once a patient has been deemed to have mild bleeding, the evaluation may be completed on an outpatient basis. Many of these patients have rectal outlet bleeding, which is defined as the intermittent passage of small amounts of blood secondary to an anorectal condition. Anorectal conditions associated with rectal outlet bleeding include hemorrhoids, anal abrasions, anal fissures, ulcers, polyps, tumors, and proctitis.

In the younger patient (<50 years of age), evaluation should proceed with anoscopy and flexible sigmoidoscopy. In the event that the source of bleeding is not identified, an air-contrast barium enema should be performed.

In older patients (≥50 years of age), a full colonoscopy should be performed even if the history is suggestive of hemorrhoids. The increased risk of colonic polyps and tumors in this age group behooves the clinician to perform colonoscopy over the combination of flexible sigmoidoscopy and barium enema.

End of Section.

STEP 10: *What are the Results of the Nasogastric Aspirate?*

Recall that brisk upper gastrointestinal bleeding can result in hematochezia. In fact, 11% of patients presenting with hematochezia are found to have an upper gastrointestinal etiology. When an upper gastrointestinal lesion presents with hematochezia, hemodynamic instability is almost always present.

A nasogastric tube should be placed followed by aspiration to ensure that an upper gastrointestinal source is not present in the patient thought to have a severe lower gastrointestinal bleed. It is important to note that a nonbloody aspirate does not exclude an upper gastrointestinal etiology, especially if the aspirate does not contain bile. In fact, 15% of patients with an upper gastrointestinal source of bleeding will have a nonbloody aspirate.

If the nasogastric aspirate is bloody, proceed to the section on hematemesis and/or melena.

If the nasogastric aspirate is nonbloody, **Proceed to Step 11**.

STEP 11: *Does the Patient Need to Have an Upper Endoscopy?*

As discussed in Step 10, a nonbloody nasogastric aspirate does not exclude an upper gastrointestinal lesion manifesting with hematochezia. The clinician should consider performing upper endoscopy if the patient is hemodynamically unstable or there is any uncertainty about whether the patient has an upper or lower gastrointestinal bleed.

If the upper endoscopy reveals the etiology of the hematochezia, *Stop Here.*

If the upper endoscopy does not reveal the etiology of the hematochezia, *Proceed to Step 12.*

STEP 12: *Has the Bleeding Stopped or Slowed Down?*

Which test to perform in the evaluation of the patient with hematochezia depends on whether there is continued bleeding.

If the patient is bleeding rapidly, *Proceed to Step 13.*

When the bleeding has slowed down or stopped, the initial diagnostic procedure of choice is colonoscopy. Almost all sources of colonic blood loss can be diagnosed by colonoscopy. Performing the procedure within several hours of bleeding is not useful if an adequate bowel preparation has not been done. The yield of colonoscopy is improved if colonoscopy is done soon after an adequate bowel preparation. In most cases, colonoscopy should be performed within 12-24 hours after presentation.

Merely finding a lesion at colonoscopy does not mean that it is the culprit. A lesion is likely to be the source of the bleeding if any of the following criteria are met:

- Active bleeding is present
- Nonbleeding visible vessel in an ulcer (in the absence of other lesions that could cause the bleeding)
- Adherent clot in a single diverticulum or ulcerative lesion along with the following:
  1. Clot is resistant to washing
  2. Fresh blood is noted nearby
  3. No other lesion present that could account for the bleeding

If the colonoscopy is unrevealing, the clinician should consider whether the patient satisfies the definition of obscure bleeding. The American Gastroenterological Association has defined obscure bleeding as "bleeding of unknown origin that persists or recurs after a negative initial or primary endoscopy (colonoscopy and/or upper endoscopy) result." In those patients with hematochezia who have not yet had an upper endoscopy, it may be worthwhile to perform the procedure to exclude an upper gastrointestinal lesion. The reader is referred to Step 12 in the chapter on Hematemesis and/or Melena *on page 270* for more information regarding the evaluation of obscure bleeding.

End of Section.

> **STEP 13:** *What Test Should be Performed in the Patient Who is Bleeding Rapidly From the Lower Gastrointestinal Tract?*

Choices available to the clinician in the evaluation of the patient who is bleeding rapidly from the lower gastrointestinal tract include the following:

- Colonoscopy
- Angiography
- Exploratory laparotomy with intraoperative endoscopy

Some endoscopists are reluctant to perform colonoscopy in these patients, mainly because of concern that the blood will not allow the colon to be adequately visualized. Although profuse bleeding precludes bowel cleansing, the clinician should realize that blood is a cathartic so the colon may actually be free of stool. The diagnostic accuracy of colonoscopy is approximately 80% in patients with lower gastrointestinal bleeding. Findings noted during the colonoscopy may be categorized into one of the groups listed in the box below.

Diagnostic Categories in Emergency Colonoscopy for Acute Severe Bleeding
Acutely bleeding lesions
Fresh blood in an area, nonbloody contents proximally
Fresh adherent clot
Fresh blood in an area, unable to prove nonbloody contents proximally
Failure to localize bleeding

Adapted from Forde K and Treat M, "Colonoscopy for Lower Gastrointestinal Bleeding," *Surgical Endoscopy*, Dent T, Strodel W, Turcotee J, et al (eds), Chicago, IL: Year Book Medical, 1985, 261-74.

Angiography is considered to be complementary to colonoscopy in the evaluation of patients with lower gastrointestinal bleeding. It is recommended in the following situations:

- Colonoscopy is not available
- Colonoscopy is unsuccessful (failure to localize bleeding, visual field obscured by blood)

Angiography is not only useful in diagnosis but may also allow for therapeutic intervention to halt the bleeding.

If bleeding persists despite colonoscopy and angiographic intervention, emergency surgery should be considered.

REFERENCES

Clinical Practice of Gastroenterology, Brandt LJ (ed), Philadelphia, PA: Current Medicine, Inc, 1999, 652.

DeMarkles MP and Murphy JR, "Acute Lower Gastrointestinal Bleeding," *Med Clin North Am*, 1993, 77(5):1085-100.

Farrell JJ and Friedman LS, "Gastrointestinal Bleeding in Older People," *Gastroenterol Clin North Am*, 2000, 29(1):1-36.

Forde K and Treat M, "Colonoscopy for Lower Gastrointestinal Bleeding," *Surgical Endoscopy*, Dent T, Strodel W, Turcotee J, et al (eds), Chicago, IL: Year Book Medical, 1985, 261-74.

Isaacs KL, "Severe Gastrointestinal Bleeding," *Clin Geriatr Med*, 1994, 10(1):1-17.

Jensen DM and Machicado GA, "Colonoscopy for Diagnosis and Treatment of Severe Lower Gastrointestinal Bleeding. Routine Outcomes and Cost Analysis," *Gastrointest Endosc Clin N Am*, 1997, 7(3):477-98.

Manten HD and Green JA, "Acute Lower Gastrointestinal Bleeding. A Guide to Initial Management," *Postgrad Med*, 1995, 97(4):154-7.

Miller LS, Barbarevech C, and Friedman LS, "Less Frequent Causes of Lower Gastrointestinal Bleeding," *Gastroenterol Clin North Am*, 1994, 23(1):21-52.

Peter DJ and Dougherty JM, "Evaluation of the Patient With Gastrointestinal Bleeding: An Evidence Based Approach," *Emerg Med Clin North Am*, 1999, 17(1):239-61.

Talbot-Stern JK, "Gastrointestinal Bleeding," *Emerg Med Clin North Am*, 1996, 14(1):173-84.

Vernava AM, Moore BA, Longo WE, et al, "Lower Gastrointestinal Bleeding," *Dis Colon Rectum*, 1997, 40(7):846-58.

Zuccaro G, "Management of the Adult Patient With Acute Lower Gastrointestinal Bleeding," *Am J Gastroenterol*, 1998, 93(8):1202-8.

HEMATOCHEZIA

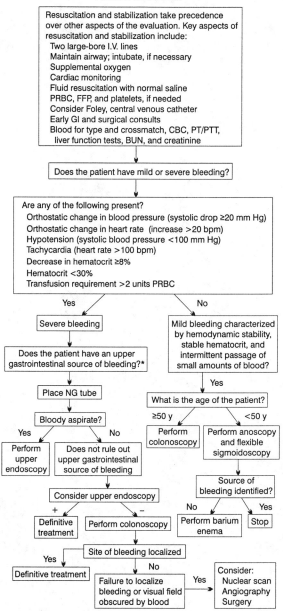

Resuscitation and stabilization take precedence over other aspects of the evaluation. Key aspects of resuscitation and stabilization include:
  Two large-bore I.V. lines
  Maintain airway; intubate, if necessary
  Supplemental oxygen
  Cardiac monitoring
  Fluid resuscitation with normal saline
  PRBC, FFP, and platelets, if needed
  Consider Foley, central venous catheter
  Early GI and surgical consults
  Blood for type and crossmatch, CBC, PT/PTT, liver function tests, BUN, and creatinine

Does the patient have mild or severe bleeding?

Are any of the following present?
  Orthostatic change in blood pressure (systolic drop ≥20 mm Hg)
  Orthostatic change in heart rate (increase >20 bpm)
  Hypotension (systolic blood pressure <100 mm Hg)
  Tachycardia (heart rate >100 bpm)
  Decrease in hematocrit ≥8%
  Hematocrit <30%
  Transfusion requirement >2 units PRBC

Yes — Severe bleeding

No — Mild bleeding characterized by hemodynamic stability, stable hematocrit, and intermittent passage of small amounts of blood?

Does the patient have an upper gastrointestinal source of bleeding?*

Place NG tube

Bloody aspirate?

Yes — Perform upper endoscopy

No — Does not rule out upper gastrointestinal source of bleeding

Consider upper endoscopy

+ Definitive treatment

− Perform colonoscopy

Yes (Mild bleeding) — What is the age of the patient?

≥50 y — Perform colonoscopy

<50 y — Perform anoscopy and flexible sigmoidoscopy

Source of bleeding identified?

No — Perform barium enema

Yes — Stop

Site of bleeding localized

Yes — Definitive treatment

No — Failure to localize bleeding or visual field obscured by blood

Yes — Consider:
  Nuclear scan
  Angiography
  Surgery

*11% of patients presenting with hematochezia have an upper gastrointestinal source of bleeding.

HEMATURIA

STEP 1: *What is Hematuria?*

Hematuria is defined as the presence of blood in the urine. It may either be gross or microscopic. When it is gross, it understandably causes considerable anxiety in both patients and clinicians alike. In particular, there is concern that the hematuria may be caused by a serious condition (ie, malignancy). It is important to realize, however, that the causes of gross and microscopic hematuria are the same. Therefore, a thorough evaluation is necessary regardless of whether the patient presents with gross or microscopic hematuria.

If the patient complains of gross hematuria, *Proceed to Step 2.*

If the patient has microscopic hematuria, *Proceed to Step 3.*

STEP 2: *Does the Patient Truly Have Gross Hematuria?*

Because there are other causes of a red or brown urine, the clinician must verify the presence of hematuria prior to embarking on an evaluation, which, at times, can be very extensive. A variety of substances may cause urine discoloration that mimics gross hematuria. This is known as pseudohematuria, the causes of which are listed in the following box.

Causes of Pseudohematuria	
Medications	Vegetable dyes
Analgesics	Beets
Phenacetin	Blackberries
Phenazopyridine	Paprika
Antimicrobials	Rhubarb
Rifampin	
Antimalarials	Antiseptics
Laxatives	Cresols
Anthraquinone (cascara, senna)	Mercurochrome
Chemotherapeutic agents	Phenols
Daunorubicin	Povidone-iodine
Doxorubicin	
Miscellaneous	Metabolic
Deferoxamine	Porphyrins
Dilantin	Urate crystalluria
Levodopa	
Methyldopa	
Phenothiazines	

To distinguish between pseudohematuria and gross hematuria, it is necessary to obtain a urinalysis.

Proceed to Step 3

STEP 3: *What are the Results of the Urine Dipstick for Blood?*

A positive urine dipstick test for blood is usually noted in both gross and microscopic hematuria. False-negative test results may be seen in the following situations:

- Ingestion of large amounts of vitamin C (>200 mg/day)
- Contamination of the urine specimen container with formaldehyde

It is important to realize, however, that a positive urine dipstick test for blood is not synonymous with hematuria because there are other causes of a positive test. The causes of a positive urine dipstick test for blood are listed in the following box.

Causes of a Positive Urine Dipstick Test for Blood	
False-positive reaction	Hemoglobinuria (hemolysis)
Hematuria	Myoglobinuria (muscle injury)

To distinguish between these possibilities, it is necessary to perform urine microscopy.

Proceed to Step 4

STEP 4: *What are the Results of Urine Microscopy?*

To differentiate between the causes of a positive urine dipstick test for blood, it is necessary to perform urine microscopy. Hematuria is present when microscopic analysis of the urine reveals the presence of red blood cells. Normal urine contains a small number of red blood cells. Just what constitutes the upper limit of normal, however, is widely debated. Although a consensus definition of hematuria is lacking, many authorities consider the presence of >3 red blood cells per high power field to be abnormal.

When the urine dipstick test is positive for blood but urine microscopy is negative for red blood cells, the clinician should suspect one of the following:

- Hemoglobinuria
- Myoglobinuria
- Lysis of red blood cells in the urine

When a patient with a positive urine dipstick test for blood but negative urine microscopy for red blood cells is encountered, it is essential to exclude hemoglobinuria (hemolysis) and myoglobinuria. The following table provides information in differentiating myoglobinuria and hemoglobinuria from hematuria.

	Urine Dipstick	Urine RBC	Serum Supernatant	LDH	Bilirubin	CPK
Hematuria	(+)	(+)	Clear	NL	NL	NL
Hemoglobinuria	(+)	(−)	Pink	Increased	Increased	NL
Myoglobinuria	(+)	(−)	Clear	NL	NL	Increased

Adapted from Desai SP and Isa-Pratt S, *Clinicians's Guide to Laboratory Medicine*, Hudson, OH: Lexi-Comp Inc, 2000, 525.

Once hemoglobinuria and myoglobinuria have been excluded, the clinician should consider the possibility that the discrepancy between the urine dipstick test result and the number of red blood cells seen during microscopy reflects red blood cell lysis. Red blood cells are more likely to lyse in hypotonic urine (specific gravity <1.008) or highly alkaline urine (pH >6.5). Red blood cell lysis should not be ignored because it may signify the presence of true hematuria.

Because of the limitations of the urine dipstick test for blood, every patient thought to have hematuria, whether gross or microscopic, should have microscopic analysis of the urine to verify the presence of hematuria.

If the patient has hemoglobinuria or myoglobinuria, *Stop Here.*

If the patient has hematuria, *Proceed to Step 5.*

STEP 5: *What are the Causes of Hematuria?*

The causes of hematuria are either intrarenal or extrarenal. Intrarenal hematuria can be of glomerular or nonglomerular origin. The nonglomerular causes of intrarenal hematuria include:

Intrarenal Causes of Nonglomerular Hematuria	
Familial	Papillary necrosis
Medullary cystic or sponge disease	Analgesic abuse
Polycystic kidney disease	Diabetes mellitus
Hydronephrosis	Obstructive uropathy
Malignancy	Sickle cell disease or trait
Metabolic	Trauma
Hypercalciuria	Vascular
Hyperuricosuria	Malignant hypertension
	Renal infarct
	Renal vein thrombosis

The glomerular causes of intrarenal hematuria include:

Intrarenal Causes of Glomerular Hematuria	
Primary	Secondary
Alport's syndrome	Anti-GBM disease
Focal segmental glomerulosclerosis	Hemolytic-uremic syndrome
IgA nephropathy	Henoch-Schönlein purpura
Membranous nephropathy	Mixed essential cryoglobulinemia
Membranoproliferative	Postinfectious glomerulonephritis
glomerulonephritis	Systemic lupus erythematosus
Minimal change disease	Vasculitis
Rapidly progressive glomerulonephritis	
Thin basement membrane disease	

The extrarenal causes of hematuria include:

Extrarenal Causes of Hematuria	
Bleeding Disorder	Malignancy
Infection	Prostatic adenocarcinoma
Cystitis	Transitional cell cancer of the urinary tract
Prostatitis	Medications
Schistosomiasis	Anticoagulants
Tuberculosis	Cyclophosphamide
Urethritis	Stones
	Trauma

Proceed to Step 6

STEP 6: *Are There Any Clinical Clues to Suggest the Etiology of the Hematuria?*

While there are many causes of hematuria, a thorough history and physical examination can be invaluable in elucidating the etiology.

Historical Clues	Condition Suggested
Burning, urgency, frequency	Urinary tract infection
Painless gross hematuria	Noninfectious origin Urinary tract malignancy
Initial gross hematuria that clears with voiding	Anterior urethral source
Initial clear urine followed by terminal gross hematuria	Prostatic source of bleed
Urinary blood clots	Nonglomerular hematuria
Weight loss	Urinary tract malignancy
Recurrent loin or lumbar pain in female	Loin pain – hematuria syndrome
Hemoptysis	Goodpasture's syndrome SLE
Arthritis / arthralgia	Vasculitis Henoch-Schönlein purpura SLE
Rash	Vasculitis Henoch-Schönlein purpura SLE
Flank pain	Upper urinary tract calculi Ureteral colic from blood clots Ureteral colic from sloughed renal papillae (papillary necrosis) Renal infarction
Medication history	Anticoagulant therapy Aspirin NSAIDs Cyclophosphamide

(Continued)

(continued)

Historical Clues	Condition Suggested
Radiation therapy	Hemorrhagic cystitis
Recent contact or noncontact sports	Exercise-related hematuria
Foreign travel	Schistosomiasis; malaria
Recent upper respiratory infection	Poststreptococcal glomerulonephritis IgA nephropathy MPGN
African-American background	Sickle cell trait
Family history of hematuria and/or renal disease	Sickle cell hemoglobinopathy Alport's syndrome Benign familial hematuria Polycystic kidney disease
Family history of deafness and/or ocular defects	Alport's syndrome

Clues in the physical examination that point to the etiology of the hematuria are listed in the following table.

Physical Exam Finding	Condition Suggested
Elevated blood pressure	Glomerular disease
Fever	Infectious origin Acute prostatitis Acute cystitis Acute pyelonephritis
Palpable kidney	Renal cell cancer
Flank tenderness	Acute pyelonephritis Ureteral calculi
Palpable bladder after voiding	Incomplete bladder emptying from outflow obstruction BPH Urethral stricture Prostate cancer Acute prostatitis
Peripheral edema	Glomerular disease
Mass on pelvic examination	Cancer of vagina or uterus invading the bladder
Tenderness on rectal examination	Acute prostatitis
Mass on rectal examination	Prostate cancer Rectal cancer invading the bladder

If clinical clues are suggestive of a particular disease, the clinician can tailor the investigation accordingly.

If clinical clues are not present, ***Proceed to Step 7.***

STEP 7: *Does the Patient Have a Urinary Tract Infection?*

Dysuria, urinary frequency, and fever are common complaints in patients with a urinary tract infection. However, urinary tract infections may be asymptomatic as well. As a result, in every patient presenting with gross or microscopic hematuria, the possibility of a urinary tract infection should be entertained. The presence of pyuria and bacteriuria supports the diagnosis. A urine culture is not needed in every case of urinary tract infection. For example, it is not necessary in the female presenting with an uncomplicated urinary tract infection.

If obtained, a urine culture usually reveals growth of a single organism. A negative urine culture, in the presence of pyuria, should prompt consideration of tuberculosis or urethritis.

At the completion of a course of antibiotic therapy, urinalysis should be repeated several times to ensure resolution of the hematuria.

If hematuria resolves after appropriate antibiotic therapy, **Stop Here**.

If hematuria persists, **Proceed to Step 8**.

STEP 8: *What are the Results of the PT and PTT?*

If the PT and PTT are normal, **Proceed to Step 9**.

Hematuria may be the result of a systemic bleeding disorder. In most cases, there will be manifestations of bleeding elsewhere. Documentation of a normal PT and PTT will help exclude this possibility.

Hematuria that develops during anticoagulation also deserves mention here. Hematuria is not uncommon in patients being treated with heparin or Coumadin®, but other etiologies must be ruled out before attributing hematuria solely to anticoagulation therapy.

Proceed to Step 9

STEP 9: *Does the Patient Have Sickle Cell Trait / Disease?*

Patients with sickle cell trait are usually asymptomatic, but occasionally, painless hematuria may occur. A hemoglobin electrophoresis should be performed to exclude this diagnosis in African-American patients presenting with hematuria. Of note, in the older patient with sickle cell trait, hematuria should not be merely attributed to the sickle cell trait. Rather, an investigation (outlined below) should be done to exclude other more serious etiologies.

Proceed to Step 10

STEP 10: *Is the Hematuria of Glomerular or Nonglomerular Origin?*

The following support a glomerular origin of the hematuria:

- Red blood cell casts
- Dysmorphic or "distorted" red blood cells
- Protein excretion >500 mg/day

292

It is important to note that the absence of these features does not exclude hematuria of glomerular origin.

If the hematuria is glomerular in origin, ***Proceed to Step 11***.

If the hematuria is nonglomerular in origin, ***Proceed to Step 12***.

STEP 11: *What Tests Should be Obtained to Determine the Etiology of Glomerular Hematuria?*

The differential diagnosis of glomerular hematuria is long and has been described earlier in this section. Definitive diagnosis can only be established by renal biopsy. However, the need for renal biopsy is controversial. There is no evidence to suggest that renal biopsy will alter treatment or prognosis in this group of patients unless the patient has hypertension, decreased renal function, or proteinuria. In the absence of these features, the clinician should evaluate the patient periodically with the following tests:

- Blood pressure
- Serum BUN and creatinine
- Creatinine clearance
- 24-hour urine collection for protein

The development of hypertension, renal insufficiency, or worsening protein-uria should prompt consideration of a renal biopsy.

Depending on the patient's clinical presentation, other tests may be helpful in elucidating the etiology of the hematuria. These laboratory abnormalities and their associated disease states are listed in the following table:

Laboratory Abnormalities	Condition Suggested
Decreased C3 level	SLE Cryoglobulinemia Poststreptococcal glomerulonephritis Postinfectious glomerulonephritis Membranoproliferative glomerulonephritis
Positive ANA	SLE
Positive antistreptolysin O (ASO) Positive anti-DNase B Positive antihyaluronidase Positive antistreptokinase	Poststreptococcal glomerulonephritis
Positive ANCA	Wegener's glomerulonephritis Microscopic polyarteritis Idiopathic crescentic necrotizing glomerulonephritis
Positive anti-GBM	Anti-GBM nephritis Goodpasture's syndrome
Increased cryoglobulins	Cryoglobulinemia
Positive hepatitis C antibody	Hepatitis C associated membranoproliferative glomerulonephritis

End of Section.

STEP 12: *What are the Results of the Intravenous Pyelography Study (IVP)?*

Intravenous pyelography (IVP) is the test of choice in evaluating the patient with nonglomerular hematuria. There are, however, some investigators who argue that the sensitivity of ultrasound is equivalent to that of IVP in the detection and characterization of masses in the renal parenchyma, and that it should replace IVP as the gold standard. However, IVP appears to be superior in detection of subtle abnormalities in the renal collecting system, and in the detection of urothelial malignancies of the upper urinary tract. As a result, IVP continues to be the initial test of choice.

If the IVP is positive, *Stop Here*.

If the IVP is negative, *Proceed to Step 13*.

STEP 13: *Which Patients Should Have a Cystoscopy?*

Many investigators have questioned the role of cystoscopy in the younger patient with nonglomerular hematuria. While there is no doubt that cystoscopy is the gold standard in the detection of bladder malignancy, the likelihood of finding a malignant lesion in the younger patient is quite low. As a result, cystoscopy is recommended in the younger patient (<40 years of age) only if one or more of the following risk factors for bladder cancer are present:

Risk Factors for Bladder Cancer	
Cigarette smoking	Occupational exposure
Cyclophosphamide	Aniline dyes
Pelvic irradiation	Aromatic amines
Urinary schistosomiasis	Benzidine

If these factors are not present in the patient <40 years of age, *Proceed to Step 15*.

Cystoscopy should be performed in the younger patient with risk factors for bladder cancer or in the older patient with nonglomerular hematuria.

If cystoscopy is positive, *Stop Here*.

If cystoscopy is negative, *Proceed to Step 14*.

STEP 14: *What are the Results of the Urine Cytology?*

Diagnosis can be established in the majority of patients who receive a full evaluation (ie, IVP, cystoscopy). However, in a minority of patients, a diagnosis cannot be established. Unfortunately, there are no consensus guidelines as to how these patients should be further evaluated. Should cystoscopy and IVP be performed again? If so, when and how often should these tests be performed?

There are no easy answers to these questions. Some studies have found that hematuria can predate the diagnosis of bladder cancer by many years. It is possible, then, that patients with hematuria who have had a negative initial evaluation are at increased risk for bladder cancer in the future. It seems reasonable to manage these patients in consultation with a urologist. In most cases, these patients will have a repeat evaluation.

It is also important to send the urine for cytology in the patient with a negative evaluation. Occasionally, urine cytology may be positive in the patient with unexplained hematuria. Such a patient may have a very superficial bladder cancer or carcinoma *in situ*. These lesions may not have been grossly evident during cystoscopy. Multiple biopsies and washings may aid in establishing the diagnosis.

In the event that repeat evaluation is unrevealing, consideration should be given to hypercalciuria, hyperuricosuria, and mild glomerulopathy as the cause of hematuria. A 24-hour urine collection for uric acid and calcium can establish the diagnosis of hyperuricosuria and hypercalciuria, respectively. Treatment with thiazide diuretics or allopurinol for hypercalciuria or hyperuricosuria, respectively, may lead to the resolution of hematuria. If the 24-hour urine collection is unrevealing, then a mild glomerulopathy may be present. The most common glomerular diseases include IgA nephropathy, thin basement membrane disease, and Alport's syndrome.

End of Section.

> **STEP 15: *What are the Results of the 24-Hour Urine Collection for Calcium and Uric Acid?***

In younger patients without risk factors for bladder cancer, it is not necessary to do cystoscopy. In these patients, the most likely diagnoses include hyper-calciuria, hyperuricosuria, or a mild glomerulopathy. Hypercalciuria and hyperuricosuria can be diagnosed with a 24-hour urine collection for calcium and uric acid, respectively. Treatment with thiazide diuretics and allopurinol can lead to resolution of hematuria if hypercalciuria and hyperuricosuria are the suspected etiologies. If the 24-hour urine collection is unrevealing, then the patient likely has a glomerular lesion. Glomerular diseases that often present with isolated hematuria include IgA nephropathy, thin basement membrane disease, and Alport's syndrome.

End of Section.

REFERENCES

Ahmed Z and Lee J, "Asymptomatic Urinary Abnormalities. Hematuria and Proteinuria," *Med Clin North Am*, 1997, 81(3):641-52.

Bryden AA, Paul AB, and Kyriakides C, "Investigation of Haematuria," *Br J Hosp Med*, 1995, 54(9):455-8.

Desai SP and Isa-Pratt S, *Clinicians's Guide to Laboratory Medicine,* Hudson, OH: Lexi-Comp Inc, 2000, 525.

Fogazzi GB and Ponticelli C, "Microscopic Hematuria Diagnosis and Management," *Nephron*, 1996, 72(2):125-34 (review).

Grossfeld GD and Carroll PR, "Evaluation of Asymptomatic Microscopic Hematuria," *Urol Clin North Am*, 1998, 25(4):661-76.

Hall CL, "The Patient With Haematuria," *Practitioner*, 1999, 243(1600):564-6, 568, 570-1.

McCarthy JJ, "Outpatient Evaluation of Hematuria: Locating the Source of Bleeding," *Postgrad Med*, 1997, 101(2):125-8, 131.

Rockall AG, Newman-Sanders AP, al-Kutabima, et al, "Haematuria," *Postgrad Med J*, 1997, 73(857):129-36.

Thaller TR and Wang LP, "Evaluation of Asymptomatic Microscopic Hematuria in Adults," *Am Fam Phys*, 1999, 60(4):1143-52, 1154.

Webb JA, "Imaging in Haematuria," *Clin Radiol*, 1997, 52(3):167-71 (review).

HEMATURIA

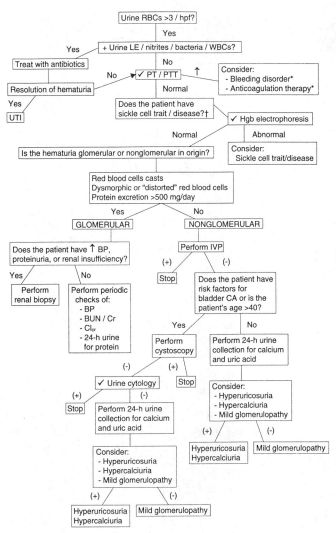

*Hematuria that occurs in the patient with an elevated PT/PTT may be the result of anticoagulation therapy or a bleeding disorder. However, an underlying structural etiology cannot be excluded.

†Sickle cell trait/disease may be the sole cause of hematuria; however, this diagnosis must be one of exclusion.

HEMOPTYSIS

STEP 1: *Does the Patient Have Hemoptysis?*

Hemoptysis refers to the expectoration of blood from a source below the vocal cords. Not all expectorated blood originates from the respiratory tract. At times, it may be difficult to differentiate blood originating from the gastrointestinal tract from hemoptysis. The features listed in the following table may allow the clinician to make the distinction between hematemesis and hemoptysis.

	Hemoptysis	Hematemesis
Appearance	Bright red (at times, frothy)	Dark red/brown
pH	Alkaline	Acidic
Mixed with _____	Mixed with sputum containing white blood cells	Mixed with food particles
Respiratory symptoms	Often present	Usually absent
Dyspepsia	Usually absent	Often present

It may also be difficult to separate an upper (source above the vocal cords) from a lower respiratory tract source of bleeding. Once again, a thorough history and physical examination is the key. In patients with a lower respiratory tract source of bleeding, the expectoration of blood often follows coughing.

When the patient complains of blood pooling in the mouth or the need to clear the throat, the clinician should suspect an upper airway source of bleeding. Particularly helpful is a history of epistaxis, which is very suggestive of an upper airway source. A nasopharyngeal source should be suspected when patients complain of hemoptysis that primarily occurs in the morning after sleeping or worsens in the supine position.

It is important to look carefully at the mouth, nose, and pharynx because, in some cases, a source of bleeding may be obvious upon inspection of these areas. When there is uncertainty as to whether the patient has an upper or lower respiratory source of bleeding, the clinician may elect to consult ENT for rhinoscopy and laryngoscopy.

If the patient has hematemesis, proceed to the chapter on Hematemesis *on page 259*.

If the patient has an upper respiratory tract source of bleeding, ***Stop Here.***

If the patient has hemoptysis, ***Proceed to Step 2.***

STEP 2: *Does the Patient Have Massive Hemoptysis?*

Uncommonly, hemoptysis may be massive. When present, massive hemoptysis is a potentially life-threatening condition. In these patients, the airways and alveoli may become filled with blood, leading to respiratory failure or asphyxiation.

Just what satisfies the definition of massive hemoptysis continues to be debated. Although a widely accepted definition is not available, some consider the expectoration of over 100 mL/24 hours to represent massive hemoptysis. Others maintain that massive hemoptysis is not present until at least 600 mL has been expectorated in a 24-hour period. However, the actual amount of blood expectorated can be difficult to determine clinically. Reasons why the history is often inaccurate in determining the amount of blood lost include the following:

- Patients are often unreliable in quantifying the amount of blood loss

- Expectoration of blood is usually accompanied by sputum, making it difficult to determine how much of expectorated volume is blood

- Blood that is coughed up may be swallowed

Therefore, it may be wise to define massive hemoptysis as that which leads or has the potential to lead to an embarrassment in pulmonary function and gas exchange. It is important to identify patients with massive hemoptysis because it is an emergency, requiring rapid diagnosis and management.

If the patient does not have massive hemoptysis, **Proceed to Step 3.**

If the patient has massive hemoptysis, **Proceed to Step 10.**

STEP 3: What are the Causes of Hemoptysis?

The many causes of hemoptysis are listed in the following box.

Causes of Hemoptysis	
Airway diseases	Parenchymal disease
Malignancy	Infection
Bronchial carcinoma	Aspergilloma
Metastatic malignancy	Lung abscess
Other primary lung cancers	Pneumonia
Inflammatory diseases	(bacterial, fungal, parasitic)
Acute bronchitis	Tuberculosis
Bronchiectasis	Inflammatory disorders
Chronic bronchitis	Behcet's syndrome
Foreign body	Goodpasture's syndrome
Trauma	Henoch-Schönlein purpura
Vascular-bronchial fistula	Idiopathic pulmonary
	hemosiderosis
Cryptogenic	Systemic lupus erythematosus
	Wegener's granulomatosis
Vascular disorders	Coagulopathy
Arteriovenous malformation	Anticoagulant use
Congestive heart failure (LV failure)	Thrombocytopenia
Mitral stenosis	Iatrogenic
Pulmonary artery rupture	Percutaneous lung biopsy
(from Swan-Ganz catheter)	Transbronchial lung biopsy
Pulmonary embolism / infarction	Miscellaneous
	Catamenial
	Cocaine

Despite the large number of conditions that may be associated with hemoptysis, the clinician should realize that the majority of cases are caused by a few of these conditions. Over the years, many studies have been done to determine how common the above causes are in patients presenting with hemoptysis. The results of these studies can be pooled together, yielding information about the final diagnoses in patients presenting with hemoptysis. The following table summarizes the data from these studies.

Final Diagnosis	Approximate Percentage of Cases Attributed to the Diagnosis (%)
Malignancy	25
Cryptogenic	20
Bronchiectasis	18
Miscellaneous	14
Bronchitis	13
Bacterial pneumonia	5
Tuberculosis	5

Adapted from *Comprehensive Respiratory Medicine*, Albert R, Spiro S, and Jett J (eds), St Louis, MO: Mosby, 1999, 4.17.3.

Proceed to Step 4

STEP 4: *Are There Any Historical Clues That Point to the Etiology of the Hemoptysis?*

Historical clues that may point to the etiology of the hemoptysis are listed in the following table.

Historical Clue	Condition Suggested
Tobacco use	Bronchial carcinoma
Recurrent hemoptysis in younger nonsmoking adult	Carcinoid
Known malignancy	Metastatic lung disease Primary lung cancer
Asbestos exposure	Bronchial carcinoma
Recent trauma	Trauma
Alcoholism	Aspiration pneumonia Lung abscess Foreign body
Illicit drug use	Aspiration pneumonia Lung abscess Foreign body
Loss of or impairment in consciousness	Aspiration pneumonia Foreign body Lung abscess
Swallowing disorder	Aspiration pneumonia Foreign body Lung abscess
Risk factors for pulmonary embolism	Pulmonary embolism / infarction
History of deep venous thrombosis	Pulmonary embolism / infarction
Weight loss	Lung abscess Malignancy Tuberculosis

(continued)

(continued)

Historical Clue	Condition Suggested
Fever	Lung abscess Pneumonia
Hematuria	Goodpasture's syndrome Other types of vasculitis Wegener's granulomatosis
Pleuritic chest pain	Pneumonia Pulmonary embolism / infarction
History of rheumatic fever	Mitral stenosis
Immigrant or traveler from Asia, Middle East, or South America	Hyatid cyst Paragonimiasis
Paroxysmal nocturnal dyspnea Orthopnea	Congestive heart failure (LV failure) Mitral stenosis
Occurring with menstruation	Catamenial (Endometriosis)
Chronic cough productive of sputum	Bronchiectasis Chronic bronchitis
Foul-smelling sputum	Lung abscess Necrotizing pneumonia
Sinusitis	Wegener's granulomatosis
History of cavitary or bullous disease secondary to tuberculosis, fungal infection, sarcoidosis, or COPD	Aspergilloma

Some of the more common causes of hemoptysis are discussed in further detail below.

Neoplasm

Malignancy is a common cause of hemoptysis, occurring in up to 30% of cases. Most of these cases are due to bronchial carcinoma, particularly squamous cell carcinoma because of its propensity to affect central airways. Typically, the hemoptysis associated with bronchial carcinoma is characterized by at least several weeks of coughing up blood-streaked sputum. In the patient with lung cancer, hemoptysis does not imply advanced or metastatic disease. In some, the tumor is resectable.

Other pulmonary malignancies that can cause hemoptysis, albeit less commonly, include bronchial carcinoid, hamartoma, and adenoma. Bronchial carcinoid should be more of a consideration in the nonsmoking younger adult who presents with recurrent hemoptysis.

Metastases to the lung are usually not associated with hemoptysis because most metastatic lesions tend to be peripheral. However, certain malignancies including melanoma, breast, colorectal, and kidney cancer have a tendency to metastasize to the bronchi. In these cases, hemoptysis may occur in the setting of metastatic disease.

Kaposi's sarcoma, which is mainly a concern in HIV patients, may also be associated with hemoptysis.

Infection

Bacterial, viral, fungal, and parasitic infections of the lung may be associated with hemoptysis. Although hemoptysis may be a clinical symptom of any bacterial pneumonia, its presence should prompt the clinician to consider *S.*

pneumoniae, S. aureus, P. aeruginosa, K. pneumoniae, and anaerobic organisms. Viral infections are a rare cause of hemoptysis with the exception of varicella pneumonia.

Of the different types of fungal infections of the lung, an aspergilloma or mycetoma (fungus ball) has the highest frequency of associated hemoptysis. In fact, hemoptysis occurs in up to 50% of cases. Hemoptysis may also occur in other fungal infections of the lung, particularly those that are angio-invasive. These include aspergillosis and mucormycosis.

Tuberculosis is a major cause of hemoptysis worldwide. Hemoptysis may accompany shortness of breath, fever, and night sweats in patients with cavitary disease. In patients who have a history of treated tuberculosis, hemoptysis may occur because of reactivation, bronchiectasis, mycetoma, or development of a scar carcinoma. Massive hemoptysis is also a concern in patients with tuberculosis, particularly in those who have rupture of a Rasmussen's aneurysm.

Hemoptysis, developing in immigrants who have emigrated to North America, should warrant consideration of paragonimiasis and hyatid cyst. The same considerations are important in travelers returning to North America.

Vascular Disorders

Vascular disorders causing hemoptysis include pulmonary embolism/infarction, arteriovenous malformation, mitral stenosis, congestive heart failure, pulmonary artery rupture, and aortic aneurysm. Hemoptysis accompanied by pleuritic chest pain may be appreciated in patients with pulmonary embolism, particularly when infarction occurs.

Hemoptysis due to mitral stenosis has become less common as the prevalence of rheumatic fever has decreased. Nevertheless, in some cases, hemoptysis is the initial presentation of mitral stenosis.

The expectoration of blood-tinged sputum may also occur in patients with congestive heart failure. When severe, the sputum may be pink and frothy.

On occasion, hemoptysis may be due to an aortic aneurysm which ruptures into the tracheobronchial tree.

Arteriovenous malformations may be congenital or acquired. Congenital lesions may occur alone or as part of the Osler-Weber-Rendu syndrome (hereditary hemorrhagic telangiectasia). Acquired lesions are usually iatrogenic or due to trauma. Both congenital and acquired arteriovenous malformations may be associated with hemoptysis.

Acute Bronchitis

Inflammatory disease of the bronchi such as acute bronchitis is a common cause of hemoptysis. Most commonly, acute bronchitis is due to viral infection with coronavirus, rhinovirus, adenovirus, and influenza being the leading etiologies. Bacterial bronchitis may be due to *M. pneumoniae, C. pneumoniae*, and *B. pertussis*. A nonproductive cough is common early in the course, often giving way to the expectoration of purulent sputum. Hemoptysis may also occur. It is important, however, to exclude other causes of hemoptysis in these patients.

Bronchiectasis

In the past, symptoms of bronchiectasis would occur in childhood, the result of infection due to measles, pertussis, necrotizing pneumonia, and tuberculosis. With widespread immunization and readily available antibiotics, bronchiectasis has become much less of a problem. Currently, most cases are due to some underlying anatomic or functional abnormality. Nearly 50% of patients have cystic fibrosis.

The hallmark of bronchiectasis is a cough productive of purulent sputum. Sputum production tends to be worse in the morning, mainly because it accumulates during the night while the patient is recumbent. Not uncommonly, patients have exacerbations due to viral infection, bacterial infection, or bronchial plugging. These exacerbations may be characterized by fever, worsening cough, increased sputum production, and shortness of breath. Hemoptysis, which was a more common feature of bronchiectasis in the past, may also be appreciated.

Trauma

Hemoptysis can occur in both penetrating and nonpenetrating injuries of the chest wall.

Proceed to Step 5

STEP 5: *Are There Any Clues in the Patient's Physical Examination That Point to the Etiology of the Hemoptysis?*

Clues in the patient's physical examination that point to the etiology of the hemoptysis are listed in the following table.

Physical Examination Finding	Condition Suggested
Saddle nose	Wegener's granulomatosis
Nasal septal perforation	Wegener's granulomatosis
Oral ulceration	Behcet's syndrome
Genital ulceration	Behcet's syndrome
Uveitis	Behcet's syndrome
Cutaneous nodules or pustules	Behcet's syndrome
Telangiectasias of lip, buccal mucosa, skin	Hereditary hemorrhagic telangiectasia
Unilateral leg edema	Deep venous thrombosis (pulmonary embolism/infarction)
Scattered ecchymoses Multiple petechiae	Coagulopathy
Clubbing	Bronchial carcinoma Bronchiectasis Lung abscess
Bronchial breath sounds	Pneumonia
Localized wheeze	Bronchial carcinoma Foreign body
Pleural rub	Pneumonia Pulmonary embolism / infarction

(continued)

Physical Examination Finding	Condition Suggested
Diastolic murmur	Mitral stenosis
Ventricular gallop	Congestive heart failure (LV failure)
Localized decrease in breath sounds	Bronchial carcinoma Foreign body

Proceed to Step 6

STEP 6: *What are the Results of the Laboratory Studies?*

Laboratory tests that are useful in the patient presenting with hemoptysis include the following:

- Hemoglobin
- Urinalysis
- BUN, creatinine
- Platelet count
- PT, PTT

Proceed to Step 7

STEP 7: *What are the Results of the CXR?*

The first imaging test performed in the evaluation of hemoptysis is usually the chest radiograph. Chest radiographic findings and their diagnostic significance are listed in the following table.

Chest Radiograph Finding	Condition Suggested
Nodule(s) or mass(es)	Amyloidosis Bronchial carcinoma Fungal infection Lung abscess Other malignancy Wegener's granulomatosis
Atelectasis	Bronchial carcinoma Broncholithiasis Foreign body Other malignancy
Hilar / mediastinal lymphadenopathy	Amyloidosis Bronchial carcinoma Fungal infection Mycobacterial infection Other malignancy Sarcoidosis
Dilated peripheral airways	Bronchiectasis
Air-space consolidation	Alveolar hemorrhage Bronchiolitis obliterans with organizing pneumonia Pneumonia Pulmonary contusion

(Continued)

(continued)

Chest Radiograph Finding	Condition Suggested
Reticulonodular densities	Amyloidosis Lymphangioleiomyomatosis Lymphangitic carcinoma Sarcoidosis
Cavity	Bronchial carcinoma Fungal infection Lung abscess Mycetoma Mycobacterial infection
Hilar/mediastinal calcification	Broncholithiasis Previous mycobacterial or fungal infection

Adapted from *Comprehensive Respiratory Medicine*, Albert R, Spiro S, and Jett J (eds), St Louis, MO: Mosby, 1999, 4.17.3.

When a chest radiograph is obtained, an abnormal or localizing finding is noted in about 60% of cases. A normal or nonlocalizing chest radiograph is obtained in about 40% of cases. The term "nonlocalizing" refers to the presence of abnormal but nonspecific findings. Chest radiographic findings that are considered to be nonlocalizing are listed in the following box.

Chest Radiographic Findings Considered to be Nonlocalizing	
Cardiomegaly	Increased peribronchial markings
Hilar fullness	Minimal granulomatous changes
Hyperinflation	Tortuous aorta

Chest radiographic findings considered to be localizing are listed in the following box.

Chest Radiographic Findings Considered to be Localizing	
Cavity	Mass
Localized atelectasis	Pleural effusion

This categorization of the chest radiographic findings into localizing and nonlocalizing is important in estimating the patient's risk of having a malignancy. Less than 5% of cases with nonlocalizing or normal chest radiographs are subsequently found to have malignancy. When localizing findings are present, however, malignancy is diagnosed in close to 40% of cases.

At this point in the patient's evaluation, the clinician should decide if the history, physical examination, and CXR are suggestive of a diagnosis. In particular, the clinician should determine the likelihood of the following conditions:

- Pulmonary embolism
- Pneumonia
- Congestive heart failure

If one of the above conditions are likely, then the clinician should direct the work-up accordingly. In the patient suspected of having pulmonary embolism, the clinician may elect to perform ventilation-perfusion lung scanning. Echocardiogram may be warranted in the patient whose clinical presentation is suggestive of congestive heart failure. Sputum Gram's stain/culture and blood culture are reasonable tests in the patient with pneumonia.

If the patient's presentation raises concern for congestive heart failure, pneumonia, or pulmonary embolism, the clinician should tailor the work-up accordingly.

In all other patients, the clinician should base further testing on the results of the CXR.

If the CXR is normal or nonlocalizing, *Proceed to Step 8*.

If the CXR is abnormal or localizing, *Proceed to Step 9*.

STEP 8: *Does the Patient Need to Have Fiberoptic Bronchoscopy?*

A normal or nonlocalizing chest radiograph is not uncommon in patients presenting with hemoptysis, occurring in 20% to 30% of cases. Causes of hemoptysis that may present with a normal chest radiograph are listed in the following box.

Causes of Hemoptysis that May Present with a Normal Chest Radiograph	
Acute bronchitis	Bronchiectasis
Arteriovenous malformation	Chronic bronchitis
Bleeding diathesis/coagulopathy	Endobronchial tuberculosis
Bronchial adenoma	Foreign body
Bronchial carcinoma	Pulmonary embolism
Bronchial endometriosis	

A concern that all clinicians have in this setting is the possibility of bronchial carcinoma that was not apparent on the CXR. Should all of these patients undergo bronchoscopy?

Those who oppose performing bronchoscopy in all these patients maintain that malignancy is found in <5% of patients with normal or nonlocalizing chest radiographic findings. They argue that many of these patients have a benign condition such as acute bronchitis. In an effort to address this issue, some authorities have proposed criteria for bronchoscopy in patients with hemoptysis and normal or nonlocalizing chest radiographic findings. Factors that favor a bronchoscopic examination include the following:

- Age >40 years
- History of hemoptysis >1 week
- History of tobacco smoking
- Chronic cough
- Anemia
- Weight loss

Bronchoscopy reveals the presence of lung cancer in 33% of patients with hemoptysis who have one or more of the above factors. Currently available data suggest that in the absence of these factors, the clinician may elect to forgo bronchoscopy unless the patient develops recurrent episodes of hemoptysis. In the absence of recurrent episodes of hemoptysis, the clinician may still wish to perform bronchoscopy if any of the following hold true:

- Patient requires reassurance that malignancy is not present
- Adequate follow-up cannot be assured

In these cases, the clinician may wish to perform a CT scan prior to bronchoscopy. CT scan and bronchoscopy are considered to be complementary tests in the evaluation of hemoptysis. Of particular concern in patients with a normal or nonlocalizing chest radiograph is the ability of the CT scan to identify endobronchial lesions that may represent malignancy. Studies have revealed that false-negative results are uncommon unless the endobronchial lesion is <2 mm in diameter. Lesions that are this small are unlikely to give rise to clinically apparent bleeding.

CT scanning has been found to be superior to the chest radiograph in the detection of abnormalities in the following areas:

- Mediastinum
- Central airways
- Peripheral airways
- Lung parenchyma

The CT scan will identify an abnormality in nearly 50% of patients who have a normal or nonlocalizing chest radiograph. In these cases, the more common findings noted on CT scan include bronchiectasis, pulmonary nodule, and cavitary disease.

End of Section.

STEP 9: *What are the Results of the CT Scan?*

Even when the CXR is localizing or abnormal, CT scan is often necessary for the following reasons:

- CT scan may identify a new source of hemoptysis
- CT scan may provide more information about an abnormality detected on the chest radiograph

In many of these cases, bronchoscopy will be necessary to obtain a tissue diagnosis. In these cases, the yield of the bronchoscopic study will be increased if a CT scan is performed first. This is largely due to the fact that the results of the CT scan can help guide the bronchoscopic examination, especially when bronchial and transbronchial biopsies are planned. The yield of biopsy will be optimized in patients who have a CT scan preceding bronchoscopy. In other cases, the CT scan findings may suggest that it is preferable to perform percutaneous needle biopsy rather than bronchoscopy.

End of Section.

STEP 10: *What are the Causes of Massive Hemoptysis?*

Although any cause of hemoptysis can result in massive hemoptysis, the more common causes are listed in the following box.

Common Causes of Massive Hemoptysis	
Tuberculosis	Bronchial carcinoma
Bronchiectasis	Lung abscess
Mycetoma	Vascular-bronchial fistula

Proceed to Step 11

STEP 11: *Is the Patient Stable Hemodynamically and is the Airway Adequately Controlled?*

Patients with massive hemoptysis should be placed in the intensive care unit. The early management of these patients should revolve around the following two questions:

1. Is there any compromise in the patient's oxygenation?
2. How brisk is the bleeding?

When bleeding is brisk or oxygenation is compromised, the clinician should consider endotracheal intubation, preferably with a size 8 or larger caliber endotracheal tube. These considerations should preclude any evaluation in the patient with massive hemoptysis.

Once the patient has been stabilized, the clinician should do the following:

- Consult pulmonary specialist
- Consult thoracic surgery
- Place patient in lateral decubitus position with bleeding side down (if site of bleeding is known)

Proceed to Step 12

STEP 12: *Should the Patient Have Fiberoptic or Rigid Bronchoscopy?*

All patients with massive hemoptysis should have bronchoscopy. It is better to intubate patients with massive hemoptysis prior to bronchoscopy for the following reasons:

- Optimizes airway control
- Allows for effective suctioning if the rate of bleeding accelerates
- Allows for easy removal and reinsertion of the bronchoscope should the suction channel become occluded

Bronchoscopy is important in localizing the site of bleeding. Localization of the bleeding site, which requires visualization of fresh bleeding, is higher in patients who are actively bleeding. Therefore, bronchoscopy should be performed as soon as possible in patients who are actively bleeding. In those who have stopped bleeding, most authorities recommend early bronchoscopy in an effort to increase the yield of the procedure. Not uncommonly, however, bronchoscopy is unrevealing in the absence of active hemorrhage.

There is some debate as to whether clinicians should perform fiberoptic or rigid bronchoscopy in the patient presenting with massive hemoptysis. The differences between fiberoptic and rigid bronchoscopy are listed in the following table.

	Fiberoptic Bronchoscopy	Rigid Bronchoscopy
Anesthesia	Light sedation	General anesthesia
Performed Rapidly	Yes	No
Suctioning	Not as good as rigid	Better than fiberoptic
Visualization of Airways	Excellent	Relatively poor visualization of the lobar and segmental bronchi

Because of the advantages listed in the above table, most authorities recommend fiberoptic over rigid bronchoscopy in the evaluation of massive hemoptysis. However, the clinician may elect to perform rigid bronchoscopy in patients with particularly brisk bleeding, especially if the fiberoptic approach is unlikely to be successful. In addition, rigid bronchoscopy is a consideration in any patient with a suboptimal fiberoptic study.

If the bleeding site is localized, *Proceed to Step 13.*

If the bleeding site is not localized, *Proceed to Step 14.*

STEP 13: *What are the Results of Arteriography?*

Once the bleeding site has been localized, the clinician should then focus on efforts to cease the bleeding and prevent aspiration of the blood into the major airways. The inflation of a balloon catheter under guidance of fiberoptic or rigid bronchoscopy can help protect the airways from the aspiration of blood. Once inflated, the balloon can remain in place for up to a few days. During this time, the patient can be stabilized and plans can be made for more definitive therapy such as arteriographic embolization or surgery.

It is important to understand that endobronchial tamponade described above is only a temporizing measure. Arteriographic embolization and surgical resection are the two major methods available to clinicians to control ongoing hemorrhage. Traditionally, surgery was the treatment of choice but the mortality of 30% that accompanies the surgical treatment of massive hemoptysis has prompted investigators to look more closely at other techniques. In particular, there has been much focus on arteriography.

Recall that the lungs have a dual blood supply, being fed by both the pulmonary and bronchial circulation. Because over 90% of massive hemoptysis cases are due to bleeding from the bronchial circulation, arteriography of the bronchial vessels should be initially performed. Exception to this rule are in patients suspected of having pulmonary embolism, arteriovenous malformation, Rasmussen's aneurysms, iatrogenic pulmonary artery tears (perforation of Swan-Ganz catheter) in which case pulmonary arteriography should be performed first. If findings are consistent with a bleeding lesion, the clinician may elect to perform embolization.

Surgical resection may be indicated if there is failure to control the bleeding using medical and arteriographic techniques. It is also a consideration when arteriography is unavailable.

Once the bleeding has stopped, either spontaneously or by embolization, it is important to identify the cause of the massive hemoptysis. Correctly identifying the cause of the hemoptysis will help prevent recurrence. Recurrence is common, occurring in 10% to 20% of patients who are successfully treated with arteriographic embolization.

End of Section.

STEP 14: *What are the Results of Arteriography?*

When a bleeding site is not localized by bronchoscopy, arteriography should be performed. Although the lungs have a dual blood supply, over 90% of massive hemoptysis cases are due to bleeding from the bronchial circulation. As a result, arteriography of the bronchial circulation should be initially performed. The clinician may elect, however, to perform pulmonary arteriography if there is considerable suspicion for bleeding from the pulmonary circulation, as in the following conditions:

- Pulmonary embolism
- Pulmonary arteriovenous malformations
- Rasmussen's aneurysm
- Iatrogenic pulmonary artery rupture (eg, perforation of Swan-Ganz catheter)

Arteriography not only allows localization of the bleeding site but also permits embolization during the procedure to halt the bleeding.

Once the bleeding stops, spontaneously or through embolotherapy, it behooves the clinician to determine the etiology of the massive hemoptysis. Appropriate treatment of the cause will help prevent recurrence, which has been reported in 10% to 20% of patients who have undergone successful embolotherapy.

REFERENCES

Cahill BC and Ingbar DH, "Massive Hemoptysis. Assessment and Management," *Clin Chest Med*, 1994, 15(1):147-67.

Colice GL, "Hemoptysis. Three Questions That Can Direct Management," *Postgrad Med*, 1996, 100(1):227-36 (review).

Comprehensive Respiratory Medicine, Albert R, Spiro S, and Jett J (eds), St Louis, MO: Mosby, 1999, 4.17.3.

Dweik RA and Stoller JK, "Role of Bronchoscopy in Massive Hemoptysis," *Clin Chest Med*, 1999, 20(1):89-105.

Jean-Baptiste E, "Clinical Assessment and Management of Massive Hemoptysis," *Crit Care Med*, 2000, 28(5):1642-7 (review).

Liebler JM and Markin CJ, "Fiberoptic Bronchoscopy for Diagnosis and Treatment," *Crit Care Clin*, 2000, 16(1):83-100.

Marshall TJ, Flower CD, and Jackson JE, "The Role of Radiology in the Investigation and Management of Patients With Haemoptysis," *Clin Radiol*, 1996, 51(6):391-400 (review).

Tasker AD and Flower CD, "Imaging the Airways. Hemoptysis, Bronchiectasis, and Small Airways Disease," *Clin Chest Med*, 1999, 20(4):761-73.

HEMOPTYSIS

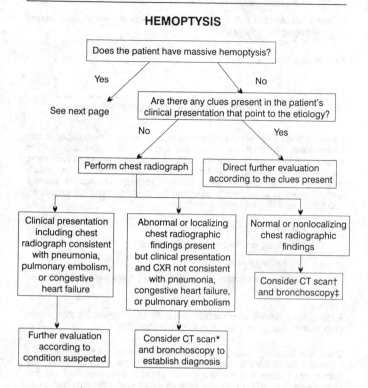

Does the patient have massive hemoptysis?

Yes → See next page

No → Are there any clues present in the patient's clinical presentation that point to the etiology?

No → Perform chest radiograph

Yes → Direct further evaluation according to the clues present

Clinical presentation including chest radiograph consistent with pneumonia, pulmonary embolism, or congestive heart failure

Abnormal or localizing chest radiographic findings present but clinical presentation and CXR not consistent with pneumonia, congestive heart failure, or pulmonary embolism

Normal or nonlocalizing chest radiographic findings

Consider CT scan† and bronchoscopy‡

Further evaluation according to condition suspected

Consider CT scan* and bronchoscopy to establish diagnosis

*CT scan is often necessary even when chest radiographic findings are abnormal or localizing. Reasons for this include the following:
  - CT scan may identify a new source of hemoptysis
  - CT scan may provide more information about an abnormality detected on chest radiograph
  - Yield of bronchoscopy is often increased if CT scan is performed first
†CT scan is superior to the chest radiograph in the detection of abnormalities in the mediastinum, central airways, peripheral airways, and lung parenchyma. An abnormality will be identified in nearly 50% of patients who have a normal or nonlocalizing chest radiograph.
‡Bronchoscopy is not indicated in all patients with normal or nonlocalizing chest radiographs. Many of these patients have acute bronchitis, but since malignancy is a concern in patients with hemoptysis who have normal or nonlocalizing chest radiographs, experts have proposed criteria for bronchoscopy in these patients. Factors favoring bronchoscopy include age >40 years, history of hemoptysis >1 week, history of tobacco smoking, chronic cough, anemia, and weight loss. In those who have had a CT scan, bronchoscopy may be indicated depending upon the abnormalities identified.

HEMOPTYSIS

(continued)

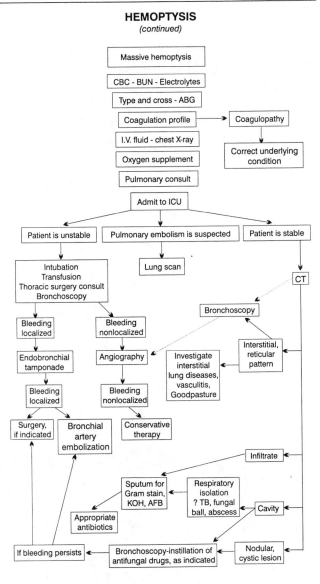

Note: ◄······· indicates, if nondiagnostic

Adapted and modified with permission from Jean-Baptiste E, "Clinical Assessment and Management of Massive Hemoptysis," *Crit Care Med*, 2000, 28(5):1642-7 (review).

HIRSUTISM

STEP 1: *What is Hirsutism?*

Hirsutism is a commonly encountered problem. In the United States, it affects approximately 5% of women. It is defined as excessive growth of hair in androgen-dependent skin sites. These sites include upper lip, chin, chest, areola, linea alba, lower back, buttocks, abdomen, inner thighs, and external genitalia.

Although most patients with hirsutism have a benign underlying condition, on occasion, a serious cause may be present. In addition, the emotional impact of hirsutism in women cannot be taken lightly. As such, hirsutism should never be dismissed as merely a cosmetic problem.

Proceed to Step 2

STEP 2: *Does the Patient Have Normal Hair Growth?*

Hair is present on the upper lip in 33% of women during the reproductive years. Up to 10% have hair on the chin or sideburn area. Whether there is hair growth in these areas depends on familial, race, and ethnic factors. In terms of race, Caucasians have more facial and body hair than do Asians, Native Americans, and African Americans. Even among Caucasians, there are differences in hair growth, with those of Mediterranean ancestry having heavier hair growth than those of Nordic origin.

Age is also a factor in hair growth. Facial hair tends to increase with advancing age, particularly after menopause. With this wide range of normal hair growth, it can be quite challenging for clinicians to differentiate normal hair growth from true hirsutism. What clinicians should be particularly vigilant about is whether the hair growth thought to be excessive is severe or if it is accompanied by signs of virilization. In these settings, hirsutism may be a manifestation of a serious underlying disorder.

One way to gauge severity is based on the Ferriman and Gallwey grading system, which will be discussed in further detail later in this chapter. This grading system assesses the degree of hirsutism based upon the physical examination. Unfortunately, many women remove unwanted hair prior to seeking medical attention, limiting the usefulness of this grading system. The clinician should take this into account when estimating severity of the hirsutism based on physical examination.

If the patient has normal hair growth, *Stop Here.*

If the patient has excessive hair growth, *Proceed to Step 3.*

STEP 3: *Does the Patient Have Hypertrichosis?*

Prior to embarking on an evaluation of hirsutism, the clinician should ensure that the patient does not have hypertrichosis. There are two types of hair in adults: terminal and vellus. Vellus hair is long, fine, soft, and unpigmented. The excessive growth of vellus hair is known as hypertrichosis. It varies from hirsutism not only in the type of hair (vellus versus terminal) but also in the location of the hair growth. Hypertrichosis is characterized by hair growth evenly over the body whereas the hair growth of hirsutism only occurs in androgen-dependent areas. It is important to make this distinction because the causes of hypertrichosis are different from that of hirsutism. The causes of hypertrichosis are listed in the following box.

Causes of Hypertrichosis	
After severe head injury	Medications
Anorexia nervosa	Corticosteroids
Congenital	Cyclosporine
Dermatomyositis	Diazoxide
Hypothyroidism	Hexachlorobenzene
Malnutrition	Minoxidil
Porphyria	Penicillamine
	Phenytoin
	Psoralens
	Streptomycin

If the patient has hypertrichosis, **Stop Here.**

If the patient has hirsutism, **Proceed to Step 4.**

STEP 4: *What are the Causes of Hirsutism?*

The causes of hirsutism are listed in the following box.

Causes of Hirsutism	
Acromegaly	Medications
Congenital adrenal insufficiency	Anabolic steroids
21-hydroxylase deficiency	Cyclosporine*
11-β-hydroxylase deficiency	Danazol
3-β-hydroxysteroid dehydrogenase	Diazoxide*
deficiency	Minoxidil*
Cushing's syndrome	Oral contraceptives
Hyperprolactinemia	Penicillamine
Hyperthecosis	Phenothiazines derivatives
Idiopathic	Phenytoin
Neoplasm	Progestins
Adrenal	(19-nortestosterone derivatives)
Adenoma	Psoralens*
Carcinoma	Streptomycin
Ovarian	Testosterone
Polycystic ovarian syndrome	

*These medications are more commonly associated with hypertrichosis than hirsutism.

Proceed to Step 5

STEP 5: *What is the Frequency of the Causes Listed Above in Adult Hirsute Women?*

The approximate frequency of some of the causes of excessive hair growth in adult hirsute women is shown in the following table.

Condition	Frequency
Adrenal	
Congenital adrenal hyperplasia	
21-hydroxylase deficiency	1%
11-β-hydroxylase deficiency	<1%
3-β-hydroxysteroid dehydrogenase deficiency	<1%
Cushing's syndrome	<1%
Androgen-secreting adrenal tumor	<1%
Ovarian	
Severe insulin resistance	1%
Androgen-secreting ovarian neoplasms	<1%
Combined adrenal and ovarian	95%
Polycystic ovarian syndrome	
Idiopathic hirsutism	
Exogenous androgens	
Anabolic steroids	<1%
Postmenopausal androgen therapy	1%

Adapted from Rittmaster RS, "Hirsutism," *Lancet*, 1997, 349(9046):191-5 (review).

Proceed to Step 6

STEP 6: *Are There Any Clues in the History That Point to the Etiology of the Hirsutism?*

Clues in the patient's history that point to the etiology of the hirsutism are listed in the following table.

Historical Clue	Condition Suggested
Weight loss	Adrenal or ovarian tumor
Peripubertal onset Irregular menses Little or no progression of hirsutism Obesity	Polycystic ovarian syndrome
Ashkenazi Jew Hispanic Yugoslav Italian Eskimo	Consider late-onset congenital adrenal hyperplasia
Offending medication	Medication-induced hirsutism
Rapid progression of hirsutism	Adrenal or ovarian tumor
Peripubertal onset with slow progression	Suggests benign cause
Galactorrhea	Hyperprolactinemia

(Continued)

(continued)

Historical Clue	Condition Suggested
Enlargement of hands and feet (eg, ring becoming too tight) Arthralgias Excessive sweating	Acromegaly
Athlete	Consider anabolic steroids
Positive family history	Polycystic ovarian syndrome Idiopathic hirsutism Late-onset congenital adrenal hyperplasia
Diabetes mellitus	Polycystic ovarian syndrome
Easy bruising	Cushing's syndrome
Muscle weakness	Cushing's syndrome

Proceed to Step 7

STEP 7: *Are There Any Clues in the Patient's Physical Examination That Point to the Etiology of the Hirsutism?*

The Ferriman-Gallwey scoring system grades the amount of hair growth in nine different areas of the body. Each area is scored from 1 to 4 for a maximum score of 36. When the score exceeds 8, hirsutism is said to be present. The method used to evaluate the severity of the hirsutism is shown in the following diagram.

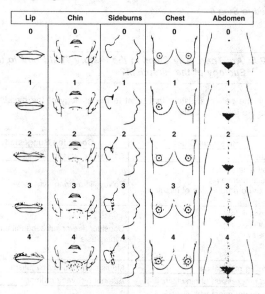

Method of determining degree of hirsutism by hair growth in areas responsive to sex hormone. Score of 8 or more considered beyond normal growth in adult women.

Clues in the patient's physical examination that point to the etiology of the hirsutism are listed in the following table.

Physical Examination Finding	Condition Suggested
Deepening of voice Temporal balding Acne Increased muscle mass Decreased breast size Clitoromegaly	Virilization
Purple abdominal striae	Cushing's syndrome
Thin skin	Cushing's syndrome
Galactorrhea	Hyperprolactinemia
Proximal muscle weakness	Cushing's syndrome
Truncal or centripetal obesity	Cushing's syndrome
Facial plethora	Cushing's syndrome
Dorsocervical hump	Cushing's syndrome
Acanthosis nigricans (brown to black velvety-feeling hyperpigmentation noted on skin of axilla, groin, or neck)	Associated with insulin resistance*
Abdominal mass	Adrenal carcinoma
Ovarian enlargement	Ovarian tumor Polycystic ovarian syndrome
Hypertension	Hirsute women tend to have higher systolic and diastolic blood pressures
Headache Visual field defects	Pituitary tumor (Cushing's disease, acromegaly, prolactinoma)
Greasiness of the skin Coarse features Increased breadth of the nose Thickening of the lips Macroglossia Spade-like hands with sausage-shaped fingers	Acromegaly

*Acanthosis nigricans is commonly noted in obese women who have the polycystic ovarian syndrome. It is a sign of insulin resistance rather than hyperandrogenism.

Proceed to Step 8

STEP 8: *Are There Any Features in the Patient's Clinical Presentation Suggestive of a Serious Cause of Hirsutism?*

Although polycystic ovarian syndrome and idiopathic hirsutism account for about 95% of cases, the clinician must be able to recognize features in the patient's clinical presentation that are suggestive of the less common but potentially serious underlying etiologies such as ovarian or adrenal cancer. These features are listed in the following box.

Clinical Features in the Hirsute Patient That Point to a Serious Underlying Condition	
Abrupt onset of hirsutism	Recent onset of menstrual irregularity
Onset of hirsutism that is not prepubertal	Severe hirsutism*
	Virilization (see box below)
Rapid progression of hirsutism	

*A Ferriman-Gallwey score exceeding 15 is considered by some authorities to represent severe hirsutism.

As indicated in the above box, virilization that accompanies hirsutism is worrisome for a serious underlying cause. Signs of virilization are listed in the following box.

Features of Virilization	
Acne	Decreased breast size
Clitoromegaly*	Increased muscle mass
Crown balding	(especially shoulder girdle)
Deepening of the voice	Loss of female body contour
	Temporal hair recession

*One way to determine if the patient has clitoromegaly is to calculate the clitoral index. This index is calculated by multiplying the vertical and horizontal dimensions of the clitoris. 95% of normal women have a clitoral index that is less than 35 mm^2. An index exceeding 100 mm^2 is very suggestive of a serious underlying disease. Alternatively, the clitoral length may be used, with a value exceeding 10 mm consistent with the presence of clitoromegaly.

In addition, the clinician should determine if the patient has signs and symptoms of Cushing's syndrome. These signs and symptoms are considered in the following box.

Signs and Symptoms of Cushing's Syndrome	
Acne	Hypertension
Central obesity	Hypokalemic metabolic alkalosis
Facial plethora	Proximal muscle weakness
Hirsutism	Psychiatric disorders
Hyperglycemia	Spontaneous ecchymoses
Hyperpigmentation	Wide purple striae

Adapted from Desai SP and Isa-Pratt S, *Clinician's Guide to Laboratory Medicine,* Hudson, OH: Lexi-Comp, Inc, 2000.

If the patient has signs and symptoms of Cushing's syndrome, *Proceed to Step 9.*

If the patient has any clinical features that point to a serious underlying condition (other than Cushing's syndrome), *Proceed to Step 10.*

If the patient does not have any clinical features that point to a serious underlying condition (including Cushing's syndrome), *Proceed to Step 13.*

> ### STEP 9: *What are the Results of the 24-Hour Urine Collection for Cortisol?*

Although Cushing's syndrome is an unusual cause of hirsutism, it needs to be considered, particularly when symptoms and signs of Cushing's syndrome are present. Indeed, most patients with Cushing's syndrome will have characteristic features of steroid excess. The evaluation of the patient suspected of having Cushing's syndrome begins with a 24-hour urine collection for cortisol. Levels exceeding 250-300 µg/day confirms that the patient has Cushing's syndrome. Further evaluation is directed at determining the source of the corticosteroid excess.

End of Section.

> ### STEP 10: *What are the Results of Hormonal Testing?*

When factors are present in the patient's clinical presentation that are suggestive of a serious underlying condition, the clinician should obtain the following tests:

- Testosterone
- Dehdyroepiandrosterone sulfate (DHEA-S)

An elevated serum testosterone level suggests an ovarian cause of hirsutism while an elevated serum DHEA-S level is indicative of an adrenal cause.

If the serum DHEA-S and/or testosterone levels exceed 700 µg/dL and 200 ng/dL, respectively, ***Proceed to Step 11.***

If the serum DHEA-S and testosterone levels are below 700 µg/dL and 200 ng/dL, respectively, ***Proceed to Step 12.***

> ### STEP 11: *Does the Patient Have an Adrenal or Ovarian Tumor?*

A serum DHEA-S level exceeding 700 µg/dL in a hirsute woman should prompt the clinician to consider an adrenal tumor. Both adenomas and carcinomas of the adrenal gland are associated with hirsutism. In these patients, the evaluation begins with a CT or MRI of the adrenal gland. If an adrenal lesion is identified, the size of the lesion may provide a clue as to whether the patient has an adrenal adenoma or carcinoma. When compared to adrenal carcinoma, adenomas tend be smaller. Not uncommonly, adrenal carcinomas reach a large size before diagnosis. Many carcinomas have metastasized by the time of detection. It is important to realize that an elevation of the DHEA-S level to above 700 µg/dL is not specific for an adrenal tumor. Benign conditions can, at times, be associated with such an elevation. In the event that the imaging tests are unrevealing, benign causes of hirsutism should be considered.

A serum testosterone level exceeding 200 ng/dL in a hirsute woman warrants consideration of an ovarian tumor. In many cases, physical examination may reveal a unilateral adnexal mass. Regardless of whether the pelvic exam is consistent with an ovarian neoplasm, these patients should have an ultrasound or CT of the pelvis in an effort to identify an ovarian tumor. When the imaging tests are normal, the clinician should consider the following possibilities:

- False-Negative Imaging Test

  The absence of an ovarian mass on imaging studies does not exclude the diagnosis because small ovarian tumors have been found at the time of laparoscopy or laparotomy in patients with an unremarkable ultrasound or CT study of the pelvis. In cases where the clinician has a high suspicion for an ovarian neoplasm, the clinician may wish to consider laparoscopy or laparotomy.

- Adrenal Neoplasia

  Also worth considering is the possibility of an adrenal cancer. Recall, that the DHEA-S level is markedly elevated in most patients with adrenal cancer. However, some adrenal cancers are associated with normal DHEA-S levels, perhaps due to a loss in their ability to sulfate DHEA. In these types of adrenal cancer, only the testosterone level may be elevated. CT or MRI imaging of the adrenal glands can help exclude this possibility.

When results of the imaging tests are normal, the clinician should consider benign causes of hirsutism. Marked elevations in the serum testosterone level are not specific for ovarian neoplasia. In fact, the insulin resistance that is found in many patients with polycystic ovarian syndrome can cause an elevation in the serum testosterone level to this degree. The benign causes of hirsutism are considered in Step 13.

End of Section.

STEP 12: *What are the Considerations in the Patient Who Has Serum DHEA-S and Testosterone Levels < 700 µg/dL and 200 ng/dL, Respectively?*

It is important to realize that serum DHEA-S and testosterone levels <700 µg/dL and 200 ng/dL, respectively, do not definitively exclude adrenal or ovarian malignancy. However, in the absence of virilization or rapid onset of hirsutism, it is not necessary to pursue further evaluation with imaging studies.

Other possibilities include the following:

- Polycystic ovarian syndrome
- Late-onset congenital adrenal hyperplasia
- Idiopathic hirsutism
- Hyperprolactinemia

In the above conditions, serum testosterone and DHEA-S levels may be normal or elevated (with the exception of idiopathic hirsutism in which levels are always normal). These conditions are discussed further in Step 13.

End of Section.

> **STEP 13:** *What are the Possibilities in the Patient Who Has No Factors Suggestive of a Serious Underlying Etiology?*

Possibilities in the hirsute patient who has no features suggestive of a serious underlying etiology include the following:

Polycystic Ovarian Syndrome

In the United States, polycystic ovarian syndrome affects 5% of women. Patients with the polycystic ovarian syndrome may present with a wide range of clinical manifestations. Features present in the classic syndrome include obesity, anovulation, hirsutism, and bilaterally enlarged, multicystic ovaries. These features, as well as others, are listed in the following box.

Features of the Polycystic Ovarian Syndrome	
Acne	Infertility
Bilateral polycystic ovaries*	Obesity
Hirsutism	Oligomenorrhea / amenorrhea

*The diagnosis of the polycystic ovarian syndrome does not require ultrasound to assess ovarian structure.

The hirsutism of polycystic ovarian syndrome typically begins around the time of menarche. In contrast to ovarian and adrenal tumors, the progression of the hirsutism is slow.

Supportive of the diagnosis is an LH to FSH ratio that exceeds 2.5. Women with normal ovulation usually have a ratio less than 1.0. A ratio exceeding 2.5, however, is not always present in patients with polycystic ovarian syndrome. Indeed, an elevated LH level is neither sensitive nor specific for the diagnosis. Total testosterone levels are elevated in 40% to 60% of patients.

Late-Onset Congenital Adrenal Hyperplasia

Although many patients with congenital adrenal hyperplasia present at an early age, some patients present in adolescence or young adulthood. Late-onset congenital adrenal hyperplasia is an uncommon cause of hirsutism. There are, however, certain ethnic groups in which hirsutism, due to late congenital adrenal hyperplasia, is more common. These groups include Ashkenazi Jews, Italians, Yugoslavs, and Hispanics. Late-onset congenital adrenal hyperplasia is clinically indistinguishable from polycystic ovarian syndrome and idiopathic hirsutism.

In late-onset congenital adrenal hyperplasia, one of several enzymes may be deficient, leading to the accumulation of cortisol precursors. Some of the cortisol precursors have androgenic activity which can lead to hirsutism. The most common form of late-onset congenital adrenal hyperplasia is 21-hydroxylase deficiency, which is thought to account for about 1% of all cases of hirsutism. Establishing a diagnosis of late-onset congenital adrenal hyperplasia is not always necessary because the management of the condition does not differ from other causes of benign hirsutism such as polycystic ovarian syndrome or idiopathic hirsutism. However, if there is a family history of congenital adrenal hyperplasia or the patient is insistent on establishing the diagnosis, testing is available.

To establish the diagnosis of 21-hydroxylase deficiency, a serum 17-hydroxyprogesterone level should be obtained, preferably between the hours of 7 and 9 AM. A level that exceeds 45 nmol/L corroborates the diagnosis while a value below 7 nmol/L excludes this possibility. When levels are intermediate, the clinician can repeat the test before and one hour after the administration of 250 mcg of cosyntropin. The diagnosis is established if the stimulated value exceeds 45 nmol/L.

Idiopathic Hirsutism

Idiopathic hirsutism is a diagnosis of exclusion. Excessive hair growth usually starts shortly after puberty and is characterized by slow progression. Not uncommonly, the hirsutism is accompanied by acne. A family history of hirsutism is common. Hormonal testing is not necessary but, if performed, will reveal normal serum levels of testosterone and DHEA-S. Some consider idiopathic hirsutism to be a mild variant of the polycystic ovarian syndrome.

Medications

The medications that can cause hirsutism are listed in the box in Step 4. In athletes, the clinician should suspect the use of anabolic steroids. Alternatively, hirsutism may be a side effect of prescription medications, many of which are listed in the box in Step 4.

Hyperprolactinemia

In hirsute women with irregular menses and/or galactorrhea, a serum prolactin level should be obtained to evaluate for hyperprolactinemia. Although hyperprolactinemia is associated with hirsutism, the excessive hair growth tends to be mild. Of note, patients with polycystic ovarian syndrome may have elevated serum prolactin levels. Polycystic ovarian syndrome, however, should be a diagnosis of exclusion in hyperprolactinemic patients. First and foremost are efforts to exclude more serious causes of hyperprolactinemia such as pituitary tumor or hypothalamic disease.

REFERENCES

Ahmed B and Jaspan JB, "Hirsutism: A Brief Review," *Am J Med Sci*, 1994, 308(5):289-94.

Chang RJ and Katz SE, "Diagnosis of Polycystic Ovary Syndrome," *Endocrinol Metab Clin North Am*, 1999, 28(2):397-408.

Davis S, "Syndromes of Hyperandrogenism in Women," *Aust Fam Physician*, 1999, 28(5):447-51.

de Berker D, "The Diagnosis and Treatment of Hirsutism," *Practitioner*, 1999, 243(1599):493-8, 501 (review).

Desai SP and Isa-Pratt S, *Clinician's Guide to Laboratory Medicine,* Hudson, OH: Lexi-Comp, Inc, 2000.

Gilchrist VJ and Hecht BR, "A Practical Approach to Hirsutism," *Am Fam Phys*, 1995, 52(6):1837-46.

Kalve E and Klein JF, "Evaluation of Women With Hirsutism," *Am Fam Phys*, 1996, 54(1):117-24 (review).

Marshburn PB and Carr BR, "Hirsutism and Virilization. A Systematic Approach to Benign and Potentially Serious Causes," *Postgrad Med*, 1995, 97(1):99-102, 105-6.

Rittmaster RS, "Hirsutism," *Lancet*, 1997, 349(9046):191-5 (review).

Sakiyama R, "Approach to Patients With Hirsutism," *West J Med*, 1996, 165(6):386-91.

Watson RE, Bouknight R, and Alguire PC, "Hirsutism: Evaluation and Management," *J Gen Intern Med*, 1995, 10(5):283-92 (review).

HIRSUTISM

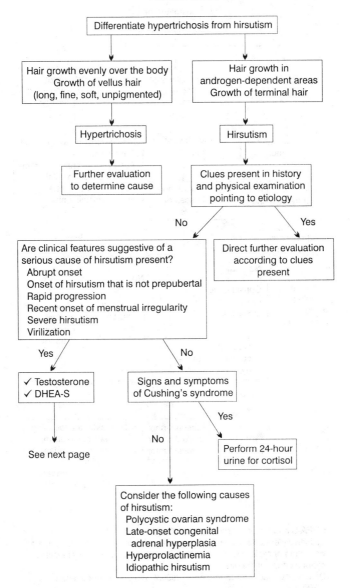

HIRSUTISM
(continued)

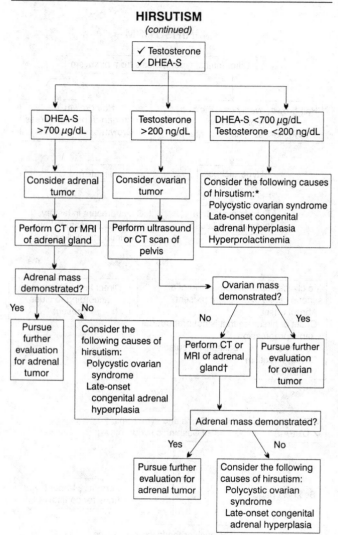

*DHEA-S and testosterone levels <700 μg/dL and 200 ng/L do not definitively exclude ovarian or adrenal tumor. However, in the absence of virilization or rapid onset of hirsutism, further evaluation rarely reveals a serious cause of the hirsutism.

†On occasion, adrenal cancer may present with testosterone levels >200 ng/dL.

HOARSENESS

STEP 1: *What are the Causes of Hoarseness?*

Hoarseness is defined as a change in normal voice quality. It is the most common symptom of laryngeal disease. Although there are many benign causes of hoarseness, the clinician should be aware of the more serious etiologies, some of which are life-threatening. The causes of hoarseness are listed in the following box.

Causes of Hoarseness	
Acute laryngitis	Laryngeal cancer
Allergic reaction	Laryngeal papilloma
Amyloidosis	Laryngitis sicca
Arthritis	Leukoplakia
Chronic laryngitis	Nasogastric tube
Diphtheritic laryngitis	Postsurgical
Epiglottitis	Psychogenic
Exposure to smoke or chemicals	Trauma
Hypopharyngeal cancer	Vocal cord granuloma
Hypothyroidism	Vocal cord nodule
Intubation	Vocal cord polyp
Intubation granuloma	Vocal cord paralysis

The evaluation of the hoarse patient begins with consideration as to the duration of the voice change. When the voice change has been present for less than two weeks, the patient is said to have acute hoarseness. Hoarseness present for more than two weeks is considered to be chronic.

If the patient has acute hoarseness, ***Proceed to Step 2.***

If the patient has chronic hoarseness, ***Proceed to Step 5.***

STEP 2: *What are the Causes of Acute Hoarseness?*

The causes of acute hoarseness are listed in the following box.

Causes of Acute Hoarseness
Acute laryngitis
Allergic reactions
Diphtheritic laryngitis
Epiglottitis
Exposure to smoke or chemicals
Intubation
Nasogastric tube
Trauma

Proceed to Step 3

> **STEP 3:** *Are There Any Clues in the Patient's History That Point to the Etiology of the Acute Hoarseness?*

Clues in the patient's history that may point to the etiology of the acute hoarseness are listed in the following table.

Historical Clue	Condition Suggested
Severe throat pain Inability to swallow secretions	Epiglottitis
Recent intubation	Injury to vocal cord mucosa Intubation granuloma
Nasogastric tube	Associated with inflammation in area of cricoid, arytenoids, and cricoarytenoid joints
Exposure to toxic fumes or smoke	Exposure to smoke or chemicals
Blunt or penetrating trauma	Trauma (can cause a variety of laryngeal injuries)
Symptoms of upper respiratory tract infection	Acute laryngitis
Angioedema or anaphylaxis	Allergic reaction

The causes of acute hoarseness are discussed in further detail below.

Acute Laryngitis

Acute laryngitis is the most common cause of acute hoarseness in adults. In most cases, the hoarseness is just one manifestation of an upper respiratory tract infection. Cough often accompanies the change in the voice quality. Affected individuals may also complain of considerable pain in the throat and laryngeal area. Most cases are due to a viral infection. However, bacterial superinfection may occur.

Epiglottitis

Although epiglottitis is more common in children, it does occur in adults. The initial symptoms of epiglottitis are similar to that of pharyngitis. Sore throat, cough, and fever are all quite common. Soon after the onset of these symptoms, there is rapid progression to severe throat pain, air hunger, restlessness, and inability to swallow secretions. Upper airway obstruction is a major concern in these patients.

Direct examination of the epiglottis may precipitate sudden respiratory obstruction. As a result, suspicion of this diagnosis should warrant an examination of the epiglottis only when personnel are available to quickly establish an airway should the need arise. The lateral neck radiograph may reveal a markedly swollen epiglottis.

Diphtheritic Laryngitis

Diphtheritic laryngitis is caused by the organism, *Corynebacterium diphtheriae*. It is a rare cause of laryngitis in the United States since vaccination is so widespread. The disease, however, does continue to occur in epidemics throughout certain parts of the world.

Signs and symptoms of a generalized systemic illness such as fever and malaise are usually present. Most patients have signs and symptoms of diphtheritic pharyngitis which may include slight pain on swallowing, moderately reddened and swollen tonsils, and a white or gray membrane. The membrane extends beyond the tonsils to involve the faucial pillars and soft palate. It is difficult to wipe the membrane off but, if successful, a bleeding surface will be left behind. The lymph nodes, particularly the jugulodigastric chain, are enlarged and tender.

Nearly 10% of patients with diphtheritic pharyngitis have concomitant laryngeal disease. Hoarseness suggests laryngeal involvement. Of major concern is the development of laryngeal obstruction.

Intubation

Even a brief period of intubation can result in serious injury to the mucosa of the vocal cords. Patients may complain of hoarseness, cough, and neck pain immediately or shortly after extubation. In most cases, the normal voice returns as the injury resolves. In some cases, however, the injury may be permanent. The intubation granuloma, a well known complication of intubation, should be suspected when hoarseness persists after intubation. In these cases, granulomas form over the medial surface of the arytenoid cartilage.

Nasogastric Tube

The placement of a nasogastric tube can lead to inflammation of the cricoid, arytenoids, and cricoarytenoid joints. This inflammation may manifest with hoarseness and pain. In some cases, subglottic stenosis may develop.

Exposure to Smoke or Chemicals

Trauma to the larynx from the inhalation of chemical toxins may result in acute symptoms of cough, burning sensation, hoarseness, epiphora, and asphyxia. Examples include exposure to smoke in fires and escaping gases or steams in industrial explosions.

Laryngeal Trauma

The larynx may be injured in patients who have suffered blunt or penetrating injury to the neck. Because of the close proximity to the cervical spine, pharynx, and upper esophagus, laryngeal injuries seldom occur alone. Fracture dislocation of the cervical spine should always be a major consideration in any patient who has suffered neck trauma. Unrecognized cervical fractures can lead to serious neurologic deficits.

The symptoms will vary depending on the severity of the neck injury. With mild blunt trauma, hemorrhage may occur in the glottic and supraglottic larynx. Fracture of the thyroid cartilage or contusion of the recurrent laryngeal nerve may result from severe blunt trauma.

Symptoms of laryngeal injury include hoarseness, dysphagia, dyspnea, hemoptysis, and neck swelling. Physical examination may reveal a patient in respiratory distress. Swelling may be noted over the larynx. Loss of the normal prominence of the Adam's apple warrants consideration of a fracture of the thyroid cartilage. Subcutaneous cervical emphysema may also be appreciated.

Soft tissue x-ray films of the neck may be helpful in assessing laryngeal injury due to trauma. Free air in the neck suggests a diagnosis of a laryngotracheal tear. Films of the cervical spine should also be obtained.

Allergic Reaction

Recurrent angioedema or true anaphylaxis can lead to laryngeal edema manifesting as hoarseness. There may be rapid progression to stridor and upper airway obstruction.

Proceed to Step 4

STEP 4: *Has the Hoarseness Resolved?*

Since most patients with acute hoarseness are suffering from acute laryngitis, it is reasonable to treat symptomatically for two weeks with voice rest and increased hydration. Many of the inflammatory and infectious conditions causing hoarseness will resolve within this time period. When hoarseness persists after two weeks of conservative therapy, the patient is considered to have chronic hoarseness. Chronic hoarseness requires further evaluation to elucidate the cause. In particular, benign causes of chronic hoarseness must be differentiated from malignancy.

If the hoarseness resolves with two weeks of conservative therapy, *Stop Here.*

If the hoarseness persists despite two weeks of conservative therapy, *Proceed to Step 5.*

STEP 5: *What are the Causes of Chronic Hoarseness?*

The causes of chronic hoarseness are listed in the following box.

Causes of Chronic Hoarseness	
Amyloidosis	Laryngitis sicca
Arthritis	Leukoplakia
Chronic laryngitis	Postsurgical
Exposure to smoke or chemicals	Psychogenic
Hypopharyngeal cancer	Vocal cord granuloma
Hypothyroidism	Vocal cord nodule
Intubation granuloma	Vocal cord paralysis
Laryngeal cancer	Vocal cord polyp
Laryngeal papilloma	

Proceed to Step 6

STEP 6: *Are There Any Clues in the History That Point to the Etiology of the Chronic Hoarseness*

Clues in the patient's history that may point to the etiology of the chronic hoarseness are listed in the following table.

Historical Clue	Condition Suggested
Cigarette smoking	Chronic laryngitis Laryngeal cancer Leukoplakia
Vocal abuse or misuse	Vocal cord nodule Vocal cord polyp Chronic laryngitis Vocal cord granuloma (contact ulcer)
Symptoms and signs consistent with allergic rhinitis or chronic sinusitis	Associated with hoarseness*
History of radiation therapy to the head and neck	Scarring of the vocal cords
Intubation	Intubation granuloma
Cough Hemoptysis Weight loss Fever Night sweats	Tuberculosis
History of rheumatoid arthritis	Ankylosis of cricarytenoid joints Rheumatoid nodules of the vocal cords
History of neurologic condition	Neurologic disorder resulting in hoarseness#
Dry hair Dry skin Weight gain Fatigue	Hypothyroidism
Bitter taste Halitosis upon awakening Dry or coated mouth Substernal burning sensation precipitated or worsened by bending, lying down, etc.	Chronic laryngitis secondary to reflux
History of head and neck surgery such as carotid endarterectomy, thyroidectomy, tonsillectomy, endolaryngeal surgery	Damage or injury to vagus, recurrent laryngeal nerve, or larynx
Medication history	Hoarseness secondary to medication use†
Exposure to smoke or chemicals	Exposure to smoke or chemicals
Alcohol abuse	Risk factor for laryngeal cancer Leukoplakia Drying effect on laryngeal mucosa

*Allergic rhinitis and chronic sinusitis are often associated with hoarseness. They are usually not the sole cause of the hoarseness. The inflammation, reactive glottic edema, repetitive throat clearing, and alterations in the mucosal secretions of the upper respiratory tract that accompany these conditions are thought to contribute to the change in voice quality.

#Neurologic conditions associated with hoarseness include Parkinson's disease, myasthenia gravis, Shy-Drager syndrome, muscular dystrophy, amyotrophic lateral sclerosis, benign essential tremor, Huntington's disease, pseudobulbar palsy, and multiple sclerosis.

†A number of different medications can have effects on the quality of the voice. Medications that can commonly affect voice quality include antihistamines, decongestants, diuretics, α-adrenergic antagonists, cough suppressants, selective serotonin reuptake inhibitors, phenothiazines, chemotherapeutic agents, inhaled steroids, vitamin C, retinoic acid derivatives, and tricyclic antidepressants. Many of these medications cause drying and thickened secretions. Voice change due to medications should be a diagnosis of exclusion.

Proceed to Step 7

STEP 7: *What are the Results of the Laryngeal Examination?*

There are several techniques available for visualization of the larynx. These techniques include the following:

Indirect Laryngoscopy

With indirect laryngoscopy, patient cooperation is essential. After asking the patient to open the mouth widely, the tongue is grasped with gauze. A laryngeal mirror is then advanced above the tongue and against the soft palate. A light is then focused on the mirror and proper angling of the mirror allows the clinician to visualize the larynx. It is best to avoid stimulating the base of the tongue and posterior pharyngeal wall so as not to provoke the gag reflex. The procedure may be difficult, however, in patients having a sensitive gag reflex.

Indirect laryngoscopy is often the first procedure performed because the equipment is readily available in the otolaryngologist's office. In addition, the procedure is quick and inexpensive, allowing the clinician a rapid, gross examination of the larynx. Subtle lesions, however, may be missed.

Fiberoptic Laryngoscopy

Fiberoptic laryngoscopy can overcome the limitations of indirect laryngoscopy, particularly in those who have a sensitive gag reflex. In this technique, the scope is passed through the nose after the administration of topical anesthesia to the nasal cavity and pharynx. The flexibility of the scope allows for excellent views of the epiglottis, larynx, and parts of the pyriform sinus and hypopharynx. It does, however, require more time to perform than indirect laryngoscopy.

Direct Laryngoscopy

General anesthesia is usually required with direct laryngoscopy. The mucous membranes and anatomic structures of the larynx and hypopharynx are well visualized during this procedure.

If laryngoscopy reveals a structural lesion, ***Proceed to Step 8.***

If laryngoscopy reveals vocal cord paralysis, ***Proceed to Step 9.***

If laryngoscopy is normal, ***Proceed to Step 13.***

STEP 8: *What Structural Lesions of the Larynx May be Identified by Laryngoscopy?*

The structural lesions that may be identified by laryngoscopy are discussed in further detail below.

Chronic Laryngitis

Chronic inflammation of the larynx from a variety of causes can lead to chronic laryngitis. The most common cause of chronic laryngitis is cigarette smoking. Other causes include vocal abuse or misuse, and inhalation of irritants such as chemicals or dusts.

Another common cause of chronic laryngitis is reflux laryngitis. The heartburn that is characteristic of gastroesophageal reflux disease is often absent in patients with reflux laryngitis. As a result, it is important for the clinician to ask about other symptoms associated with laryngopharyngeal reflux such as chronic cough, postnasal drip, thick throat mucus, throat-clearing, and throat burning or tickling. Improvement in voice quality with antireflux precautions and acid suppressive therapy supports the diagnosis.

In contrast to acute laryngitis, chronic laryngitis is seldom caused by infection. On occasion, chronic inflammation of the larynx may be due to tuberculosis. In most cases of laryngeal tuberculosis, active pulmonary disease is readily apparent. Hoarseness and pain in the patient presenting with signs and symptoms of pulmonary tuberculosis should prompt consideration of concomitant laryngeal involvement. Most other causes of chronic laryngitis are not associated with pain. When signs and symptoms of pulmonary tuberculosis are not present, the diagnosis is not usually made until the laryngeal lesion has been biopsied

Other infections that may cause chronic laryngitis include histoplasmosis, blastomycosis, candidiasis, syphilis, and leprosy. Syphilis is a rare cause of hoarseness but, when it does occur, symptoms of laryngeal involvement usually manifest in the secondary or tertiary stage of syphilis.

Vocal Cord Nodule

Nodules that develop at the junction of the anterior third and middle third of the vocal cord are known as vocal cord nodules. Vocal abuse is a contributing factor in many patients. In fact, vocal cord nodules may be referred to as singer's nodules or nodes when they occur in professional users of voice such as preachers and singers. Screamer's nodule is another term used synonymously with vocal cord nodule.

Vocal Cord Polyp

Vocal abuse also seems to be a factor in the development of vocal cord polyps. In contrast to vocal cord nodules, polyps are usually unilateral and are located in the free margin of the vocal cord.

Vocal Cord Granuloma (Contact Ulcer)

Professional users of voice are also prone to develop vocal cord granulomas. Also known as contact ulcers, vocal cord granulomas manifest with hoarseness and pain. At times, the pain may radiate to the ear.

Laryngitis Sicca

Laryngitis sicca, also known as atrophic laryngitis, is characterized by marked crusting and irritation of the larynx. Symptoms of laryngitis sicca include hoarseness, chronic cough, and mild throat discomfort.

Intubation Granuloma

Hoarseness is not uncommon in patients who have been intubated. After extubation, the voice returns to normal as the injury resolves. However, in some patients, hoarseness persists. Intubation granuloma is one common cause of persistent hoarseness in patients who have recently been intubated.

Exposure to Smoke or Chemicals

Exposure to smoke in fires or gases or steams in industrial explosions may give rise to both acute and chronic symptoms. Chronic symptoms include hoarseness, cough, frequent need to clear the throat, and sensation of dryness.

Arthritis

The cricoarytenoid joint may be involved in up to 25% of patients with rheumatoid arthritis. The hallmarks of this type of arthritis are hoarseness and pain worsened by swallowing.

Hypothyroidism

On occasion, hoarseness may be the initial manifestation of hypothyroidism. In most cases, however, other signs and symptoms of hypothyroidism are present. Laryngoscopy may reveal diffusely dull and thickened vocal cords. Confirmation of the diagnosis rests upon the results of the thyroid function tests.

Laryngeal Papilloma

Benign tumors of the larynx are rare. Among these benign tumors, laryngeal papillomas are the most common. Unlike children, adult-onset laryngeal papillomas tend to be solitary. On occasion, laryngeal papillomas may lead to upper airway obstruction. Upper airway obstruction is more common in children. Because there is a concern that papillomas may undergo malignant degeneration in adults, surgical removal is usually recommended. After removal, laryngeal papillomas frequently recur.

Leukoplakia

Whitish plaques or patches of the laryngeal mucosa are known as leukoplakia. A leukoplakic lesion may be premalignant or malignant. Therefore, histologic evaluation of the lesion is necessary to define the lesion. Only by biopsy can a premalignant lesion be differentiated from carcinoma in situ or invasive carcinoma.

Hypopharyngeal Cancer

Hypopharyngeal cancer may involve any of the following three regions:

- Piriform sinus
- Posterior pharyngeal wall
- Postcricoid region

In nearly 50% of cases, patients will present with neck lymphadenopathy, especially involving the nodes at the angle of the jaw. Often accompanying the lymphadenopathy are symptoms of dysphagia and pain radiating to the ear. With extension of the cancer to the larynx or the recurrent laryngeal nerve, patients may complain of hoarseness or difficulty in breathing. Endoscopic examination is necessary to establish the diagnosis.

Laryngeal Cancer

Accounting for almost 2% of all malignancies, most cases of laryngeal cancer are squamous cell carcinomas. Risk factors for laryngeal cancer include smoking and alcohol abuse. It is useful to divide the larynx into three regions:

supraglottic (region above the vocal cords), glottic (region of the vocal cords) and subglottic (region below the vocal cords). The presentation of laryngeal cancer will differ depending on the location of the lesion:

- Glottic carcinoma

  Hoarseness is an early complaint in patients with glottic carcinomas since properly functioning vocal cords are integral in the production of a normal voice.

- Supraglottic carcinoma

  Supraglottic carcinoma tends to present with hoarseness late in the disease course. The initial symptom is often an awareness of something in the throat. At times, patients complain of swallowing difficulty. Late in the course of the disease, patients may complain of hoarseness.

- Subglottic carcinoma

  Hoarseness is also a late finding in patients with subglottic carcinomas. In fact, airway obstruction may occur before hoarseness.

Cervical lymph node enlargement may be appreciated in patients with laryngeal cancer. Supraglottic carcinomas tend to metastasize more frequently to the cervical lymph nodes than glottic or subglottic carcinomas.

End of Section.

STEP 9: *What is the Etiology of the Vocal Cord Paralysis?*

Although vocal cord paralysis may be unilateral or bilateral, unilateral paralysis is more commonly encountered. Not all patients with unilateral vocal cord paralysis are symptomatic. The presence of symptoms depends on how close the paralyzed vocal cord is to the midline. When the paralyzed vocal cord is very close to the midline, there is often no change in the voice.

Since the etiology of the vocal cord paralysis involves a lesion of the vagus nerves or one of its branches, usually the recurrent laryngeal nerve, the goals of the evaluation are to answer the following questions:

- Where is the lesion?
- What is the lesion?

To answer the above questions, it is necessary to first understand the innervation of the larynx.

Proceed to Step 10

STEP 10: *What is the Neuroanatomy of the Vagus Nerve and Its Branches?*

The innervation of the larynx is provided by the vagus nerve and its branches. The motor fibers of the vagus nerve originate in the nucleus ambiguus. These fibers are carried in the vagus nerve as it travels in the posterior fossa. In its course through the posterior fossa, the vagus nerve is in close proximity to cranial nerves IX, XI, and XII. Within the jugular foramen, it lies together with cranial nerves IX and XI in the carotid sheath between the artery and the internal jugular vein. Upon leaving the jugular foramen, the vagus nerves descends into the thorax, giving rise to the recurrent laryngeal nerve.

The left recurrent laryngeal nerve hooks around the aortic arch to ascend along the tracheoesophageal groove. Before entering the larynx, the left recurrent laryngeal nerve is intimately related to the thyroid gland.

After arising from the vagus nerve, the right recurrent laryngeal nerve hooks around the subclavian artery. It then ascends in the tracheoesophageal groove before entering the larynx.

Proceed to Step 11

STEP 11: *What are the Causes of Unilateral Vocal Cord Paralysis?*

Once the neuroanatomy of the vagus nerve and its branches is understood, identifying the cause of the unilateral vocal cord paralysis becomes much easier. The causes are listed in the following box.

Causes of Unilateral Vocal Cord Paralysis	
Intracranial conditions*	Miscellaneous
Base of the skull	Postsurgical
Tumors of the jugular foramen†	Anterior cervical disc surgery
Trauma	Cardiac surgery
Neck	Carotid surgery
Thyroid disease (especially cancer)	Esophagectomy
Trauma	Mediastinal surgery
Esophageal malignancy	Mediastinoscopy
Tracheal malignancy	Neck dissection for head and
Subclavian aneurysm (on right)	neck cancer
Tumors high in the neck	Thymectomy
Chest	Thyroid surgery
Bronchogenic carcinoma	Tracheal surgery
Esophageal malignancy	Valve repair
Tracheal malignancy	Neuropathy
Lymphoma	Diabetes mellitus
Aortic aneurysm	Lead or mercury poisoning
Left atrial dilatation	Syphilis
	Sarcoidosis
	Viral

* Intracranial conditions such as cerebrovascular accidents, brainstem tumor, or high skull-base tumors do not present with unilateral vocal cord paralysis alone. In these conditions, other neurologic symptoms or cranial nerve deficits are usually present as well.

† In the jugular foramen, the vagus nerve is closely related to cranial nerves IX and XI. As a result, a mass lesion involving the jugular foramen will involve not only the vagus nerve but these other cranial nerves as well.

In the following table, the frequency of the etiologies of unilateral vocal cord paralysis are listed based upon a literature review of approximately 1000 patients.

Condition	Frequency
Malignancy	35.8%
Postsurgical	24.6%
Idiopathic	14.3%
Medical / inflammatory	13.3%
Intracranial	6%
Trauma	6%

Adapted from Terris DJ, Arnstein DP, and Nguyen HH, "Contemporary Evaluation of Unilateral Vocal Cord Paralysis," *Otolaryngol Head Neck Surg*, 1992, 107(1):84-90 (review).

Proceed to Step 12

STEP 12: *What Evaluation is Necessary in Patients With Unilateral Vocal Cord Paralysis?*

Since malignancy is the most common cause of unilateral vocal cord dysfunction, efforts should be focused on the identification of malignancy, which may be present anywhere along the vagus nerve and its branches. To identify a malignancy, the following imaging tests may be needed.

- CXR
- CT or MRI of skull base, neck, and chest

If the history and physical examination in conjunction with appropriate imaging studies fail to elucidate the cause, the patient may be considered to have idiopathic unilateral vocal cord paralysis. Idiopathic unilateral vocal cord paralysis is not uncommon, occurring in up to 33% of cases.

End of Section.

STEP 13: *What are the Possibilities in the Patient With Hoarseness Who Has an Unremarkable Larynx Examination?*

When the laryngeal examination is unremarkable, the clinician should give consideration to the following conditions:

- Psychogenic Dysphonia

  Psychogenic dysphonia is one possibility in the chronically hoarse patient who has a normal laryngeal examination. In these patients, environmental stress may play a role in the development of the hoarseness. A common type of functional voice disorder is dysphonia plicae ventricularis, which is often psychologically based. In this condition, closure of the false vocal cords over the true vocal cords results in occlusion of the larynx. Occluding the larynx manifests clinically as muffling of the voice. In some cases, however, dysphonia plicae ventricularis occurs as a complication of chronic laryngitis.

- Endocrine Dysphonia

  Endocrine disorders, particularly acromegaly and hypothyroidism, may present with chronic hoarseness. In most cases, other features of acromegaly or hypothyroidism are present. Appropriate endocrinologic testing confirms the diagnosis.

- Neurogenic Dysphonia

- Medications (see table in Step 6)

- Normal Aging

  With aging, the voice may become tremulous and weak. Laryngeal examination may be unremarkable but careful examination may reveal bowing of the vocal cords secondary to atrophy of the vocalis muscles.

REFERENCES

Banfield G, Tandon P, and Solomons N, "Hoarse Voice: An Early Symptom of Many Conditions," *Practitioner*, 2000, 244(1608):267-71 (review).

Benninger MS, Crumley RL, Ford CN, et al, "Evaluation and Treatment of the Unilateral Paralyzed Vocal Fold," *Otolaryngol Head Neck Surg*, 1994, 111(4):497-508.

Berke GS and Kevorkian KF, "The Diagnosis and Management of Hoarseness," *Compr Ther*, 1996, 22(4):251-5 (review).

Garrett CG and Ossoff RH, "Hoarseness: Contemporary Diagnosis and Management," *Compr Ther*, 1995, 21(12):705-10.

Rosen CA, Anderson D, and Murry T, "Evaluating Hoarseness: Keeping Your Patient's Voice Healthy," *Am Fam Phys*, 1998, 57(11):2775-82 (review).

Terris DJ, Arnstein DP, and Nguyen HH, "Contemporary Evaluation of Unilateral Vocal Cord Paralysis," *Otolaryngol Head Neck Surg*, 1992, 107(1):84-90 (review).

HOARSENESS

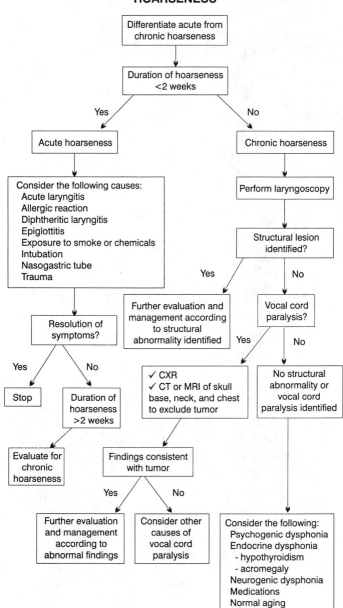

JAUNDICE

STEP 1: *What are the Causes of Jaundice?*

Hyperbilirubinemia of sufficient magnitude may manifest as jaundice. Jaundice refers to a yellowing of the skin. Yellowing of the sclera is known as icterus. As a general rule, jaundice can be appreciated when the serum bilirubin exceeds 2.5 mg/dL. The causes of jaundice are listed in the following box.

Causes of Jaundice	
Unconjugated Hyperbilirubinemia	
Crigler-Najjar syndrome	Hemolysis
Drug-induced	Ineffective erythropoiesis
Gilbert's syndrome	Resorption of hematoma
Conjugated Hyperbilirubinemia	
Hepatocellular diseases	
Alcoholic hepatitis	Hepatotoxins
α_1-antitrypsin deficiency	Ischemia
Autoimmune hepatitis	Medications
Cirrhosis	Rotor's syndrome
Dubin-Johnson syndrome	Viral hepatitis (acute or chronic)
Hemochromatosis	Wilson's disease
Hepatic vein thrombosis	
Cholestatic diseases	
Intrahepatic	Extrahepatic
Alcoholic hepatitis	AIDS cholangiopathy
Benign recurrent intrahepatic cholestasis	Biliary malformation
	Choledocholithiasis
Cholestasis of pregnancy	Malignancy
Drug-induced	Ampullary
Postoperative jaundice	Cholangiocarcinoma
Primary biliary cirrhosis	Duodenal
Systemic infection	Lymphoma
Total parenteral nutrition	Metastases to portal lymph nodes
Viral hepatitis	Pancreatic
	Pancreatic pseudocyst
	Pancreatitis
	Primary sclerosing cholangitis

Proceed to Step 2

STEP 2: *Does the Patient Have Conjugated or Unconjugated Hyperbilirubinemia?*

The evaluation of jaundice begins with the determination of whether the hyperbilirubinemia is conjugated or unconjugated. There are several ways of making this distinction:

- Other liver function test abnormalities

  The causes of unconjugated hyperbilirubinemia are not typically associated with other liver function test abnormalities. In contrast, most cases of conjugated hyperbilirubinemia are accompanied by other liver function test abnormalities.

- Urine dipstick for bilirubin

  Of the two types of bilirubin, only conjugated bilirubin is water soluble. As a result, a positive urine dipstick for bilirubin signifies the presence of conjugated hyperbilirubinemia.

- Foam test

  When normal urine is shaken, the foam appears white. In the presence of bilirubinuria, however, the foam will be yellow. Because the yellow color characteristic of conjugated hyperbilirubinemia may be subtle, it is useful to compare the specimen with the white foam of a normal urine specimen.

- Serum bilirubin fractionation

  A predominantly conjugated hyperbilirubinemia is said to exist when 30% or more of the serum bilirubin is in the conjugated form.

If the patient has unconjugated hyperbilirubinemia, **Proceed to Step 3**.

If the patient has conjugated hyperbilirubinemia, **Proceed to Step 9**.

STEP 3: *What are the Causes of Unconjugated Hyperbilirubinemia?*

The approach to the patient presenting with unconjugated hyperbilirubinemia is more easily understood if one considers the steps involved in bilirubin metabolism. Close to 80% of the serum bilirubin originates from the breakdown of senescent red blood cells. The remainder is derived from the metabolism of other proteins containing heme as well as the destruction of red blood cell precursors in the bone marrow (ineffective erythropoiesis). The unconjugated bilirubin then travels to the liver. Uptake of bilirubin occurs at the liver cell followed by conjugation. Conjugation is catalyzed by the enzyme, UDP-glucuronyl transferase. Therefore, a process that leads to or affects any of the following steps in bilirubin metabolism can lead to unconjugated hyperbilirubinemia:

- Increased production of bilirubin
- Impaired hepatic uptake of bilirubin
- Impaired conjugation of bilirubin

The causes of unconjugated hyperbilirubinemia are listed in the box below.

Causes of Unconjugated Hyperbilirubinemia	
Increased production	**Impaired hepatic uptake**
Hemolysis	Medications
Ineffective erythropoiesis	Gilbert's syndrome
Resorption of large hematoma	**Impaired conjugation**
	Crigler-Najjar syndrome
	Gilbert's syndrome

Proceed to Step 4

> **STEP 4:** *Does the Patient Have Unconjugated Hyperbilirubinemia Secondary to Hemolysis?*

With hemolysis, the degradation of hemoglobin in large amounts overwhelms the liver's ability to excrete it. Because the liver has a remarkable capacity to excrete bilirubin, the hyperbilirubinemia that accompanies hemolysis is characteristically mild. The serum bilirubin is usually <5 mg/dL in patients with hemolysis. Only when the hemolysis is superimposed on underlying liver disease or the hemolytic disease involves the liver (eg, sickle cell anemia) will the bilirubin level rise above 5 mg/dL. Other laboratory test abnormalities that support the presence of hemolysis include the following:

- Anemia
- Reticulocytosis
- Increased LDH
- Decreased haptoglobin
- Urine hemosiderin

In many cases, the etiology of the hemolysis is known. In other cases, a thorough history, physical examination, and other laboratory testing will establish the diagnosis.

If the patient has unconjugated hyperbilirubinemia secondary to hemolysis, **Stop Here**.

If the patient does not have unconjugated hyperbilirubinemia secondary to hemolysis, **Proceed to Step 5**.

> **STEP 5:** *Does the Patient Have Unconjugated Hyperbilirubinemia Secondary to Ineffective Erythropoiesis?*

Ineffective erythropoiesis refers to the increased destruction of red blood cells or red blood cell precursors in the bone marrow. Disorders associated with ineffective erythropoiesis are listed in the following box.

Causes of Ineffective Erythropoiesis	
Dyserythropoietic porphyria	Sideroblastic anemia
Folate deficiency	Thalassemia
Lead poisoning	Vitamin B_{12} deficiency
Severe iron deficiency anemia	

The history and physical examination may direct the clinician to one of the above causes of ineffective erythropoiesis. As a general rule, the above conditions are not characterized by serum bilirubin levels in excess of 4 mg/dL unless there is concomitant liver disease.

If the patient has unconjugated hyperbilirubinemia secondary to ineffective erythropoiesis, **Stop Here**.

If the patient does not have unconjugated hyperbilirubinemia secondary to ineffective erythropoiesis, **Proceed to Step 6**.

STEP 6: *Does the Patient Have Unconjugated Hyperbilirubinemia Secondary to Decreased Hepatic Uptake of Bilirubin?*

This is an uncommon cause of unconjugated hyperbilirubinemia but may be noted with the use of certain medications. These medications include the following:

- Rifampin

- Probenecid

- Flavaspidic acid

- Some radiographic contrast agents (bunamiodyl)

Resolution of the unconjugated hyperbilirubinemia typically occurs within 48 hours of drug discontinuation. Another cause of impaired hepatic uptake of bilirubin is Gilbert's syndrome. However, since Gilbert's syndrome is a heterogeneous disorder characterized by defects of bilirubin conjugation as well, it will be discussed shortly.

If the patient has unconjugated hyperbilirubinemia secondary to decreased hepatic uptake of bilirubin, *Stop Here*.

If the patient does not have unconjugated hyperbilirubinemia secondary to decreased hepatic uptake of bilirubin, *Proceed to Step 7*.

STEP 7: *Does the Patient Have Unconjugated Hyperbilirubinemia Secondary to the Crigler-Najjar Syndrome?*

There are two types of Crigler-Najjar syndrome. Type I Crigler-Najjar syndrome is characterized by the absence of UDP-glucuronyltransferase activity. As a result, unconjugated hyperbilirubinemia develops immediately after birth. Infants often have impressive elevations in the serum bilirubin level. Left untreated, all affected patients will die of kernicterus. The only treatment is liver transplantation.

In type II Crigler-Najjar syndrome, also known as Arias disease, affected individuals have about 10% of the normal UDP-glucuronyltransferase activity. While most develop jaundice before the age of 1 year, some may not until later in life. It is unusual for affected individuals to present after the age of 10 years. The serum bilirubin levels typically range between 10-20 mg/dL. Therapy is usually not needed but, in those at risk for kernicterus, phenobarbital can decrease the bilirubin level.

If the patient has unconjugated hyperbilirubinemia secondary to the Crigler-Najjar syndrome, *Stop Here*.

If the patient does not have unconjugated hyperbilirubinemia secondary to the Crigler-Najjar syndrome, *Proceed to Step 8*.

STEP 8: *Does the Patient Have Gilbert's Syndrome?*

In outpatients, the most common cause of unconjugated hyperbilirubinemia is Gilbert's syndrome. Gilbert's syndrome is found in 3% to 8% of the Caucasian population. Inherited in an autosomal dominant pattern, this syndrome typically manifests during or after adolescence. Jaundice usually develops with the following precipitants:

- Intercurrent illness
- Exercise
- Stress
- Fatigue
- Alcohol use
- Fasting
- Nicotinic acid intake

The diagnosis should be suspected in younger patients who present with unconjugated hyperbilirubinemia but no other liver function test abnormalities. Defects in hepatic uptake and/or conjugation of bilirubin have been described in patients with Gilbert's syndrome.

A diagnosis of Gilbert's syndrome can be established in the patient who has the features listed in the following box.

Features of Gilbert's Syndrome	
No bilirubinuria	Normal MCV
Normal alkaline phosphatase	Normal peripheral blood smear
Normal AST/ALT	Normal reticulocyte count
Normal GGT	Unconjugated hyperbilirubinemia
Normal hemoglobin	

In most cases, the presence of the features listed above are sufficient to establish the diagnosis. If there is any uncertainty, the clinician can elect to perform either one of the following tests:

- Nicotinic acid stress test

    When nicotinic acid is given intravenously, an increase in serum bilirubin by more than >18 µmol/L has been found to have 100% sensitivity and specificity in the diagnosis of Gilbert's syndrome. One hour before the intravenous administration of nicotinic acid, 100 mg of indomethacin is recommended to prevent flushing.

- Caloric restriction test

    A rise in the serum bilirubin to greater than two times the upper limit of normal after two days of caloric restriction (400 kcal/day) is consistent with Gilbert's syndrome. Other causes of hyperbilirubinemia may be associated with a lesser rise in the serum bilirubin.

The following table offers a comparison between Gilbert's syndrome and the two types of Crigler-Najjar syndrome.

	Gilbert's Syndrome	Crigler-Najjar Syndrome (Type I)	Crigler-Najjar Syndrome (Type II)
Incidence	3% to 8%	Very rare	Uncommon
Inheritance Pattern	Autosomal dominant	Autosomal recessive	Autosomal recessive
Serum Bilirubin	<5 mg/dL	Usually >20 mg/dL	Usually <20 mg/dL
Response to Phenobarbital	Decrease in serum bilirubin	No response	Decrease in serum bilirubin
Prognosis	Normal	Death in infancy	Usually normal
Treatment	None needed	Liver transplantation	Phenobarbital if serum bilirubin markedly increased

Making the diagnosis of Gilbert's syndrome can obviate an unnecessary and expensive work-up. The patient can then be reassured that their illness is benign.

End of Section.

> **STEP 9:** *What are the Causes of Conjugated Hyperbilirubinemia?*

The causes of conjugated hyperbilirubinemia are listed in the following box.

Causes of Conjugated Hyperbilirubinemia

Hepatocellular disease

Alcoholic hepatitis	Hepatotoxins
α_1-antitrypsin deficiency	Hepatic vein thrombosis
Autoimmune hepatitis	Ischemia
Cirrhosis	Rotor's syndrome
Drug-induced	Viral hepatitis
Dubin-Johnson syndrome	Wilson's disease
Hemochromatosis	

Cholestasis

Extrahepatic	Intrahepatic
AIDS cholangiopathy	Alcoholic hepatitis
Biliary malformation	Benign recurrent intrahepatic
Choledocholithiasis	cholestasis
Malignancy	Cholestasis of pregnancy
Ampullary	Drug-induced
Cholangiocarcinoma	Postoperative hyperbilirubinemiaa
Duodenal	Primary biliary cirrhosis
Lymphoma	Systemic infection
Metastases to portal lymph nodes	Total parenteral nutrition
Pancreatic	Viral hepatitis
Pancreatic pseudocyst	
Pancreatitis	
Primary sclerosing cholangitis	

The initial step in elucidating the etiology of the conjugated hyperbilirubinemia is consideration of the other liver function tests.

If the conjugated hyperbilirubinemia is not accompanied by other liver function test abnormalities, **Proceed to Step 10**.

If the conjugated hyperbilirubinemia is accompanied by other liver function test abnormalities, **Proceed to Step 11**.

STEP 10: Does the Patient Have Conjugated Hyperbilirubinemia Secondary to Dubin-Johnson or Rotor's Syndrome?

When the conjugated hyperbilirubinemia is not accompanied by other liver function test abnormalities, consideration should be given to the Dubin-Johnson and Rotor's syndrome. Both are inherited disorders that typically become apparent in childhood. Serum bilirubin levels typically range between 2-5 mg/dL. The following table offers a comparison between these two congenital disorders.

	Dubin-Johnson Syndrome	Rotor's Syndrome
Incidence	Uncommon	Rare
Inheritance Pattern	Autosomal recessive	Autosomal recessive
Bilirubin	Usually between 2-5 mg/dL	Usually between 2-5 mg/dL
Plasma Sulfobromophthalein Disappearance	Slow initial disappearance with frequent secondary rise at 1.5-2 hours	Very slow disappearance without secondary rise
Oral Cholecystography	Faint or nonvisualization	Usually normal visualization
Liver Histology	Coarse pigment in centrilobular hepatocytes	Normal
Prognosis	Normal	Normal
Treatment	No specific treatment	No specific treatment

End of Section.

STEP 11: Are There Any Historical Clues That Point to the Etiology of the Conjugated Hyperbilirubinemia?

When other liver function test abnormalities are present in the patient with conjugated hyperbilirubinemia, the clinician should consider the causes of hepatobiliary disease. Clues in the patient's history that may point to the etiology of the hepatobiliary disease are listed in the following table.

Historical Clue	Disease Suggested
Anorexia	Viral hepatitis
	Malignancy
Arthritis	Viral hepatitis
	Autoimmune hepatitis
	Primary sclerosing cholangitis
	Sarcoidosis
	Hemochromatosis

(Continued)

Historical Clue	Disease Suggested
Pregnancy	Intrahepatic cholestasis of pregnancy Acute fatty liver of pregnancy Pre-eclampsia
Light stools	Cholestasis
Anorexia Myalgias Malaise	Viral hepatitis (prodrome)
History of COPD	α_1-antitrypsin deficiency
Right shoulder or subcapsular pain	Choledocholithiasis
Pruritus	Cholestasis
Aversion to cigarettes	Viral hepatitis
Weight loss	Malignancy Alcoholic hepatitis End stage liver disease or cirrhosis
Fever / chills	Cholangitis Viral hepatitis Amebic abscess Alcoholic hepatitis Drug-induced hepatitis
RUQ tenderness	Alcoholic hepatitis Viral hepatitis Amebic abscess Choledocholithiasis / cholangitis
Pain in epigastric / RUQ region radiating to back Pain worsened by recumbency	Pancreatitis Pancreatic cancer
History of cholecystectomy	Retained common bile duct stone Biliary stricture
Receiving total parenteral nutrition	Cholestasis secondary to total parenteral nutrition
Alcohol use	Alcoholic hepatitis
History of inflammatory bowel disease	Primary sclerosing cholangitis

Recent surgery	Postoperative jaundice:
	   Benign postoperative cholestasis
	   Inhalational anesthetic
	   Impaired hepatic perfusion
	   Blood transfusion
	   Occult sepsis

Family history of jaundice	Dubin-Johnson syndrome Rotor's syndrome Benign recurrent intrahepatic cholestasis
After transplantation Accompanied by rash and diarrhea	Graft-vs-host disease
Medications (including herbal and over-the-counter)	Drug-induced hepatitis or cholestasis
Daycare centers Institutions for the retarded Sharing drug paraphernalia Travel to endemic area Engaging in oral-anal sex Ingestion of raw shellfish	Hepatitis A (risk factors)

(Continued)

Historical Clue	Disease Suggested
Intravenous drug abuse Hemodialysis patients Sharing razor blades / toothbrushes Tattooing Body piercing Acupuncture Healthcare worker History of blood transfusion High-risk sexual activity	Hepatitis B (risk factors)
Intravenous drug abuse Hemophilia History of blood transfusion Healthcare worker	Hepatitis C (risk factors)

Proceed to Step 12

STEP 12: *Are There Any Clues in the Physical Examination That Point to the Etiology of the Conjugated Hyperbilirubinemia?*

Clues in the physical examination that point to the etiology of the conjugated hyperbilirubinemia are listed in the following table.

Physical Examination Finding	Disease Suggested
Wasting	Advanced liver disease Malignancy
Needle track or skin popping	Intravenous drug abuse (risk factor for viral hepatitis)
Skin excoriations	Cholestasis
Generalized lymphadenopathy	Lymphoma
Supraclavicular lymphadenopathy	Gastric malignancy
Spider angiomas Gynecomastia Parotid enlargement Testicular atrophy Paucity of axillary and pubic hair Dupuytren's contracture	Chronic liver disease or cirrhosis
Palpable abdominal mass	Malignancy
Pulsatile liver	Tricuspid regurgitation (congestive hepatopathy)
Palpable gallbladder (Courvosier's sign)	Malignant biliary duct obstruction
Xanthomas	Primary biliary cirrhosis
Hyperpigmentation	Hemochromatosis Primary biliary cirrhosis
Abdominal scar in midline or right upper quadrant	Prior biliary surgery (suggestive of retained stone or biliary stricture)

(Continued)

(continued)

Physical Examination Finding	Disease Suggested
Kayser-Fleischer ring	Wilson's disease
Fever	Acute cholangitis
	Alcoholic hepatitis
	Viral hepatitis
	Amebic abscess
	Pancreatitis

Proceed to Step 13

STEP 13: *Does the Patient Have Conjugated Hyperbilirubinemia Secondary to Hepatocellular Injury or Cholestasis?*

Consideration of the other liver function test abnormalities allows hepatocellular injury to be distinguished from cholestasis, which is defined as an impairment in bile flow. Specifically, the transaminase (AST and ALT) and alkaline phosphatase levels need to be obtained. The information in the table below allows the clinician to differentiate hepatocellular from cholestatic liver injury.

	Alkaline Phosphatase	Transaminases
Hepatocellular injury	Normal or <3 X normal	>400 U/L (acute) <300 U/L (chronic)
Cholestasis	>4 X normal	<300 U/L

At times, it can be difficult to make the distinction between hepatocellular injury and cholestasis because the laboratory test abnormalities described above may overlap.

If the patient has cholestasis, *Proceed to Step 14.*

If the patient has hepatocellular injury, *Proceed to Step 18.*

STEP 14: *Does the Patient Have Extrahepatic or Intrahepatic Cholestasis?*

Cholestasis refers to an impairment in bile flow. As such, it may be intrahepatic or extrahepatic. It is important to make this distinction because prompt drainage is often necessary in patients with extrahepatic cholestasis. In contrast, drainage usually has no role in the management of intrahepatic cholestasis and, if performed, may result in increased morbidity and mortality.

The history and physical examination may provide clues as to whether the patient has extrahepatic (also known as obstructive jaundice) or intrahepatic cholestasis. These clues are described in the following table.

	Extrahepatic Cholestasis (Obstructive Jaundice)	Intrahepatic Cholestasis
Historical Clues	Abdominal pain Fever Shaking, chills Prior biliary surgery Older age	Anorexia, malaise, myalgias (suggestive of viral prodrome) Known infectious exposure Receipt of blood products Use of intravenous drugs Exposure to known hepatotoxin Family history of jaundice
Physical Examination Clues	High fever Abdominal tenderness Palpable abdominal mass Abdominal scar	Ascites Stigmata of chronic liver disease Prominent abdominal veins Gynecomastia Spider angiomas Asterixis Encephalopathy

Imaging with ultrasound or CT scan plays a prominent role in differentiating between extrahepatic and intrahepatic cholestasis. The demonstration of dilated bile ducts establishes the presence of extrahepatic cholestasis. Of note, mild dilatation of the common bile duct is commonly appreciated in postcholecystectomy patients. The advantages and disadvantages of these two radiologic tests in the evaluation of cholestasis are listed in the following table.

	Ultrasound	CT Scan
Noninvasive	Yes	Yes
Portable	Yes	Yes
Operator-Dependent	Yes	No
Expensive	No (relative to CT scan)	Yes
Sensitivity	55% to 91%	63% to 96%
Specificity	82% to 95%	93% to 100%
Contrast	No	Yes
Exposure to Radiation	No	Yes

If dilated bile ducts are demonstrated on ultrasound or CT, **Proceed to Step 15.**

If dilated bile ducts are not demonstrated on ultrasound or CT but high suspicion for extrahepatic cholestasis remains, **Proceed to Step 16.**

If bile ducts are not dilated on ultrasound or CT and suspicion for extrahepatic cholestasis is low, **Proceed to Step 17.**

STEP 15: *What are the Causes of Extrahepatic Cholestasis?*

The causes of extrahepatic cholestasis are listed in the following box.

Causes of Extrahepatic Cholestasis	
Choledocholithiasis	Pancreatitis
Biliary stricture	Pancreatic pseudocyst
Malignancy	Biliary malformation
Cholangiocarcinoma	Atresia
Pancreatic carcinoma	Choledochal cyst
Ampullary carcinoma	Primary sclerosing cholangitis
Duodenal carcinoma	AIDS cholangiopathy
Lymphoma	
Metastases to portal lymph nodes	

The presentation of the more common causes of extrahepatic cholestasis are considered below.

Choledocholithiasis

Patients with choledocholithiasis often present with signs and symptoms of biliary colic. The abdominal pain is steady, often lasting several hours in duration. Most patients complain of pain in the epigastrium and/or right upper quadrant.

Other patients with choledocholithiasis may seek medical care because of cholangitis, which results from infection in the setting of biliary obstruction. Charcot's triad of right upper quadrant pain, jaundice, and fever may be present in up to 75% of patients. Reynold's pentad includes this triad in combination with altered mental status and hypotension.

Soon after an attack of choledocholithiasis, the transaminases are markedly elevated. This is a transient finding, however, that is followed by a rise in the alkaline phosphatase. Rarely does the alkaline phosphatase exceed five times the upper limit of normal. Bilirubin rises in parallel, typically ranging between 2-14 mg/dL. Higher levels of alkaline phosphatase and/or bilirubin should prompt the clinician to consider malignancy. Ultrasound and CT have a sensitivity of about 20% and 50%, respectively, in the detection of common bile duct stones. In contrast, the sensitivity of ERCP is approximately 90%. It offers the clinician some therapeutic options as well including sphincterotomy and stone extraction.

Cholangiocarcinoma

Cholangiocarcinoma is a rare tumor that typically presents in middle age. There is a higher incidence of this malignancy in Southeast Asia, perhaps a reflection of an association with the liver fluke, *Clonorchis sinensis*. Cholangiocarcinoma is also associated with primary sclerosing cholangitis and biliary cysts. Nonspecific symptoms such as weight loss and fatigue are quite common while pain is uncommon. Cholangitis is unusual in these patients. The investigation of a patient suspected of having cholangiocarcinoma begins with either an ultrasound or CT scan. Of the two imaging modalities, CT scan usually provides more information. Confirmation of the diagnosis requires histologic analysis of cytologic brushings performed during an ERCP or PTC. While the sensitivity of the brushings is only 30%, a forceps biopsy in conjunction with brushings improves the sensitivity to 70%.

Pancreatic Cancer

Abdominal pain is a frequent complaint in patients with pancreatic cancer. Poor localization of the pain is not uncommon. The pain is typically constant with radiation from the upper abdomen to the back. There is usually a positional difference in the intensity of the pain; it is worse when supine but better when sitting up and leaning forward. Careful questioning of the patient usually reveals that the pain preceded the jaundice. Weight loss is almost invariably present. Diabetes mellitus is present in >60% of patients with pancreatic cancer. In a small percentage of patients, acute pancreatitis may be the initial presentation of the disease.

Physical examination typically reveals a jaundiced patient. Palpation of a mass argues for a lesion in the body or tail of the pancreas. In cases characterized by malignant biliary obstruction, the gallbladder may become distended and palpable (Courvosier's sign).

Abnormal laboratory tests are not uncommon at the time of presentation but, unfortunately, the abnormalities are often nonspecific. Mild elevations may be noted in the amylase and lipase concentrations. While both transaminases and alkaline phosphatase are often elevated, the alkaline phosphatase is often disproportionately so.

While ultrasound may detect a pancreatic cancer, more often, the utility of the test is poor because of overlying intraluminal gas. Even if the pancreas is not adequately visualized, ultrasound may provide important information such as the presence of biliary dilatation, which is suggestive of malignant biliary obstruction. CT scan can detect a pancreatic mass with an 80% sensitivity. ERCP is even better, exhibiting a 90% sensitivity in the diagnosis of pancreatic cancer. ERCP may demonstrate the double duct sign, which refers to a rather abrupt obstruction of both the common bile and pancreatic ducts. This finding is almost pathognomonic for pancreatic cancer. ERCP can also enable the clinician to obtain cytologic samples, yielding a sensitivity of nearly 40%. In recent years, endoscopic ultrasound has gained popularity because of its greater than 90% sensitivity in the diagnosis of pancreatic cancer. FNA of a mass can be performed with the guidance of endoscopic ultrasound.

Ampullary Tumor

Ampullary tumors are uncommon malignancies that can be benign (adenoma) or malignant (adenocarcinoma). While most malignant tumors originate from the mucosa of the ampulla of Vater, some ampullary tumors may arise from the pancreas, distal common bile duct, or duodenum. Jaundice, often cyclic, is the most common initial manifestation. Other symptoms include abdominal pain, nausea, vomiting, melena, and anorexia. The silver stool sign of Thomas, appreciated in <5% of patients, derives its appearance from acholic stools mixed with blood. Courvosier's sign may be appreciated in approximately 30% of patients.

Metastases to Portal Lymph Nodes (Porta Hepatis)

There are a number of malignancies that may metastasize to the periductal lymph nodes. With sufficient enlargement of the nodes in the porta hepatis, extrahepatic cholestasis may ensue. Tumors that have been reported to do so include colon cancer, breast cancer, gastric cancer, and melanoma. Lymphoma is also a consideration.

Primary Sclerosing Cholangitis (PSC)

Primary sclerosing cholangitis refers to bile duct injury in the absence of an apparent cause. It needs to be differentiated from secondary sclerosing cholangitis which occurs in the patient with a known predisposition. The injury to the bile ducts may take the form of inflammation, fibrosis, and strictures. PSC, a disease that has a predilection for young males, typically presents with pruritus, fatigue, and jaundice. Cholangitis is rare in these patients. A helpful clue is a history of inflammatory bowel disease since nearly 75% of patients have ulcerative colitis or Crohn's disease. Laboratory tests reveal elevations of the transaminases and alkaline phosphatase, with the latter being disproportionately elevated. ERCP can confirm the diagnosis.

Pancreatitis

Jaundice may be seen in alcoholic patients who present with both pancreatitis and hepatitis. Jaundice may also occur in pancreatitis that is secondary to gallstones. In these cases, the gallstones interrupt the flow of bile and pancreatic secretions in the distal common bile duct. Biliary obstruction may also occur if the pancreatitis is associated with extensive edema or is complicated by the development of a significant fluid collection.

Epigastric pain that typically radiates to the back is the hallmark of pancreatitis. The pain usually develops over a period of several hours but can last for days. There is a characteristic positional component to the pain. Most describe a worsening of the pain with recumbency and amelioration of the pain when leaning forward after assuming a sitting position. Nausea and vomiting frequently accompany the pain of pancreatitis. A low grade fever is also common.

Physical examination reveals epigastric tenderness with or without guarding. Tachycardia and decreased bowel sounds may also be appreciated. Less commonly observed are Cullen's and Grey Turner signs, which refer to periumbilical and flank ecchymoses, respectively. Laboratory testing reveals the characteristic rise in the amylase and lipase.

Pancreatic Pseudocyst

A pseudocyst may complicate either acute or chronic pancreatitis. Pseudocysts develop in approximately 10% of patients with acute pancreatitis. While patients with pancreatic pseudocysts may be asymptomatic, many complain of persistent abdominal pain. In some patients, physical examination may reveal an abdominal mass. Jaundice is one complication of pancreatic pseudocyst that typically occurs when a pseudocyst in the pancreatic head obstructs the common bile duct. Other complications include rupture, infection, compression of contiguous structures, erosion into nearby blood vessels, and fistula formation. Ultrasound and CT can readily establish the diagnosis.

AIDS Cholangiopathy

Pruritus and abdominal pain are common symptoms in patients with AIDS cholangiopathy, a disorder often associated with sclerosing cholangitis and/or papillary stenosis. Several organisms including *Microsporidia, Cryptosporidium, I. belli,* and CMV have been implicated in the pathogenesis. Ultrasound or CT may demonstrate the biliary dilatation that is characteristic of AIDS cholangiopathy. ERCP is required to confirm the diagnosis.

Biliary Stricture

Conditions associated with the development of biliary stricture are listed in the following box.

Conditions Associated with Development of Biliary Stricture	
AIDS cholangiopathy	Malignancy
Bile duct injury from surgery	Pancreatic
Chronic pancreatitis	Cholangiocarcinoma
Mirizzi's syndrome	Gallbladder
Radiation	Ampullary
Sclerosing cholangitis	Duodenal

Choledochal Cysts

More commonly seen in the Orient, extrahepatic biliary cysts, also known as choledochal cysts, tend to have a predilection for women. Although most cysts come to clinical attention in childhood with symptoms of obstructive jaundice, it is not unusual for the initial manifestations to appear in adulthood, usually in the form of pancreatitis or recurrent cholangitis. Intrahepatic biliary cysts (Caroli's syndrome) commonly present in young adulthood with fever. Abdominal pain and/or jaundice may be present. The diagnosis of both extrahepatic and intrahepatic biliary cysts requires imaging with ultrasound, CT, and cholangiography.

End of Section.

STEP 16: *What are the Results of ERCP or PTC?*

In patients strongly suspected of having extrahepatic cholestasis, the absence of biliary duct dilatation on ultrasound or CT should not prompt the clinician to discard this possibility. ERCP and PTC are invasive tests that should be considered when noninvasive testing (ultrasound or CT) is negative or equivocal in a patient likely to have extrahepatic cholestasis. ERCP and PTC have a sensitivity and specificity of 99% in the detection of ductal obstruction. In addition, the precise nature, extent, and location of the obstruction can be determined.

If the ERCP or PTC establishes the presence of extrahepatic cholestasis, *Proceed to Step 15.*

If the ERCP or PTC does not establish the presence of extrahepatic cholestasis, *Proceed to Step 17.*

STEP 17: *What is the Approach to the Patient With Intrahepatic Cholestasis?*

When imaging studies do not reveal biliary dilatation, intrahepatic cholestasis is likely. The causes of intrahepatic cholestasis are listed in the following box.

Causes of Intrahepatic Cholestasis	
Alcoholic hepatitis	Postoperative cholestasis
Benign recurrent intrahepatic cholestasis	Primary biliary cirrhosis
	Systemic infection
Drug-induced	Total parenteral nutrition
Intrahepatic cholestasis of pregnancy	Viral hepatitis

Common causes of intrahepatic cholestasis are discussed below.

Primary Biliary Cirrhosis

Primary biliary cirrhosis, a disease of unknown etiology, is a chronic chole-static illness. Nearly half of all patients are diagnosed at a time when they are asymptomatic. In these cases, the illness comes to clinical attention because of an elevated alkaline phosphatase level. Those who are symptomatic commonly complain of pruritus and fatigue. Approximately 25% of patients present with jaundice. Excoriations and hyperpigmentation of the skin may occur as a result of the frequent scratching.

The laboratory test abnormality that is the hallmark of the disease is the elevated alkaline phosphatase. While serum bilirubin levels are often normal at the time of presentation, hyperbilirubinemia develops in over 50% as the illness becomes more advanced. Antimitochondrial antibodies can be detected in 95% of patients. Serum protein electrophoresis may reveal IgM hypergammaglobulinemia. Imaging has a role in excluding extrahepatic causes of cholestasis in patients suspected of having primary biliary cirrhosis. The definitive diagnosis of primary biliary cirrhosis requires liver biopsy.

Viral Hepatitis

Cholestasis is not common in patients with viral hepatitis but may occur with any viral cause of hepatitis. It is more commonly appreciated in patients with hepatitis A. EBV and CMV are also considerations in the patient presenting with cholestasis thought to be secondary to a viral etiology.

In these patients, symptoms of acute viral hepatitis including fever, anorexia, and right upper quadrant pain are usually present. Jaundice and pruritus usually follow the onset of these symptoms. Early in the illness, the transaminase levels may exceed 1000 U/L but are usually less than 200 U/L by the time features of cholestasis manifest. During the cholestatic phase, the bilirubin and alkaline phosphatase levels are significantly elevated. Not uncommonly, cholestatic viral hepatitis persists for weeks to months.

Alcoholic Hepatitis

While alcoholic hepatitis usually presents with hepatocellular injury, some cases are characterized by cholestasis. In these cases, serum bilirubin and alkaline phosphatase levels are elevated out of proportion to the transaminase levels. Because patients with alcoholic hepatitis often present with fever and leukocytosis, it is necessary to exclude extrahepatic biliary obstruction.

Drug-Induced Cholestasis

Medications are a major cause of cholestasis. As such, drug-induced cholestasis should be considered in any patient with liver function test abnormalities consistent with cholestatic injury. Common offenders are listed in the following box.

Medications Commonly Associated with Cholestasis	
Amoxicillin and clavulanic acid	Oral contraceptives
Androgenic steroids	Penicillin derivatives
Cyclosporine A	Phenothiazines
Estrogens	Tamoxifen
Glyburide	

Other medications may cause a mixed picture with features of both cholestasis and hepatocellular injury. These are listed in the following box.

Medications Causing a Mixed Picture of Cholestasis and Hepatocellular Injury	
ACE inhibitors	Ketoconazole
Allopurinol	NSAIDs
Azathioprine	Oral hypoglycemic agents
Barbiturates	Penicillamine
Benzodiazepines	Phenothiazines
Clavulanic acid	Phenytoin
Erythromycin	Prochlorperazine
Fluoxetine	Propylthiouracil
H_2-blockers	Sulfonamides
Haloperidol	Tricyclic antidepressants

In most cases, cholestasis develops several weeks after starting the offending medication. In some cases, however, cholestasis has been described in patients several years after the institution of a medication. Most cases of drug-induced cholestasis come to clinical attention when abnormal liver function tests are found in an asymptomatic patient. Some patients may present with anorexia, abdominal pain, nausea, pruritus, or jaundice. Fever and rash are uncommon but, when present, should prompt the clinician to seriously consider drug-induced cholestasis.

Eosinophilia, although rare, lends support to the diagnosis. The diagnosis should be suspected in any patient who develops cholestatic liver injury within weeks to months after starting a new medication. Normalization of the liver function test abnormalities after cessation of the offending agent provides a strong argument for drug-induced cholestasis. While liver biopsy can demonstrate features consistent with drug-induced cholestasis, rarely is it diagnostic.

Total Parenteral Nutrition (TPN)

Not uncommonly, patients develop liver function test abnormalities 1-4 weeks after starting TPN. In most cases, these abnormalities resolve with time. While the most common hepatobiliary complication of TPN is steatohepatitis, cholestasis has also been reported.

Cholestatic liver disease tends to occur in patients receiving long-term TPN. Because these patients are also at risk for the development of biliary stones, it is important to exclude this possibility before attributing the cholestasis to TPN.

Systemic Infection

When jaundice develops in the febrile patient, the clinician should consider cholestasis secondary to systemic infection or sepsis. Affected patients are usually very ill. Jaundice is usually preceded by several days of symptoms and signs suggestive of infection. Both bilirubin and alkaline phosphatase levels are usually elevated.

Although cholestasis secondary to systemic infection has been well described in patients with Gram-negative enteric infections and toxic shock syndrome, it may also occur in Gram-positive infections. Extrahepatic biliary obstruction should be excluded in these patients.

Postoperative Jaundice

Jaundice occurs in approximately 1% of patients after an operative intervention requiring anesthesia. There are many causes of postoperative jaundice. In some cases, the etiology is multifactorial. Elucidating the precise etiology requires careful consideration of the temporal relationship between the onset of jaundice and the surgical procedure. Jaundice within the first few days suggests hepatic ischemia or hemolysis. In contrast, anesthetic related jaundice is unusual before the seventh postoperative day.

While postoperative jaundice may present with hepatocellular injury, in some cases, the injury is cholestatic. Bile duct injury may occur during abdominal surgery, resulting in jaundice. Such an injury should be suspected with certain surgeries such as laparoscopic cholecystectomy, other biliary tract surgery, and gastrectomy.

Cholestasis that occurs in the postoperative period is often multifactorial. Hypotension, hemorrhage, hypoxia, and sepsis are all factors that may play a role. This type of cholestatic syndrome manifesting after surgery has been referred to as benign postoperative jaundice.

Benign Recurrent Intrahepatic Cholestasis

Benign recurrent intrahepatic cholestasis is a rare condition that is characterized by recurrent episodes of acute cholestasis. Between exacerbations, patients are otherwise healthy. The onset of this illness is typically in childhood or adolescence. The episodes are characterized by symptoms of anorexia, pruritus, and jaundice. Liver function tests reveal a pattern consistent with cholestasis. After several weeks to months, the episode resolves, leaving the patient completely asymptomatic. With resolution of the illness, the liver function test abnormalities normalize. Although many have a family history of benign recurrent intrahepatic cholestasis, sporadic cases have been reported.

Intrahepatic Cholestasis of Pregnancy

Elevations in the alkaline phosphatase level are common during pregnancy because of the leakage of placental alkaline phosphatase into the serum. In the intrahepatic cholestasis of pregnancy, alkaline phosphatase elevation is accompanied by abnormalities of the GGT, transaminases, and bilirubin. This is an uncommon disorder that typically occurs late in pregnancy (70% during the 3rd trimester) and is characterized by pruritus. Jaundice occurs in about 25% of patients. Intrahepatic cholestasis of pregnancy is a benign condition that usually disappears after pregnancy. Affected individuals are at higher risk of developing a recurrence with subsequent pregnancies. A similar picture may develop when these individuals take oral contraceptives.

End of Section.

STEP 18: *What is the Etiology of the Hepatocellular Disease?*

Hepatocellular diseases associated with jaundice are listed in the following box.

Hepatocellular Diseases Associated with Jaundice	
Alcoholic hepatitis	Hepatic vein thrombosis
α_1-antitrypsin deficiency	Hepatotoxins
Autoimmune hepatitis	Ischemia
Cirrhosis	Viral hepatitis (acute or chronic)
Drug-induced	Wilson's disease
Hemochromatosis	

Some of the more common hepatocellular diseases are considered below.

Acute Viral Hepatitis

Acute viral hepatitis may manifest without any symptoms or signs. In these cases, the illness comes to clinical attention because of abnormal liver function tests along with serologic evidence of acute viral hepatitis. When symptomatic, patients with acute viral hepatitis often share some common features, irrespective of the viral etiology. Early in the course of the illness, patients may complain of malaise, fatigue, nausea, vomiting, anorexia, abdominal discomfort, and joint pain. On occasion, patients complain of losing the desire to drink alcohol or smoke cigarettes. Other complaints include low-grade fever and headache. These symptoms typically last 3-4 days but may linger for 2-3 weeks. This prodromal phase of the illness is followed by the icteric phase. During this phase, many patients note a darkening of the urine followed by stool discoloration and jaundice. It is important to realize that not all patients progress to the icteric phase (anicteric hepatitis).

Physical examination reveals a tender liver in up to 66% of patients. Fifteen percent of patients have mild splenomegaly.

At the time of clinical symptoms, patients with acute viral hepatitis usually have reached their peak AST and ALT levels. Levels may exceed 1000 U/L. Other findings include hyperbilirubinemia and a mild elevation in alkaline phosphatase. Identifying the specific viral etiology requires serologic testing. The following table lists the serologic tests (for the common causes of viral hepatitis) that should be obtained in the patient suspected of having acute viral hepatitis.

Viral Agent	Serologic Finding in Acute Viral Hepatitis
Hepatitis A	IgM anti-HAV
Hepatitis B	HBsAg IgM anti-HBc
Hepatitis C	Anti-HCV*

*Anti-HCV may not be detectable early in the course of acute hepatitis C. In these cases, it may be worthwhile to repeat the anti-HCV after a sufficient period of time has elapsed. Alternatively, the clinician may elect to obtain hepatitis C viral RNA to establish the diagnosis.

Chronic Viral Hepatitis

Jaundice is a cardinal manifestation of a number of chronic hepatocellular diseases. Chronic viral hepatitis is one such consideration. The major viral causes of chronic hepatitis are hepatitis B and C. Although patients with either chronic hepatitis B or C may recall a history of distant acute hepatitis, in many cases, no such history can be elicited. Most patients with chronic viral hepatitis are asymptomatic. Not uncommonly, chronic viral hepatitis comes to clinical attention only because of persistent liver function test abnormalities.

When symptoms are present, they are often nonspecific symptoms such as malaise, fatigue, and anorexia. Physical examination may reveal the stigmata of chronic liver disease such as prominent abdominal veins, spider angiomas, and gynecomastia. With advancing disease, patients with chronic viral hepatitis may present with jaundice and complications of portal hypertension. These complications include ascites, encephalopathy, and variceal hemorrhage. Viral serology for hepatitis B and C are necessary in patients suspected of having chronic viral hepatitis.

Alcoholic Hepatitis

Most patients with alcoholic hepatitis present with anorexia, malaise, fever, and abdominal pain. Physical examination often reveals scleral icterus, spider angiomas, and tender hepatomegaly. Portal hypertension may be evident in severe cases of alcoholic hepatitis. In these cases, the clinician may note splenomegaly, prominent abdominal veins, ascites, and encephalopathy.

Transaminase levels rarely exceed 300-400 U/L. Levels exceeding this should prompt the clinician to consider other causes of liver disease. In many cases, the AST to ALT ratio exceeds 2. Such a ratio in a patient with modest transaminase levels should always warrant consideration of alcoholic hepatitis. It is important to realize, however, that alcoholic hepatitis may present with an AST to ALT ratio <2.

Cirrhosis

The causes of cirrhosis are listed in the following box.

Causes of Cirrhosis	
Fairly Common	**Rare**
Ethanol	α_1-antitrypsin deficiency
Viral	Cystic fibrosis
Hepatitis B (with or without D)	Drug-induced
Hepatitis C	Glycogen storage diseases
Less Common	Jejunoileal bypass
Autoimmune hepatitis	Sarcoidosis
Cryptogenic cirrhosis	Wilson's disease
Hemochromatosis	
Primary biliary cirrhosis	
Primary sclerosing cholangitis	
Secondary biliary cirrhosis	

Many patients, particularly in the early stages of cirrhosis, are asymptomatic. With progression of the liver disease, nonspecific complaints of anorexia, malaise, fatigue, and weight loss may ensue. Complications of portal hypertension may occur in patients with advanced disease.

Although liver function tests may support the diagnosis, it is important to realize that they may be normal. A decreased serum albumin and an elevated prothrombin time are common in advanced disease, reflecting an impairment in hepatic synthetic function. Hypersplenism is a complication of portal hypertension and may result in anemia, thrombocytopenia, or leukopenia. Hyponatremia is a poor prognostic finding in patients with cirrhosis.

Elucidating the etiology of the cirrhosis often requires other laboratory testing. When the etiology is not clear, the clinician should consider obtaining the following tests:

Condition	Recommended Laboratory Tests
Hepatitis B	Hepatitis B surface antigen
	If positive, consider hepatitis D testing
Hepatitis C	Antibody to hepatitis C virus
	Hepatitis C viral RNA
Autoimmune hepatitis	Antinuclear antibodies
	Antismooth muscle antibodies
	Antiliver-kidney microsomal antibodies
Hemochromatosis	Ferritin
	Iron
	Total iron-binding capacity
	Transferrin
α_1-antitrypsin deficiency	Serum protein electrophoresis
Wilson's disease	Serum ceruloplasmin
Primary biliary cirrhosis	Antimichrondrial antibodies

Imaging studies are useful in providing evidence of cirrhosis or portal hypertension. In addition, complications of cirrhosis such as hepatocellular carcinoma may be detected.

Ultrasonographic findings that suggest the diagnosis of cirrhosis include the following:

- Dense reflective areas of irregular distribution and increased echogenicity
- Demonstration of a coarsely nodular liver surface
- Relatively enlarged caudate lobe
- Evidence of portal hypertension (portal vein diameter >1.4 cm, ascites, splenomegaly, portosystemic collaterals)

In addition, ultrasound may demonstrate a liver lesion, raising concern for hepatocellular carcinoma. Cirrhosis is a risk factor for the development of hepatocellular carcinoma.

CT findings may be normal in the early stages of cirrhosis. In advanced disease, the liver may be small with irregular edges and demonstrate inhomogeneous contrast enhancement. Not uncommonly, the caudate lobe is disproportionately larger than the other lobes of the liver. Findings of portal hypertension that may be demonstrated on CT include ascites, splenomegaly, and portosystemic collaterals.

Another imaging option available is 99mTc-sulfur colloid scintigraphy, which can assess liver size and blood flow. Heterogeneous uptake in the liver along with an increased uptake in the spleen and bone marrow are findings suggestive of cirrhosis. When these findings are present, a colloid shift is said to be present.

Taken together, the patient's clinical presentation, laboratory tests, and imaging studies can provide evidence that supports the diagnosis of cirrhosis. The definitive diagnosis, however, requires liver biopsy. In addition to confirming the presence of cirrhosis, the findings may point to a particular etiology, such as hemochromatosis.

Drug-Induced Liver Disease

Up to 5% of cases of jaundice in hospitalized patients are due to drug-induced liver disease. Drug-induced liver disease can take many forms including asymptomatic elevation in the transaminase levels, acute hepatitis, and fulminant hepatic failure. Most often, the clinician encounters the asymptomatic patient who has transaminase elevations secondary to a particular medication. The prevalence of hepatic enzyme elevation (in the asymptomatic patient) with various drugs is shown in the following table.

Prevalence (%)	Examples
25-50	Tacrine
20-25	Amiodarone Chlorpromazine Cisplatin 6-mercaptopurine Nicotinic acid Papaverine Phenytoin Valproate
10-20	Androgens Erythromycin estolate Etretinate Isoniazid Ketoconazole
5-10	Chenodeoxycholate Disulfiram Flucytosine Penicillamine
<5	Dantrolene Ethionamide Gold salts Quinidine Salicylates Sulfonamides Sulfonylureas Ticarcillin Tricyclic antidepressants

Adapted from *Clinical Practice of Gastroenterology*, Brandt LJ (ed), Philadelphia, PA: Current Medicine, Inc, 1999, 856.

Drug-induced liver disease can cause hepatocellular injury, cholestatic injury, or a mixed pattern. Medications that are predominantly associated with hepatocellular injury are listed in the following box.

Medications Causing Hepatocellular Injury	
Anesthetics	Antiarrhythmics
Enflurane	Amiodarone
Halothane	Procainamide
Methoxyflurane	Quinidine
Anticonvulsants	Lipid-lowering agents
Phenytoin	Nicotinic acid
Valproic acid	Statins
MAO inhibitors	Antibiotics
Analgesic	Antiviral agents
Acetaminophen	AZT
NSAIDs	Didanosine
Salicylates	Antineoplastic agents
Antithyroid	Miscellaneous
Propylthiouracil	Disulfiram
Steroids / hormonal agents	Etretinate
Diethylstilbestrol	Loratadine
Tamoxifen	Pemoline
Antihypertensives	Sulfasalazine
ACE-inhibitors	Tacrine
α-methyldopa	Tannic acid
β-blockers	Vitamin A
Hydralazine	
Verapamil	

The clinical presentation of drug-induced liver disease varies. The subclinical hepatic enzyme elevation that occurs with many different medications often does not lead to clinically significant liver disease despite continuing the offending medication. When a medication causes considerable hepatocellular necrosis, symptoms and signs resembling acute viral hepatitis may occur. In these cases, the degree of transaminase elevation may mimic that found in viral hepatitis.

A classic example is isoniazid hepatotoxicity. While subclinical hepatic enzyme elevation is more common, overt hepatitis occurs in 1% of patients receiving isoniazid. The risk of developing clinically significant hepatotoxicity increases with advancing age. The risk of hepatotoxicity is also increased when the medication is used in conjunction with rifampin or pyrazinamide.

Another example of drug-induced liver disease is acetaminophen hepatotoxicity, a major cause of fulminant hepatic failure. Characteristic of acetaminophen hepatotoxicity is a rise in the transaminase levels to >10,000 U/L.

Drug-induced liver disease should be suspected in any patient who presents with overt liver disease. Establishing the diagnosis begins with the exclusion of other causes of hepatocellular injury such as viral and alcoholic hepatitis. In drug-induced liver disease, resolution of the signs and symptoms along with normalization of the liver function test abnormalities following drug discontinuation provides a strong argument for the diagnosis. Rechallenging a patient with the suspect medication is not without risk. In patients who developed jaundice or other manifestations of liver disease, rechallenging the patient to confirm the diagnosis is not recommended. In those who had subclinical hepatic enzyme elevation, it is, however, possible to rechallenge the patient. Consultation with a hepatologist is recommended in these cases.

REFERENCES

Clinical Practice of Gastroenterology, Brandt LJ (ed), Philadelphia, PA: Current Medicine, Inc, 1999, 856.

Frank BB, "Clinical Evaluation of Jaundice. A Guideline of the Patient Care Committee of the American Gastroenterological Association," *JAMA*, 1989, 262(21):3031-4.

McGill JM and Kwiatkowski AP, "Cholestatic Liver Diseases in Adults," *Am J Gastroenterol*, 1998, 93(5):684-91.

Pasha TM and Lindor KD, "Diagnosis and Therapy of Cholestatic Liver Disease," *Med Clin North Am*, 1996, 80(5):995-1019.

Rossi RL, Traverso LW, and Pimentel F, "Malignant Obstructive Jaundice. Evaluation and Management," *Surg Clin North Am*, 1996, 76(1):63-70.

JAUNDICE

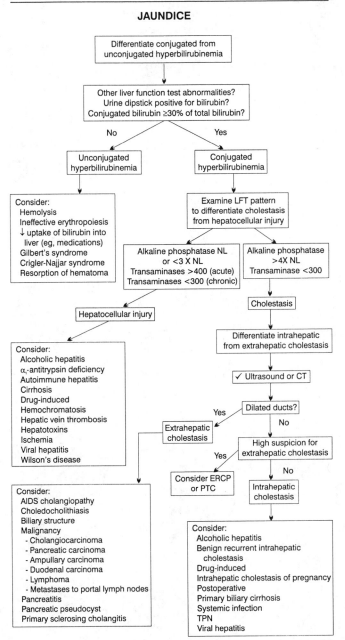

LEG SWELLING

STEP 1: *How Common is Leg Swelling?*

Leg swelling, unilateral or bilateral, is a commonly encountered problem. While many cases of leg swelling are due to benign conditions, the clinician must recognize features in the patient's presentation suggestive of more serious etiologies.

Proceed to Step 2

STEP 2: *Is the Leg Swelling Unilateral or Bilateral?*

Determination of the cause begins with consideration of whether the leg swelling is unilateral or bilateral. In patients with bilateral leg swelling, asymmetry in circumference that exceeds 1 or 2 cm is considered to be clinically significant. These patients should be evaluated for causes of unilateral leg swelling which may occur in the setting of bilateral leg swelling. If no cause of unilateral leg swelling is identified in the patient with asymmetrical bilateral leg swelling, then efforts to identify the cause of the bilateral leg swelling should be pursued.

If the leg swelling is bilateral, *Proceed to Step 3*.

If the leg swelling is bilateral, but asymmetric (difference in circumference >1 or 2 cm), *Proceed to Step 15.*

If the leg swelling is unilateral, *Proceed to Step 15*.

STEP 3: *What are the Causes of Bilateral Leg Swelling?*

The causes of bilateral leg swelling are listed in the following box.

Causes of Bilateral Leg Swelling	
Cardiac	Malnutrition
Congestive heart failure	Medications
Constrictive pericarditis	Myxedema
Pulmonary hypertension	Pregnancy
Tricuspid valve disease	Premenstrual or cyclic
Chronic venous insufficiency	Protein-losing enteropathy
Cirrhosis	Renal
Idiopathic	Acute nephritic syndrome
Inferior vena cava obstruction	Nephrotic syndrome
Lipedema	Renal failure
Lymphedema	

Proceed to Step 4

STEP 4: *Are There Any Clues in the Patient's History That Point to the Etiology of the Bilateral Leg Swelling?*

Clues in the patient's history that point to the etiology of the bilateral leg swelling are listed in the following table.

Historical Clue	Condition Suggested
Dyspnea* Orthopnea PND	Congestive heart failure
History of COPD	Pulmonary hypertension
History of alcohol abuse	Alcoholic cardiomyopathy Cirrhosis Malnutrition
History of liver disease	Cirrhosis
Diarrhea (chronic)	Protein-losing enteropathy
History of renal disease	Nephrotic syndrome Renal failure
Foamy or frothy urine	Nephrotic syndrome
Recent sore throat	Acute nephritic syndrome (PSGN)
Ascites precede edema	Cirrhosis
Edema precedes ascites	Congestive heart failure
Edema occurring during the premenstrual period	Premenstrual or cyclic edema
History of CAD or HTN	Congestive heart failure
History of hepatitis	Cirrhosis
History of jaundice	Cirrhosis
Smoky color of the urine	Acute nephritic syndrome
Congenital	Primary lymphedema
Family history of bilateral leg swelling	Lipedema Primary lymphedema
Intermittent	Premenstrual or cyclic edema
Increased abdominal girth (ascites)	Cirrhosis Congestive heart failure Constrictive pericarditis Nephrotic syndrome
Medication history	Medication-related edema (see Step 14)
Leg swelling worse in hot weather	Premenstrual or cyclic edema

*Although shortness of breath and bilateral leg swelling should prompt consideration of congestive heart failure, other possibilities to consider include nephrotic syndrome (causing pleural effusions or complicated by pulmonary embolism), angioedema (dyspnea secondary to laryngeal edema), and ascites due to any cause (secondary to diaphragmatic elevation).

Proceed to Step 5

STEP 5: *Are There Any Clues in the Patient's Physical Examination That Point to the Etiology of the Bilateral Leg Swelling?*

Clues in the patient's physical examination that point to the etiology of the bilateral leg swelling are listed in the following table.

Physical Examination Finding	Condition Suggested
Dupuytren's contracture Gynecomastia Palmar erythema Parotid gland enlargement Spider angioma Testicular atrophy	Cirrhosis

Elevated jugular venous pressure	Cardiac
	  Congestive heart failure
	  Constrictive pericarditis
	  Pulmonary hypertension
	  Tricuspid valve disease
	Renal failure

Edema of the feet and toes not present	Lipedema
S3	Congestive heart failure
Pericardial knock	Constrictive pericarditis
Periorbital edema	Nephrotic syndrome
Kussmaul's sign	Constrictive pericarditis
Prominent venous pattern in lateral flanks with cephalad drainage	Inferior vena cava obstruction

Signs of ascites:
  Bulging flanks
  Fluid wave
  Shifting dullness
	Cirrhosis
	Congestive heart failure
	Constrictive pericarditis
	Nephrotic syndrome

Proceed to Step 6

STEP 6: *What is the Jugular Venous Pressure?*

It is important to estimate the jugular venous pressure in every patient presenting with bilateral leg swelling. The jugular venous pressure reflects the right atrial pressure. An elevated jugular venous pressure suggests that the bilateral leg swelling is due to either a cardiac etiology or renal failure. All other causes of bilateral leg swelling are characterized by a normal jugular venous pressure.

If the jugular venous pressure is elevated, *Proceed to Step 7.*

If the jugular venous pressure is not elevated, *Proceed to Step 9.*

STEP 7: *Does the Patient Have Renal Failure?*

Both acute and chronic renal failure may be associated with bilateral leg swelling. Many patients with acute renal failure are oliguric. The oliguria leads to a decrease in salt and water excretion, which manifests with signs and symptoms of extracellular fluid expansion. In mild cases, physical examination may reveal bibasilar crackles, elevated jugular venous pressure, and bilateral lower extremity edema. With greater degrees of volume expansion, however, patients may develop pulmonary edema.

Chronic renal failure is also associated with volume expansion. However, many patients with stable chronic renal failure have no signs or symptoms of volume expansion. With the ingestion of large amounts of salt and water, symptoms and signs of volume excess may become apparent.

Renal failure can be distinguished from cardiac etiologies of bilateral leg swelling by measuring the serum BUN and creatinine, which usually reveal the presence of severe renal failure.

If the bilateral leg swelling is due to renal failure, *Stop Here.*

If the bilateral leg swelling is not due to renal failure, *Proceed to Step 8.*

STEP 8: What Cardiac Conditions are Associated With Bilateral Leg Swelling?

When renal failure failure has been excluded in the patient with jugular venous distention, a cardiac etiology of the bilateral lower extremity swelling is likely. Cardiac conditions associated with edema include the following:

- Constrictive pericarditis
- Congestive heart failure
- Pulmonary hypertension
- Tricuspid valve disease

When examining the jugular venous pulse, it is not sufficient to merely establish the presence of an elevated jugular venous pressure. Rather the clinician should strive to identify the waves in the jugular venous pulse. By doing so, the clinician may recognize the prominent x and y descent of constrictive pericarditis. A large cv wave would support the diagnosis of tricuspid regurgitation while a slow y descent should prompt consideration of tricuspid stenosis. Therefore, inspection of the jugular venous waveform may suggest the etiology of the bilateral leg swelling.

The cardiac conditions associated with edema will be considered below.

Congestive Heart Failure

Clues in the patient's history and physical examination that point to the presence of congestive heart failure are listed in the following table.

Type of Evidence	Highly Suggestive	Less Specific
Symptoms	Orthopnea PND	Decreased exercise tolerance Discomfort when bending Nocturnal cough
Signs	Displaced left ventricular impulse Jugular venous distention Narrow pulse pressure Pulsatile hepatomegaly Rales S3 gallop	Ascites Hypotension Peripheral edema Tachycardia

Adapted from Kannel WB and Belanger AJ, "Epidemiology of Heart Failure," *Am Heart J,* 1991, 121(3 Pt 1):951-7; also from *Primary Cardiology,* Goldman L and Braunwald E (eds), Philadelphia, PA: WB Saunders Co, 1998, 311.

In most cases of bilateral lower extremity edema secondary to congestive heart failure, left ventricular systolic dysfunction or mitral stenosis ultimately results in right-sided heart failure. With right ventricular involvement, pressures in the systemic veins and capillaries rise. This promotes the transudation of fluid into the interstitial space, which manifests as edema. Edema occurs less often in patients with diastolic dysfunction. Edema has also been reported in patients with high-output congestive heart failure. Causes of high-output congestive heart failure include anemia, hyperthyroidism, arteriovenous fistula, and beriberi.

It is important to realize that there is a poor correlation between edema and the level of the systemic venous pressure. Although edema is classically thought to be a manifestation of right-sided heart failure, it has also been noted in patients with predominantly left-sided heart failure who have only slight elevations of the systemic venous pressure.

Echocardiography is useful for confirming the diagnosis. In addition, information regarding left ventricular function, pulmonary artery pressure, and valve function can be obtained.

Constrictive Pericarditis

In constrictive pericarditis, thickening and scarring of the pericardium impedes the diastolic filling of the ventricles. The major causes of constrictive pericarditis are listed in the following box.

Causes of Constrictive Pericarditis	
Idiopathic	Postirradiation
Infectious	Postsurgical
Neoplastic	Tuberculosis

Common complaints among patients with constrictive pericarditis include fatigue, shortness of breath, abdominal discomfort, weight gain, increasing abdominal girth, and edema. In most cases, symptoms and signs develop over a period of years. However, in a minority of cases, particularly those due to trauma, surgery, and mediastinal irradiation, the clinical manifestations may develop over a few months. Physical examination findings include ascites, hepatosplenomegaly, and edema. Not well recognized is that cachexia may be encountered in patients with long-standing disease. In the latter cases, the clinician may erroneously diagnose the patient with cirrhosis.

The examination of the jugular venous pulse is important in the patient suspected of having constrictive pericarditis. Characteristic features include not only an elevation in the jugular venous pressure but also prominent x and y descents. Kussmaul's sign, which refers to the inspiratory increase in the jugular venous pressure, may be noted in some patients with constrictive pericarditis. However, it is important to realize that this sign may be elicited in other conditions such as restrictive cardiomyopathy, right ventricular infarction, right ventricular failure, and tricuspid stenosis. Auscultation of the heart may reveal the characteristic pericardial knock, a sound that is often confused with an S3. Pulsus paradoxus is an infrequent finding in patients with constrictive pericarditis.

Laboratory tests are usually unremarkable except for liver function tests which may be abnormal, reflecting hepatic congestion. The EKG is usually nonspecific. Low QRS voltage and nonspecific T wave abnormalities are not uncommon. Atrial fibrillation has been reported in about 33% of patients. CXR typically reveals a normal cardiac silhouette although, in some, the silhouette may be enlarged. Pericardial calcifications, which are suggestive of the diagnosis, are appreciated in less than 50% of cases.

Although there are some very suggestive echocardiographic findings in patients with constrictive pericarditis, no finding or combination of findings is pathognomonic for the disease. A normal study, however, argues strongly against the diagnosis. CT is very useful in the evaluation of these patients. In most patients, the CT demonstrates pericardial thickening. In fact, a normal pericardial thickness provides a strong argument against the diagnosis. Cardiac catheterization can confirm the diagnosis.

Pulmonary Hypertension

Common symptoms of pulmonary hypertension include shortness of breath, chest pain, fatigue, edema, and syncope. The chest pain of pulmonary hypertension may be exertional, closely resembling angina. Physical examination findings consistent with pulmonary hypertension are listed in the following box.

Physical Examination Findings of Pulmonary Hypertension
Ascites
Hepatic congestion with right upper quadrant tenderness
Hepatojugular reflux
Jugular venous distention
Murmur of tricuspid regurgitation
Prominent and delayed P2 (widely split S2)
Right-sided S3
Right-sided S4
Right ventricular heave

EKG findings supportive of pulmonary hypertension include the following:

- Right atrial abnormality
- Right bundle branch block or right ventricular conduction delay
- S wave in lead I
- Tall, initial R wave in V1

Cardiac catheterization is the gold standard in the diagnosis of pulmonary hypertension. However, since it is an invasive test that may carry an increased risk of death in patients with severe pulmonary hypertension, the clinician may elect to perform noninvasive testing such as echocardiography to establish the diagnosis. Once the presence of pulmonary hypertension has been confirmed, the clinician should identify the etiology of the pulmonary hypertension. The causes are listed in the following box.

Causes of Pulmonary Hypertension	
α_1-antitrypsin deficiency	Connective tissue disease
Alveolar hypoventilation	Cystic fibrosis
Central nervous system dysfunction	Hepatopulmonary syndrome
Chest wall dysfunction	Interstitial lung disease
Neuromuscular disease	Medications
Obesity	Primary pulmonary hypertension
Sleep apnea	Residence at high altitude
Chronic mountain sickness	Thromboembolic disease
Chronic obstructive pulmonary disease	Veno-occlusive disease
Congestive heart failure (left-sided)	

End of Section.

STEP 9: *What is the Serum Albumin?*

Hypoalbuminemia in the patient with bilateral leg swelling should prompt consideration of the following possibilities:

- Cirrhosis
- Malnutrition
- Nephrotic syndrome
- Protein-losing enteropathy

If the patient has hypoalbuminemia, ***Proceed to Step 10.***

If the patient does not have hypoalbuminemia, ***Proceed to Step 14.***

STEP 10: *Is There Any Protein in the Urine?*

Dipstick testing of the urine for protein is important when the nephrotic syndrome is a consideration. A positive result of the urine dipstick for protein is not synonymous with the nephrotic syndrome. It should merely prompt the clinician to obtain a 24-hour urine collection for protein, which is more accurate in quantifying the degree of proteinuria. When >3.5 grams of protein are excreted over a 24-hour time period, nephrotic range proteinuria is said to be present. The nephrotic syndrome is characterized by the features listed in the following box.

Features of the Nephrotic Syndrome	
Edema	Lipiduria
Hyperlipidemia	Proteinuria (>3.5 grams/day)
Hypoalbuminemia	

It is necessary to measure the creatinine in the urine collection to ensure that the collection was complete. If the measured creatinine falls between the values listed in the following box, then the clinician can be confident of a complete 24-hour urine collection.

Normal Creatinine Excretion Over a 24-Hour Time Period	
Female: 15-20 mg/kg	Male: 20-25 mg/kg

Values that are below the range reported in the preceding box can lead to an underestimation of the degree of proteinuria.

If the patient has the nephrotic syndrome, *Stop Here.*

If the patient does not have the nephrotic syndrome, *Proceed to Step 11.*

STEP 11: *Does the Patient Have Cirrhosis?*

The liver is a remarkable organ, having a number of different functions. One of its functions is the synthesis of various substances, including albumin. Although mild degrees of liver dysfunction may not be associated with hypoalbuminemia, with chronicity and progression to cirrhosis, the synthetic capability of the liver becomes compromised. As such, hypoalbuminemia is often found in patients with cirrhosis. Because hypoalbuminemia and edema can occur in other conditions, the clinician should become familiar with the clinical presentation of patients with cirrhosis.

The definitive diagnosis of cirrhosis can only be made when characteristic histologic findings are noted on liver biopsy. Short of that, the clinician must use the history, physical examination, laboratory data, and imaging tests to establish a clinical diagnosis. Many patients with cirrhosis are asymptomatic. Those that are symptomatic typically complain of nonspecific symptoms such as fatigue, weakness, malaise, anorexia, and weight loss. Of particular importance in the history is the identification of any risk factors for liver disease such as alcohol abuse, for example. In those who have advanced disease, complications of portal hypertension may be present. These include ascites, esophageal varices, and hepatic encephalopathy. Although the physical examination findings may be unrevealing, in some, the stigmata of chronic liver disease may be noted. These include palmar erythema, spider angioma, gynecomastia, testicular atrophy, and parotid gland enlargement.

There is no doubt that some patients with cirrhosis have a normal biochemical profile. In most patients, however, there are one or more liver function test abnormalities. Besides hypoalbuminemia, a prolonged PT may be noted, reflecting an impairment in the liver's synthetic capability. In those who have portal hypertension complicated by splenomegaly, laboratory testing may reveal leukopenia, thrombocytopenia, anemia, or a combination thereof. These findings are due to hypersplenism.

CT or ultrasound can demonstrate findings consistent with cirrhosis and portal hypertension. Once the clinical diagnosis of cirrhosis has been made, the clinician should search for the cause when the etiology is not apparent.

If the patient has cirrhosis, *Stop Here.*

If the patient does not have cirrhosis, *Proceed to Step 12.*

STEP 12: *Does the Patient Have Protein-Losing Enteropathy?*

The excessive loss of protein into the gastrointestinal lumen is known as protein-losing enteropathy. The clinical hallmarks of protein-losing enteropathy are edema and hypoproteinemia. Conditions associated with protein-losing enteropathy are listed in the box below.

Causes of Protein-Losing Enteropathy	
Acute graft-vs-host disease	Neoplasm
Bacterial overgrowth	Parasitic diseases
Celiac sprue	Pseudomembranous enterocolitis
Congenital intestinal lymphangiectasia	Retroperitoneal fibrosis
Congestive heart failure	Sarcoidosis
Constrictive pericarditis	Systemic lupus erythematosus
Crohn's disease	Tropical sprue
Eosinophilic gastroenteritis	Tuberculosis
Erosive gastroenteritis	Viral gastroenteritis
Lymphoma	Whipple's disease
Menetrier's disease	

Adapted from *Handbook of Gastroenterology*, Yamada T (ed), Philadelphia, PA: Lippincott-Raven, 1998, 321.

The diagnosis can be established by calculating the α_1-antitrypsin clearance. Elevations in the quantitative fecal α_1-antitrypsin concentration or clearance is supportive of the diagnosis.

If the patient has protein-losing enteropathy, *Stop Here.*

If the patient does not have protein-losing enteropathy, *Proceed to Step 13.*

STEP 13: *Does the Patient Have Edema Related to Malnutrition?*

Any diet severely lacking in protein may lead to hypoproteinemia and edema, especially if the nutritional deficit is long-standing. Patients who are malnourished are also at risk for thiamine deficiency, which may result in the development of beriberi heart disease.

Interestingly, malnourished patients may experience a worsening of the edema with refeeding. This is known as refeeding edema.

If the patient has edema related to malnutrition, *Stop Here.*

If the patient does not have edema related to malnutrition, *Proceed to Step 14.*

STEP 14: *What are Other Considerations in the Patient With Bilateral Lower Extremity Swelling?*

Other conditions that may be associated with bilateral lower extremity swelling are considered below. These conditions are not usually associated with hypoalbuminemia.

Pregnancy

The body's total water and sodium increase during pregnancy. In fact, nearly 80% of pregnant women will be noted to have edema. This is a normal finding.

Premenstrual Edema (Cyclic)

Excessive estrogenic stimulation during the premenstrual period can lead to the retention of sodium and water. This is known as premenstrual or cyclic edema.

Myxedema

Patients with hypothyroidism have an accumulation of hyaluronic acid in the dermis. The binding of water to hyaluronic acid results in mucinous edema, which is responsible for the thickened features and puffy appearance seen in hypothyroidism. These changes have been termed myxedema. Myxedema is particular prominent around the eyes and on the dorsa of the hands and feet. It is classically nonpitting in nature.

Lipedema

Lipedema is not a true type of edema. It really refers to the deposition of fat in the legs. Lipedema tends to spare the feet.

Lymphedema

Lymphatic obstruction may lead to lymphedema. Lymphedema is discussed in more detail in Step 22.

Chronic Venous Insufficiency

Chronic venous insufficiency is discussed in more detail in Step 23.

Medications

Medications can cause bilateral leg swelling by promoting renal sodium retention. These medications are listed in the following box.

Medications Causing or Exacerbating Bilateral Leg Swelling	
α-adrenergic antagonists	Guanethidine
β-blockers	Growth hormone
Calcium channel blockers	Hydralazine
Clonidine	Interleukin-2
Corticosteroids	Methyldopa
Cyclosporine	Minoxidil
Diazoxide	NSAIDs
Estrogens	Progestins
Fludrocortisone	Testosterone

Edema beginning shortly after the institution of a new medication should prompt consideration of medication-related edema. Resolution of the edema after discontinuation of the suspect medication establishes the diagnosis.

Idiopathic

Idiopathic edema has a strong predilection for women. This condition is characterized by periodic episodes of edema, which seem to be unrelated to the menstrual cycle. Fluctuations in weight are common with patients weighing more after prolonged periods of upright posture.

Inferior Vena Cava (IVC) Obstruction

The causes of inferior vena cava obstruction are listed in the following box.

Causes of Inferior Vena Cava Obstruction	
Abdominal aortic aneurysm	Retroperitoneal fibrosis
Congestive heart failure	Retroperitoneal lymphadenopathy
Hepatomegaly	Surgical clip
Hypercoagulable state	Thrombus extension from
Infection	lower extremities
Malignancy	Vena cava filter
Massive ascites	

Of the causes listed above, renal cell carcinoma is the most common cause of inferior vena cava obstruction.

A prominent venous pattern may be noted on inspection of the abdomen in patients with IVC obstruction. These collateral veins tend to have a predilection for the lateral flanks. Drainage occurs in a cephalad direction, irrespective of whether the veins are above or below the umbilicus. A prominent venous pattern may also be noted in patients with portal hypertension. In these patients, however, the collateral veins tend to appear around the umbilicus. Those that are above the umbilicus drain in a cephalad direction while those that are below the umbilicus drain caudally.

End of Section.

STEP 15: *What are the Causes of Unilateral Leg Swelling?*

The causes of unilateral leg swelling are listed in the following box.

Causes of Unilateral Leg Swelling	
Cellulitis	Lymphedema
Chronic venous insufficiency	Popliteal cyst
Congenital venous malformations	Reflex sympathetic dystrophy
Deep vein thrombosis (DVT)	Rupture of the medial head of the
Erythema nodosum	gastrocnemius

Proceed to Step 16

STEP 16: *Are There Any Clues in the Patient's History That Point to the Etiology of the Unilateral Leg Swelling?*

Clues in the patient's history that point to the etiology of the unilateral leg swelling are listed in the following table.

Historical Clue	Condition Suggested
Occurring within weeks of surgery	Deep vein thrombosis
Leg pain	Cellulitis Deep vein thrombosis Erythema nodosum Popliteal cyst Reflex sympathetic dystrophy Rupture of the medial head of the gastrocnemius muscle
Acute onset (hours to days)	Cellulitis Deep vein thrombosis Ruptured Baker's cyst Rupture of the medial head of the gastrocnemius
Gradual and progressive (over days to months)	Chronic venous insufficiency Lymphedema
Prolonged immobilization	Deep vein thrombosis
History of trauma	Deep vein thrombosis Reflex sympathetic dystrophy Rupture of the medial head of gastrocnemius
Previous history of thrombosis	Deep vein thrombosis
Family history of thrombosis	Deep vein thrombosis
Personal history of malignancy	Deep vein thrombosis Lymphedema
History of rheumatoid arthritis or other inflammatory joint disease	Popliteal cyst
History of saphenous venectomy for bypass surgery	Cellulitis
Onset at early age	Lymphedema
Shortness of breath	Deep vein thrombosis complicated by pulmonary embolism
Family history of leg swelling	Congenital lymphedema Milroy's disease

(continued)

Historical Clue	Condition Suggested
History of radiation therapy	Lymphedema
History of varicose veins	Chronic venous insufficiency
History of noninflammatory joint disease such as degenerative joint disease	Popliteal cyst

Proceed to Step 17

STEP 17: *Are There Any Clues in the Patient's Physical Examination That Point to the Etiology of the Unilateral Leg Swelling?*

Clues in the patient's physical examination that point to the etiology of the unilateral leg swelling are listed in the following table.

Physical Examination Finding	Condition Suggested
One to five centimeter nodules with red, smooth, shiny surface	Erythema nodosum
Brawny hyperpigmentation*	Chronic venous insufficiency
Associated with knee effusion	Popliteal cyst
Hyperesthesia	Reflex sympathetic dystrophy
Palpable cord	Deep vein thrombosis
Mass on pelvic exam	Deep vein thrombosis Pelvic cancer (extrinsic compression of vein or lymph vessels)
Mass on prostate exam	Deep vein thrombosis Prostate cancer (extrinsic compression of vein or lymph vessels)
Lymphadenopathy	Cellulitis (reactive) Lymphoma
Fever	Cellulitis Deep vein thrombosis Erythema nodosum
Raised, bluish-colored vessels isolated to calf or thigh	Congenital venous malformations
Diffuse tenderness	Cellulitis Reflex sympathetic dystrophy
Bluish-purple discoloration below the medial malleolus	Ruptured popliteal cyst Rupture of the medial head of the gastrocnemius

*The hyperpigmentation may be localized to medial aspect of ankle or diffuse throughout calf.

Proceed to Step 18

STEP 18: *Does the Patient Need to Have an Ultrasound?*

Ultrasound is a very useful test in the evaluation of the patient with unilateral leg swelling, particularly when deep vein thrombosis, popliteal cyst, and rupture of the medial head of the gastrocnemius are considerations. While some may argue that the acuity of the presentation (popliteal cyst and rupture of medial head of the gastrocnemius tend to be acute in onset) and the clinical presentation can allow the clinician to make the distinction between these and other causes of unilateral leg swelling, we only have to look at the sensitivity of the history and physical examination in the diagnosis of deep vein thrombosis to realize that our ability to make the diagnosis short of noninvasive testing is poor.

The fact that many cases of pulmonary embolism are not diagnosed until the time of autopsy underscores the importance of having a low threshold for further evaluation. As a result, one can make the argument that the patient presenting with unilateral leg swelling should have an ultrasound, unless the clinical presentation is strongly suggestive of a diagnosis other than deep vein thrombosis. In those who are clearly thought to have a cellulitis, for example, the clinician may forego the ultrasound study. In others, it may be worthwhile to exclude deep vein thrombosis before pursuing other diagnoses. The remainder of this step will discuss deep vein thrombosis, popliteal cyst, and rupture of the medial head of the gastrocnemius muscle in more detail. These are the conditions that are readily diagnosed by ultrasound.

If the patient does not require ultrasound, *Proceed to Step 19.*

Deep Vein Thrombosis

Every year, over 250,000 patients are hospitalized for management of deep vein thrombosis. Establishing the diagnosis is important because of the risk of pulmonary thromboembolism. The key to establishing the diagnosis is consideration of this possibility. In particular, the clinician should ascertain the presence of any risk factors for deep vein thrombosis. These risk factors are listed in the box below.

Risk Factors for Deep Vein Thrombosis	
Behcet's syndrome	Immobilization
Estrogen therapy	Malignancy
Homocystinuria	Pregnancy
Hypercoagulable states	Surgery
Activated resistance to protein C	Thromboangiitis obliterans
Antiphospholipid antibody syndrome	Trauma
Antithrombin III deficiency	Fractures
Dysfibrinogenemia	Spinal cord injuries
Myeloproliferative disorders	
Protein C deficiency	
Protein S deficiency	

The classic presentation of deep vein thrombosis is the acute onset of unilateral leg swelling and pain. Most commonly, patients describe pain in the calf. Physical examination may reveal pitting edema. Other common findings include tenderness and warmth. In a minority of cases, a cord may be palpable. Pain elicited during dorsiflexion of the foot (Homan's sign) is an unreliable finding. In some cases, stagnation of blood behind the thrombus may lead to discoloration of the leg secondary to deoxygenation of the blood. This may impart a cyanotic hue to the affected extremity known as *phlegmasia cerulea dolens*. In other cases, pallor of the affected extremity termed *phlegmasia alba dolens* may be noted.

Unfortunately, these signs and symptoms of deep vein thrombosis are not sufficiently sensitive or specific in the diagnosis. As such, in any patient suspected of having deep vein thrombosis, further diagnostic testing is necessary. Although venography has been considered the gold standard, at the present time, Doppler ultrasonography is recommended as the initial test of choice. The principal finding supporting the diagnosis of deep vein thrombosis is noncompressibility of vessels. In some cases, the thrombus may be directly visualized. The positive predictive value of the study for proximal deep vein thrombosis is about 95%. However, the sensitivity of the test in the diagnosis of calf thrombosis ranges from 50% to 75% with a specificity of 95%. In those cases in which the Doppler ultrasound study is negative but suspicion for deep vein thrombosis is high, the clinician may elect to perform venography.

Popliteal Cyst

A popliteal cyst is another consideration in the patient presenting with unilateral leg swelling. Because the clinical presentation of popliteal cyst mimics that of deep vein thrombosis, popliteal cyst has been termed the pseudothrombophlebitis syndrome. Reported to have an incidence of about 5%, popliteal cysts have been reported in both inflammatory and noninflammatory joint diseases. They have classically been described in patients with rheumatoid arthritis.

Calf pain and swelling are common clinical manifestations. Often present is an associated knee effusion. With rupture of the cyst, blood may track downward to the ankle by route of the fascial planes. Although arthrography is the gold standard in the diagnosis of popliteal cyst, Doppler ultrasound has been shown to have a comparable sensitivity and specificity. Furthermore, Doppler ultrasound allows popliteal cyst to be differentiated from deep vein thrombosis. MR imaging is also an excellent study in the patient with popliteal cyst.

Rupture of the Medial Head of the Gastrocnemius Muscle

The clinical presentation of rupture of the medial head of the gastrocnemius muscle is similar to that of deep vein thrombosis. The rupture tends to occur with sudden movements, particularly with dorsiflexion of the ankle while extending the knee. Dorsiflexion while the foot is planted can also precipitate a rupture. The pain is characteristically acute and located in the medial aspect of the ankle. Swelling usually increases over the next one to two days. In some cases, blood may track downward along the fascial planes, resulting in a bluish discoloration at the medial aspect of the ankle. On occasion, the medial side of the midcalf may reveal a small, sunken area which corresponds to the region where the muscle has been torn. Key to the diagnosis is the elicitation of the characteristic history along with physical examination findings previously described. If there is any uncertainty, Doppler ultrasonography may be performed to exclude deep vein thrombosis or popliteal cyst.

If the patient has deep vein thrombosis, popliteal cyst, or rupture of the medial head of the gastrocnemius muscle, **Stop Here.**

If the patient does not have deep vein thrombosis, popliteal cyst, or rupture of the medial head of the gastrocnemius muscle, **Proceed to Step 19.**

STEP 19: *Does the Patient Have Cellulitis?*

Cellulitis is an acute inflammatory condition of the skin. The etiologic organisms most commonly involved include the flora of the skin, namely *S. aureus* and *S. pyogenes*. Depending on the host and other factors, however, other organisms may be encountered. In many cases, an inciting event, often trauma, can be identified. In these instances, cellulitis may follow a laceration or puncture wound. In other cases, an underlying skin lesion such as a furuncle or ulcer may predispose to the development of cellulitis. The infection is characterized by pain, erythema, warmth, and swelling. Fever, chills, and malaise are not uncommon. Regional lymphadenopathy, usually tender, often accompanies the skin infection. Clues to the etiologic organism are listed in the following table.

Clinical Clue	Etiologic Organism Suggested
Cat bite	*Pasteurella multocida*
Dog bite	*Pasteurella multocida* *Staphylococcus intermedius* *Capnocytophaga canimorsus*
Cellulitis surrounding lacerations sustained in fresh water (rivers, lakes, streams)	*Aeromonas hydrophila*
Cellulitis after stepping on a nail (sweaty tennis shoe syndrome)	*Pseudomonas aeruginosa*
Hospitalized, immunocompromised hosts	Consider also gram-negative bacillary and fungal cellulitis
Bone renderers Fishmongers	*Erysipelothrix rhusiopathiae*
After exposure to water in aquarium or swimming pool	*Mycobacterium marinum*
Cellulitis occurring in saphenous vein donor site	Group A, C, G streptococcus
Lymphedema	Group A, C, G streptococcus
Stasis dermatitis	Group A, C, G streptococcus
Cellulitis following a traumatic wound sustained in salt or brackish inland waters	*Vibrio* species (primarily *V. vulnificus*)

It is usually difficult to establish the precise etiologic organism. On occasion, the clinician may be able to perform a Gram stain and culture, particularly where there is drainage or an open wound. In a minority of cases, blood cultures may reveal the etiologic organism. Of particular importance is the consideration of the factors listed in the preceding table, which, if present, will help guide the appropriate therapy.

It is important to realize that cellulitis may complicate other causes of leg swelling such as chronic venous insufficiency and lymphedema. In contrast to these latter conditions, cellulitis is an acute condition. With resolution of the infection, the inflammatory signs including edema will abate. When the edema does not resolve or the patient provides a history of chronic edema, the clinician should suspect chronic venous insufficiency or lymphedema.

If the patient has cellulitis, *Stop Here.*

If the patient does not have cellulitis, *Proceed to Step 20.*

STEP 20: *Does the Patient Have Erythema Nodosum?*

When erythematous, tender nodules are noted on anterior aspects of the lower leg, particularly the shins, the clinician should consider erythema nodosum. Swelling may be noted to accompany the findings of erythema nodosum. Besides complaining of skin rash, most patients experience fever, chills, and malaise. The causes of erythema nodosum are listed in the following box.

Causes of Erythema Nodosum	
Behcet's syndrome	Other bacterial infections
Drug-induced	Cat-scratch disease
Bromides	Leprosy
Oral contraceptives	Leptospirosis
Sulfonamides	*Mycoplasma pneumoniae*
Enteropathies	Tularemia
Crohn's disease	*Yersinia enterocolitica*
Ulcerative colitis	Sarcoidosis
Fungal infections	Streptococcal infections
Blastomycosis	Tuberculosis
Coccidioidomycosis	Virus and *Chlamydia* agents
Dermatophytes	Hepatitis B
Histoplasmosis	Infectious mononucleosis
Malignant disease	Lymphogranuloma venereum
Lymphoma and leukemia	Psittacosis
Postradiation therapy	

Adapted from *Dermatology in General Medicine*, Fitzpatrick TB (ed), 4th ed, New York, NY: McGraw-Hill, 1993, 1339.

Skin biopsy confirms the diagnosis. Once the diagnosis has been confirmed, the clinician should focus efforts on identifying the cause of the erythema nodosum. CXR and blood counts are always indicated. Laboratory testing may reveal a leukocytosis and elevated ESR. The patient's clinical presentation will dictate further testing which may include pharyngeal culture, ASLO titer, PPD, and virologic titers.

If the patient has erythema nodosum, **Stop Here.**

If the patient does not have erythema nodosum, **Proceed to Step 21.**

STEP 21: *Does the Patient Have Reflex Sympathetic Dystrophy?*

Reflex sympathetic dystrophy, a disease of unknown mechanism, is characterized by the features listed in the following box.

Features of Reflex Sympathetic Dystrophy	
Burning pain	Swelling
Hyperesthesia	Trophic change in the skin and bone of
Hyperhidrosis	the affected extremity

A number of precipitating factors have been identified in patients with reflex sympathetic dystrophy. Known precipitants of reflex sympathetic dystrophy are listed in the following box.

Precipitants of Reflex Sympathetic Dystrophy	
Brain tumor	Procedural
Cerebral infarction	Angiography
Cervical cord injury	Myelography
Dislocations	Venography
Fractures	Soft tissue injury
Infection	Sprains
Immobilization with cast or splint	

Often accompanying the swelling is pain, usually described as a burning or aching sensation. These symptoms typically manifest several weeks after the inciting event. At this point in the disease course, the patient is considered to be in the first stage of reflex sympathetic dystrophy. Stage 2 is characterized by induration of the edema along with coolness of the skin and hyperhidrosis. Livedo reticularis or cyanosis are other features of this stage. The pain usually persists and even the slightest of movements can exacerbate the pain. Stage 3 is characterized by skin thinning, contractures, and spread of the edema and pain proximally.

If the patient has reflex sympathetic dystrophy, **Stop Here.**

If the patient does not have reflex sympathetic dystrophy, **Proceed to Step 22.**

STEP 22: *Does the Patient Have Lymphedema?*

Lymphedema may result from any process that obstructs the lymphatic channels, leading to the inability to clear the interstitial space of protein rich fluid. Lymphedema may be unilateral or bilateral. Although classically painless, some patients may describe a dull, heavy ache in the leg. Early in the course, the edema may pit easily with pressure. With progression, the affected limb may become indurated. As the edema becomes woody in nature, pitting may no longer be appreciated.

Lymphedema may be classified into primary or secondary types, as shown in the following box.

Classification of Lymphedema	
Primary	
Congenital lymphedema	Lymphedema tarda†
Lymphedema praecox*	
Secondary	
Infection	Sarcoid
Bacterial infection (recurrent)	Surgery
Filiariasis	Trauma
Radiation	Tumor

*Lymphedema praecox mainly affects women, usually manifesting during the second and third decades of life. Evaluation of these patients usually reveals no other cause.

†When no cause is identified in the patient who develops lymphedema after the age of 35 years, the patient is said to have lymphedema tarda.

Secondary lymphedema is much more common than primary lymphedema. The most common cause of secondary lymphedema varies depending on the geographic location. In the United States, malignancy, either in and of itself, or the treatment of malignancy (surgery, radiation) is the usual cause. Tumor invasion or compression of the lymphatic vessels can result in the development of secondary lymphedema, even before the malignancy is known. The most frequent neoplastic causes of secondary lymphedema are prostate cancer and lymphoma in men and women, respectively.

In developing countries, secondary lymphedema is often caused by infection. In fact, filariasis is actually the most common cause of secondary lymphedema in the world. Another common cause of lymphedema is recurrent bacterial lymphangitis.

To determine the cause of the lymphedema, the clinician should consider obtaining ultrasound or CT of the abdomen and pelvis. These imaging studies can exclude a neoplastic cause. Other tests that are available in the evaluation of lymphedema include lymphoscintigraphy and lymphangiography.

If the patient has lymphedema, **Stop Here.**

If the patient does not have lymphedema, **Proceed to Step 23.**

STEP 23: *Does the Patient Have Chronic Venous Insufficiency?*

Edema (unilateral or bilateral) is often the initial manifestation of chronic venous insufficiency. Early in the course, the edema may be limited to an area around the malleoli. With progression, more of the leg is noted to be edematous. While chronic venous insufficiency is classically characterized by the presence of pitting edema, with progression of the disease, subcutaneous fibrosis may occur. In these advanced cases, pitting may not be appreciated.

The presence of dilated superficial veins, particularly in the medial aspect of the lower calf, is suggestive of chronic venous insufficiency. Dilation of the small veins underneath the medial malleolus, also known as the ankle flare sign, is a clue to the diagnosis. With progression of the disease, the veins become more prominent and tortuous. Not uncommonly, patients notice dilated veins in the proximal leg as well.

Although pain may be absent in chronic venous insufficiency, some may complain of limb heaviness or aching, especially after prolonged standing. Other signs of chronic venous insufficiency include brownish hemosiderin deposits in the skin and venous ulcers. Some patients may develop a pruritic dermatitis.

REFERENCES

Ciocon JO, Fernandez BB, and Ciocon DG, "Leg Edema: Clinical Clues to the Differential Diagnosis," *Geriatrics*, 1993, 48(5):34-40, 45.

Dermatology in General Medicine, 4th ed, Fitzpatrick TB (ed), New York, NY: McGraw-Hill, 1993, 1339.

Gorman WP, Davis KR, and Donnelly R, "ABC of Arterial and Venous Disease. Swollen Lower Limb-1: General Assessment and Deep Vein Thrombosis," *BMJ*, 2000, 320(7247):1453-6 (review).

Handbook of Gastroenterology, Yamada T (ed), Philadelphia, PA: Lippincott-Raven, 1998, 321.

Kannel WB and Belanger AJ, "Epidemiology of Heart Failure," *Am Heart J*, 1991, 121(3 Pt 1):951-7.

Merli GJ and Spandorfer J, "The Outpatient With Unilateral Leg Swelling," *Med Clin North Am*, 1995, 79(2):435-47.

Powell AA and Armstrong MA, "Peripheral Edema," *Am Fam Phys*, 1997, 55(5):1721-6.

Primary Cardiology, Goldman L and Braunwald E (eds), Philadelphia, PA: WB Saunders Co, 1998, 311.

Young JR, "The Swollen Leg. Clinical Significance and Differential Diagnosis," *Cardiol Clin*, 1991, 9(3):443-56.

LEG SWELLING

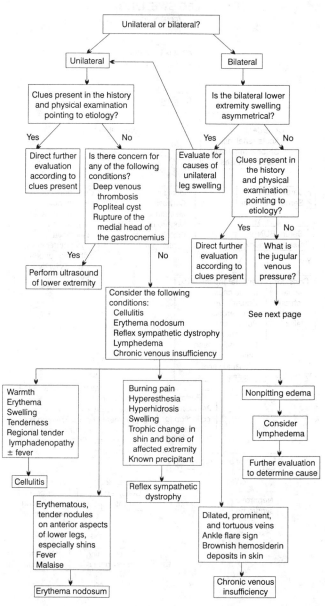

LEG SWELLING
(continued)

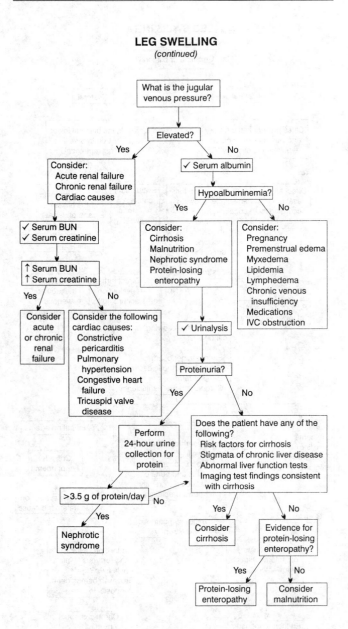

NIPPLE DISCHARGE

STEP 1: *How Common is Nipple Discharge?*

Nipple discharge is the chief complaint in approximately 5% of women presenting to specialty breast care centers. While breast pain and mass are more common manifestations of breast disease, nipple discharge should never be dismissed, especially since it can be a major source of anxiety for the patient. While most cases of nipple discharge are due to a benign process, in some cases, the nipple discharge may be a manifestation of malignant disease. In fact, about 10% of cases are linked to breast cancer. As such, a thorough evaluation is necessary to differentiate benign from malignant causes of nipple discharge.

Proceed to Step 2

STEP 2: *Does the Patient Have a True Nipple Discharge or a False (Pseudo) Discharge?*

Prior to embarking on an evaluation for nipple discharge, it is important to ensure that a nipple discharge is truly present. It is important to realize that a patient's complaint of nipple discharge does not verify that the discharge is of breast origin. A true nipple discharge is defined as fluid that leaves the breast through the lactiferous orifices after having been produced within the breast.

There are many situations in which fluid not arising within the breast may be appreciated on the surface of the nipple or areola. The skin covering the nipple areola is no different than the skin elsewhere on the body. As such, it is prone to the development of the same skin diseases that can affect other parts of the body. One example is in the patient who has eczema of the nipple or areola. In these cases, it is not uncommon to have exudation of inflammatory secretions from the skin lesions. These secretions may be mistaken for a true nipple discharge. Some dermatologic conditions associated with a false discharge are listed in the following box.

Dermatologic Conditions Associated with False (Pseudo) Nipple Discharge	
Cutaneous viral infection	Montgomery's gland infection
Herpes simplex virus	Nipple trauma
Molluscum contagiosum	Other inflammatory disorders of the skin
Eczema	Paget's disease
Infected sebaceous cyst	

Of the various causes of false nipple discharge, that due to Paget's disease deserves further mention here. A potentially life-threatening illness, Paget's disease refers to the presence of an intradermal carcinoma of the breast. Not all patients with Paget's disease have a breast mass. In fact, some only present with involvement of the skin or subcutaneous tissue of the nipple or areola (usually unilateral). Examination of the lesion often reveals it to be erosive in nature. Because the eroded surface is friable, a bloody exudate is not unusual.

In many cases, a magnifying glass is necessary to differentiate a true from false nipple discharge. A discharge that does not originate from the surface of the papilla can be considered to be a false nipple discharge. In contrast, expression of fluid from the nipple with compression supports the presence of a true nipple discharge.

It is important to distinguish a true from false nipple discharge because, with the exception of Paget's disease, a false nipple discharge is not associated with breast cancer. Although most patients with true nipple discharge do not have an underlying breast cancer, it remains a possibility. As such, it is this group of patients that requires further evaluation.

If the patient has a false nipple discharge, **Stop Here.**

If the patient has a true nipple discharge, **Proceed to Step 3.**

STEP 3: *What are the Results of the Clinical Breast Examination?*

A thorough clinical breast examination is essential in the woman presenting with nipple discharge. In particular, the clinician should search for findings that are suspicious for breast cancer. These findings include the following:

- Asymmetry
- Breast mass
- Change in breast contour
- Inverted nipple (new onset)
- Local area of redness
- Peau d'orange (indentation of skin over a mass that often looks like an orange peel)
- Skin retraction
- Supraclavicular or axillary lymphadenopathy

The likelihood of breast cancer is significantly increased when nipple discharge is accompanied by a palpable mass. One study determined that nearly 90% of patients with nipple discharge secondary to cancer had a palpable breast mass. In this study, no palpable mass was found in 13% of cancers associated with nipple discharge. In patients who do present with discharge alone, age is an important predictor of malignancy, as shown in the following table.

Age (years)	Risk of Malignancy (%)
<40	3
40-60	10
>60	32

If a breast mass is present in the patient presenting with nipple discharge, proceed to the chapter on Breast Mass / Lump *on page 37.*

If there are no findings suggestive of breast cancer, **Proceed to Step 4.**

STEP 4: *Is the Discharge Lactational?*

When worrisome physical examination findings are not present in the woman complaining of nipple discharge, the clinician should determine if the discharge is lactational. The change in hormonal milieu that accompanies pregnancy and postpartum may result in a lactational discharge. During the latter half of pregnancy, colostrum, a protein-rich fluid, accumulates within the breast. As the pregnancy progresses, the increasing accumulation of colostrum may result in its discharge from the nipples. In contrast to the milky fluid characteristic of breast milk, the typical colostrum discharge is yellowish, sticky, and opaque.

Several days after birth, colostrum gives way to the whitish fluid known as breast milk. Usually bilateral, lactational discharge may be spontaneous or nonspontaneous. On occasion, a lactational discharge may be bloody. The normal duration of milky nipple discharge after cessation of breast-feeding is a matter of some debate. Some authorities maintain that women may normally express a milky nipple discharge for up to one or two years.

If the patient has a lactational discharge, *Stop Here.*

If the patient does not have a lactational discharge, *Proceed to Step 5.*

STEP 5: *Is the Discharge Unilateral or Bilateral?*

Further evaluation of the nonlactational discharge involves determination of whether the discharge is unilateral or bilateral. A bilateral nipple discharge argues against the diagnosis of breast cancer. Although breast cancer can present with bilateral nipple discharge, such a presentation would be unusual. Although a unilateral nipple discharge raises concern for breast cancer, most cases of unilateral nipple discharge are due to benign conditions of the breast.

If the discharge is unilateral, *Proceed to Step 6.*

If the discharge is bilateral, *Proceed to Step 11.*

STEP 6: *What are the Results of Mammography?*

Diagnostic mammography should be performed in women presenting with unilateral nipple discharge. The purpose of the mammography is to assess for the presence of occult or subclinical disease. The detection of nonpalpable abnormalities raises suspicion for breast cancer. It is important to realize that false-negative results are not uncommon. In fact, mammography has been found to have a 9.5% false-negative rate for the detection of breast cancer in women with nipple discharge. Therefore, a negative mammogram does not exclude breast cancer in patients with a unilateral nipple discharge.

If the mammogram reveals findings suspicious for breast cancer, the evaluation should proceed accordingly.

If the mammogram is negative, *Proceed to Step 7.*

> ### STEP 7: *Does the Patient Have a Single-Duct or Multiple-Duct Discharge?*

The clinician should try to determine if the patient with unilateral nipple discharge has single-duct or multiple-duct discharge. To differentiate single from multiple-duct nipple discharge, it is helpful to use a magnifying glass. In cases of single-duct nipple discharge, the clinician can often identify the breast segment producing the discharge by palpation around the nipple-areolar margin. The breast segment or quadrant producing the discharge is identified when a droplet of discharge appears with palpation.

Most breast cancers begin as a unifocal process. Since these cancers typically involve one breast segment, patients usually have a single-duct discharge. When compared to the asymptomatic population, the relative risk of malignancy in patients with single-duct discharge is 4.07.

A discharge that originates from more than one duct argues against the presence of breast cancer. Multiple-duct discharge has a risk of breast cancer similar to that of the general population.

If the patient has a single-duct discharge, *Proceed to Step 8.*

If the patient has a multiple-duct discharge, *Proceed to Step 10.*

> ### STEP 8: *What is the Character of the Single-Duct Discharge?*

It is useful to note the character of the single-duct discharge. To determine the color of the discharge, it is helpful to blot the droplets of discharge on white tissue, paying particular attention to the color noted at the margins of the blot. In particular, the clinician should attempt to categorize the discharge into one of the following four groups:

- Bloody or sanguineous
- Serosanguineous
- Serous
- Watery

The cancer risk is increased if one of these types of discharge is present, as shown in the following table.

Type of Discharge	Frequency of Association with Breast Cancer (%)
Serous	6.3
Serosanguineous	11.9
Bloody or sanguineous	24
Watery	45.5

It is also worthwhile to test secretions that are not visibly bloody for the presence of heme. A positive test for heme should prompt the clinician to classify the discharge as sanguineous.

Proceed to Step 9

STEP 9: *What are the Results of the Surgical Referral?*

Surgical referral is indicated when a woman presents with a unilateral nipple discharge originating from a single duct. In some cases, the surgeon may recommend galactography. Galactography, also known as ductography, involves the injection of a small amount of water-soluble contrast material through a duct that has been catheterized. Mammography is then performed. The procedure allows the clinician to identify lesions within the ductal tree. It is important to realize that galactography cannot differentiate benign from malignant lesions. In these cases, it is not performed to establish the diagnosis but may be indicated to delineate the anatomy prior to surgical incision.

End of Section.

STEP 10: *What are the Likely Considerations in Patients Who Have Multiple-Duct Discharge?*

Malignancy is very unlikely to be the cause of multiple-duct discharge. Multiple-duct discharge should prompt consideration of duct ectasia or breast infection. The reader is encouraged to consult appropriate resources for further evaluation of the patient with unilateral, multiple-duct nipple discharge.

End of Section.

STEP 11: *Does the Patient Have Galactorrhea?*

A nipple discharge that is bilateral and originating from multiple ducts is unlikely to a manifestation of breast cancer. Bilateral, nonpeurperal milky nipple discharge should prompt the clinician to consider galactorrhea. The discharge of galactorrhea is usually induced through stimulation, nonbloody, and expressed from multiple duct openings in both breasts.

The clinician can confirm that the patient has galactorrhea by examining the discharge under the magnification of a light microscope. Galactorrhea is said to be present if fat globules are noted in specimens stained with either oil red O or Sudan IV. Alternatively, the clinician may elect to analyze the discharge for the presence of specific milk products such as casein or lactose. In usual clinical practice, however, these tests are rarely performed.

When bilateral nipple discharge is not consistent with galactorrhea, the clinician should consider benign breast diseases. These patients should be reassured that a serious cause of nipple discharge is not present.

If the patient does not have galactorrhea, benign breast disease is the most likely possibility. ***Stop here.***

If the patient has galactorrhea, ***Proceed to Step 12.***

STEP 12: *What are the Causes of Galactorrhea?*

The causes of galactorrhea are listed in the following box.

Causes of Galactorrhea
Hyperprolactinemia
Physiologic
Nipple stimulation
Pregnancy
Sleep
Strenuous exercise
Stress (physical or emotional)
Pathologic
Hypothalamic lesions
Cranipharyngioma
Metastatic neoplasms
Germinoma
Glioma
Head trauma
Encephalitis
Radiation
Surgical stalk section
Infiltrative disease
Histiocytosis X
Sarcoidosis
Tuberculosis
Pituitary lesions
Pituitary adenoma (secreting PRL)
Acromegaly
Cushing's syndrome
Empty sella syndrome
Medications
Hypothyroidism
Chronic renal failure
Irritative lesions of the chest wall
Herpes zoster
Tight fitting garments
Chest trauma
Thoracotomy
Mastectomy
Reduction mammoplasty
Spinal cord lesions
Malignancy
Lung cancer
Renal cell carcinoma
Ovarian cystic teratoma
Adrenal carcinoma
Idiopathic
Medication-related

Proceed to Step 13

STEP 13: *Is the Patient Pregnant?*

In women, especially if a history of amenorrhea is elicited, the clinician should exclude pregnancy by obtaining an hCG level.

If the patient is pregnant, *Stop Here.*

If the patient is not pregnant, *Proceed to Step 14.*

STEP 14: *Does the Patient Have Hypothyroidism?*

Galactorrhea can occur in patients with hypothyroidism. Dry skin, cold skin, coarse hair, loss of hair, weight gain, and constipation are some historical clues suggestive of the diagnosis. Physical examination findings supportive of hypothyroidism include eyelid edema, lethargy, hoarseness, and hung-up reflexes. A high TSH and low free T_4 level or free thyroxine index establishes the diagnosis.

If the patient has hypothyroidism, *Stop Here.*

If the patient does not have hypothyroidism, *Proceed to Step 15.*

STEP 15: *What is the Prolactin Level?*

It is important to realize that stress of different forms can raise the serum prolactin level. In fact, hyperprolactinemia has been noted following a general medical examination or venipuncture. In these cases, there is usually a modest elevation in the serum prolactin level. The clinician may elect to obtain a prolactin level at a time when the patient is relatively free of stress. To obtain an unstressed prolactin level, the patient should be asked to rest for up to two hours after a needle or catheter is inserted. At the end of the rest period, the prolactin level can be drawn.

If the patient has hyperprolactinemia, *Proceed to Step 16.*

If the patient does not have hyperprolactinemia, *Proceed to Step 18.*

STEP 16: *Does the Patient Have a Pituitary or Hypothalamic Cause of the Hyperprolactinemia?*

In most laboratories, the upper limit of normal for prolactin is 20-25 ng/mL. Levels exceeding 200 ng/mL are especially concerning for a prolactin-secreting pituitary adenoma. However, lower levels do not exclude the presence of a pituitary tumor. All patients with hyperprolactinemia require radiologic investigation to exclude intracranial pathology. Almost 20% of women with galactorrhea will have radiologically apparent tumors. This percentage increases to nearly 35% when women with both galactorrhea and amenorrhea are imaged. MRI is the imaging test of choice in the evaluation of hyperprolactinemia.

If the imaging test reveals a hypothalamic or pituitary mass lesion, *Stop Here.*

If the imaging test does not reveal a hypothalamic or pituitary mass lesion, *Proceed to Step 17.*

STEP 17: *Has a Pituitary Tumor Been Excluded?*

The clinician should realize that an unremarkable imaging test does not exclude the presence of a pituitary adenoma. Some adenomas (microadenomas) may be so small that they escape detection with conventional imaging tests. These patients should be seen periodically and assessed for the development of signs and symptoms of a pituitary tumor. In addition, repeat imaging is also recommended.

When the imaging tests do not reveal the etiology of the hyperprolactinemia, the clinician should also consider other causes of hyperprolactinemia. These other causes are listed in the box in Step 12. In particular, the clinician should focus on the medications that the patient is taking, as many drugs can cause hyperprolactinemia. Common medicinal causes of hyperprolactinemia are listed in the following box.

Common Medicinal Causes of Hyperprolactinemia	
Antihypertensives	Fluphenazine
Methyldopa	Haloperidol
Reserpine	Metoclopramide
Verapamil	Opiates
Chlorpromazine	Perphenazine
Cimetidine	Promazine
Domperidone	Sulpiride
Estrogens	

With medication-related hyperprolactinemia, rarely does the serum prolactin level exceed 100 ng/mL. A potential offender should not be considered causative unless the clinician documents normalization of the prolactin level and resolution of the galactorrhea with discontinuation of the suspect medication.

End of Section.

STEP 18: *What is the Cause of the Galactorrhea?*

Not all patients with galactorrhea have hyperprolactinemia. In fact, the serum prolactin level is normal in approximately 45% of patients with galactorrhea. In these cases, the clinician should consider idiopathic galactorrhea. In many of these patients, the clinician may be able to elicit a history of persistent nipple discharge since postpartum lactation. Quite often, these patients have normal menses. Regular menstrual periods and normal prolactin levels strongly argue against the possibility of a pituitary tumor. Therefore, these patients do not require CNS imaging.

In other patients with idiopathic galactorrhea, the nipple discharge may have resulted from a transient condition associated with hyperprolactinemia. In these patients, measurement of the prolactin level at the onset of the galactorrhea may have revealed an elevated level. With resolution of the cause, however, the prolactin level may have normalized. In these patients, it may take some time for the galactorrhea to disappear following normalization of the prolactin level.

Medications are a common cause of galactorrhea. Not all medication-related galactorrhea is associated with hyperprolactinemia. Therefore, a close look at the medication list may raise suspicion for medication-related galactorrhea. Resolution of the galactorrhea following discontinuation of the suspect medication establishes the diagnosis.

REFERENCES

Arnold GJ and Neiheisel MB, "A Comprehensive Approach to Evaluating Nipple Discharge," *Nurse Pract*, 1997, 22(7):96-102, 105-11.

Conry C, "Evaluation of a Breast Complaint: Is It Cancer?" *Am Fam Phys*, 1994, 49(2):445-50, 453-4.

Desai DC, Brennan EJ, and Carp NZ, "Paget's Disease of the Male Breast," *Am Surg*, 1996, 62(12):1068-72 (review).

Fiorica JV, "Nipple Discharge," *Obstet Gynecol Clin North Am*, 1994, 21(3):453-60.

Morrow M, "The Evaluation of Common Breast Problems," *Am Fam Phys*, 2000, 61(8):2371-8, 2385.

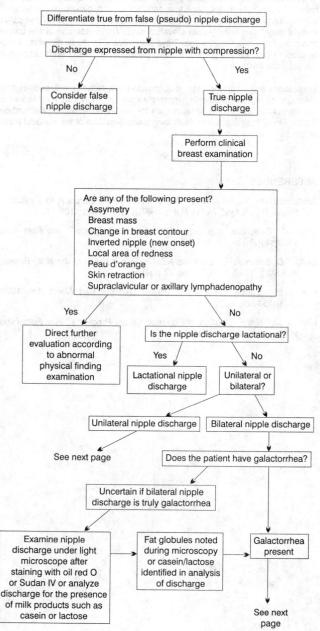

NIPPLE DISCHARGE

Differentiate true from false (pseudo) nipple discharge

↓

Discharge expressed from nipple with compression?

No → Consider false nipple discharge

Yes → True nipple discharge

↓

Perform clinical breast examination

↓

Are any of the following present?
- Assymetry
- Breast mass
- Change in breast contour
- Inverted nipple (new onset)
- Local area of redness
- Peau d'orange
- Skin retraction
- Supraclavicular or axillary lymphadenopathy

Yes → Direct further evaluation according to abnormal physical finding examination

No → Is the nipple discharge lactational?

Yes → Lactational nipple discharge

No → Unilateral or bilateral?

Unilateral nipple discharge → See next page

Bilateral nipple discharge → Does the patient have galactorrhea?

Uncertain if bilateral nipple discharge is truly galactorrhea

Examine nipple discharge under light microscope after staining with oil red O or Sudan IV or analyze discharge for the presence of milk products such as casein or lactose → Fat globules noted during microscopy or casein/lactose identified in analysis of discharge → Galactorrhea present

↓

See next page

NIPPLE DISCHARGE
(continued)

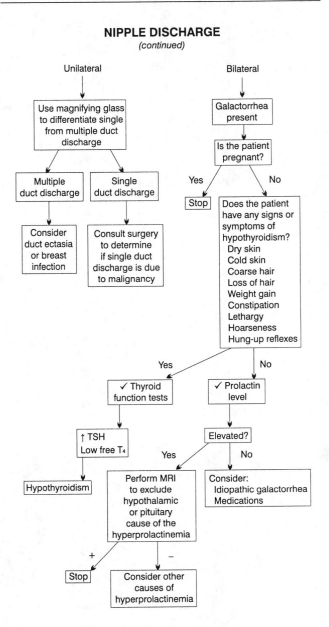

ODYNOPHAGIA

STEP 1: *What is Odynophagia?*

Pain upon swallowing is termed odynophagia. It should not be confused with dysphagia which refers to difficulty in swallowing. Although both often are present together, odynophagia may occur alone. When present, it suggests esophageal ulceration or inflammation.

Proceed to Step 2

STEP 2: *What are the Causes of Odynophagia?*

The causes of odynophagia are listed in the following box.

Causes of Odynophagia
Acute radiation esophagitis
Behcet's disease
Corrosive esophagitis
Crohn's disease
Dermatologic conditions
Benign mucous membrane pemphigoid
Bullous pemphigoid
Epidermolysis bullosa dystrophica
Pemphigus vulgaris
Esophageal cancer
Gastroesophageal reflux disease
Graft-versus-host disease
Infectious esophagitis
Candida
Cytomegalovirus
Herpes simplex virus
HIV (acute seroconversion)
Pill-induced esophagitis

Proceed to Step 3

STEP 3: *Does the Patient Have Risk Factors for Infectious Esophagitis?*

Although infectious esophagitis may occur in otherwise healthy individuals, more often, risk factors are present. In particular, infectious esophagitis tends to occur in immunocompromised patients. Risk factors for the development of infectious esophagitis are listed in the following box.

Risk Factors for Infectious Esophagitis	
Defects in immune system	Esophageal abnormalities
Advancing age	Caustic injuries
Alcoholism	Diverticula
Chemotherapy	Motility disorders
Chronic mucocutaneous candidiasis	Achalasia
Cushing's syndrome	Scleroderma
Debility	Stricture
Diabetes mellitus	Medications
HIV	Acid suppressive therapy
Malignancy	Antibiotics
Neutropenia	Corticosteroids
Organ transplantation	Immunosuppressive agents

If the patient has risk factors for the development of infectious esophagitis, **Proceed to Step 4.**

If the patient does not have risk factors for the development of infectious esophagitis, **Proceed to Step 10.**

STEP 4: *Are There Any Clues in the Patient's Clinical Presentation That Point to the Etiology of the Suspected Infectious Esophagitis?*

Although many different organisms have been documented as causes of infectious esophagitis, the major etiologic agents include the following:

- *Candida* species
- Herpes simplex virus
- Cytomegalovirus

In general, the clinical presentation of infectious esophagitis does not allow the clinician to differentiate among the three major causes. Most often, patients with infectious esophagitis report dysphagia, odynophagia, and chest pain. Weight loss occurs in 35% of patients. Heartburn and regurgitation are uncommon symptoms in patients with infectious esophagitis. The presence of severe odynophagia is a soft historical clue supportive of viral rather than *Candida* esophagitis.

Dehydration may be noted on physical examination, reflecting decreased oral intake. Fever may be noted in CMV esophagitis but typically does not occur in patients with *Candida* or herpes simplex viral esophagitis. Of the three major etiologic organisms, herpes simplex virus and *Candida* commonly involve both the esophagus and oropharynx. As such, the finding of oral thrush should raise suspicion for *Candida* esophagitis. In fact, thrush is apparent in about 66% of HIV patients with *Candida* esophagitis. Aphthous ulcerations should prompt consideration of herpes simplex virus. It is important to realize that the absence of oral thrush and aphthous ulcerations do not exclude the diagnosis of *Candida* and herpes simplex viral esophagitis, respectively.

CMV esophagitis usually does not present with concomitant oral manifestations. Instead, features suggestive of a systemic illness are often present. Up to 40% of patients with CMV esophagitis complain of fever, nausea/vomiting, and abdominal pain.

Of note, esophageal ulceration resulting in odynophagia, has been described during acute HIV seroconversion. With seroconversion, patients typically develop symptoms and signs of a systemic illness 2-3 weeks after exposure. Clinical manifestations include fever, malaise, myalgias, pharyngitis, and rash. In some cases, esophageal ulceration accompanies these manifestations. Odynophagia usually resolves several weeks later.

Proceed to Step 5

STEP 5: What Laboratory Tests Should be Obtained in the Patient Suspected of Having Infectious Esophagitis?

Laboratory testing is usually not helpful in establishing the etiology. On occasion, the following laboratory tests may be useful in pointing to the etiology of the odynophagia:

- CBC with differential

    Neutropenia, a risk factor for infectious esophagitis, may be noted on differential cell count.

- CD4 count

    In HIV patients, determination of the absolute CD4 count may be helpful. The likelihood of infectious esophagitis is increased in HIV patients with CD4 counts <200/mm^3. CMV, HSV, and idiopathic ulcerations of the esophagus are more commonly appreciated in patients with CD4 counts <100/mm^3.

Serologic testing is not useful in distinguishing between the causes. Blood cultures are only necessary in the febrile patient. In those suspected of having acute HIV seroconversion, standard antibody testing may be unrevealing. In these cases, a viral load may be necessary to corroborate the diagnosis.

Unfortunately, the clinical presentation and laboratory testing usually do not allow the clinician to distinguish between the major causes of infectious esophagitis.

Proceed to Step 6

STEP 6: Should the Patient be Treated Empirically?

In general, empiric therapy is acceptable in HIV patients because of the high frequency of *Candida* esophagitis. In these cases, treating with empiric fluconazole has been shown to have a high response rate and considerable cost savings. Studies have shown that complications prior to endoscopy are rare in patients who do not respond to antifungal therapy. In those who do respond, improvement usually occurs within a few days. If there is no symptomatic improvement after one week of therapy, further evaluation is necessary. In all other patients, the definitive diagnosis should be established prior to starting treatment.

If the patient has HIV and an empiric course of antifungal therapy for *Candida* esophagitis results in symptomatic improvement, ***Stop Here***.

If the patient has HIV but an empiric course of antifungal therapy for *Candida* esophagitis does not result in symptomatic improvement, ***Proceed to Step 7***.

If the patient does not have HIV, ***Proceed to Step 7***.

STEP 7: *Should Barium Esophagography or Endoscopy be Performed?*

Prior to the advent of endoscopy, barium esophagography was routinely performed. Findings on radiography suggestive of a particular etiologic organism are listed in the following table.

Etiologic Organism	Findings on Barium Esophagography
Candida species	Multiple plaque-like lesions
	Often linear in configuration
	Lesions can become confluent, resulting in shaggy appearance of the esophagus
HSV	Small ulcers (usually <1 cm) or
	Diffuse mucosal ulceration
CMV	Larger well-circumscribed ulcers or
	Diffuse erosive pattern

Since there is overlap in the barium esophagography findings among the major etiologic agents, endoscopy is recommended as the diagnostic test of choice. At the time of endoscopy, mucosal biopsies and cytologic studies can be performed to establish the definitive diagnosis.

Proceed to Step 8

STEP 8: *What are the Results of the Endoscopy?*

The endoscopic appearance of the major pathogens are listed in the following table.

Etiologic Organism	Endoscopic Finding
Candida species	Multiple isolated or confluent plaques
HSV	Multiple shallow ulcers
CMV	Multiple or diffuse shallow ulcers (non-HIV)
	Multiple large (>2 cm), deep ulcers (HIV)

Despite these suggestive appearances, biopsy with histopathologic examination is required to establish the definitive diagnosis. Brushings of mucosal lesions after potassium hydroxide staining is more sensitive than biopsy in the diagnosis of *Candida* infection. In contrast, biopsy is more sensitive and specific than brushings in establishing the diagnosis of viral esophagitis. Biopsy and brushings may reveal the characteristic multinucleated giant cells with inclusions (Cowdry's type A inclusions), suggestive of herpes simplex virus esophagitis. The epithelial or endothelial inclusions of CMV may also be noted on examination of brushing and biopsy specimens. Viral cultures may be necessary in some cases. Some patients may have more than one pathogen demonstrated.

If the endoscopic findings are consistent with infection, *Stop Here*.

If the endoscopic findings including histologic examination is not consistent with infection, *Proceed to Step 9*.

STEP 9: *What are Possibilities in the Patient With Endoscopic Findings Not Consistent With Infectious Esophagitis?*

The lack of endoscopic (gross and histologic) findings consistent with infectious esophagitis does not exclude the possibility of infection. The clinician should ascertain whether enough biopsies (usually 6-10 are recommended) were obtained during endoscopy. In addition, it is useful to determine if biopsies were obtained from the ulcer base or edge. The diagnostic yield for HSV esophagitis is increased when biopsies of the ulcer edge are obtained. In contrast, biopsies of the ulcer base are more likely to be revealing in patients with CMV esophagitis. If routine staining does not demonstrate the characteristic viral inclusions of CMV or HSV, the clinician should determine if the laboratory has performed immunohistochemical staining in an effort to improve the yield.

In the AIDS patient, endoscopic findings that are not consistent with infection should prompt the clinician to consider idiopathic esophageal ulceration.

In allogeneic bone marrow transplant patients, consideration should be given to chronic graft-versus-host disease. Esophageal involvement is quite common in the chronic phase of graft-versus-host disease. Establishing the diagnosis requires exclusion of all other causes of odynophagia, particularly infectious esophagitis. Graft-versus-host disease is described in further detail in Step 12.

When the evaluation does not reveal an infectious etiology, the clinician should consider the possibility that the odynophagia is the result of a noninfectious process. These causes are considered in Step 11.

End of Section.

STEP 10: *Does the Patient Have HIV?*

Many patients with HIV are not aware that they are infected. In these patients, esophageal disease secondary to HIV or opportunistic infection may be the cause of the odynophagia. In these cases, the esophageal disease may be the initial presentation of their HIV disease. As such, serologic testing for HIV is indicated in patients at risk for the infection for the following reasons:

- To prevent further transmission of the disease

- To offer appropriate medical care to infected patients unaware that they have HIV

In addition, the presence of HIV infection requires consideration of diagnoses that would be unusual in the immunocompetent individual. The CDC recommends serologic testing for HIV if the patient meets any of the criteria listed in the following box.

Indications for HIV Serologic Testing
Active tuberculosis
Current or former intravenous drug use
Hemophilia
History of receiving blood products between 1978 and 1985
History of sexually transmitted disease
Immigrant from developing country with high rate of HIV infection
Occupational exposure to blood or other at-risk body fluids (eg, healthcare workers)
Prostitution
Sexual activity with partners having risk factors for HIV
Sexual activity with partners with HIV
Signs and symptoms of HIV

If the patient has HIV, *Proceed to Step 4.*

If the patient does not have HIV, *Proceed to Step 11.*

STEP 11: *What are the Noninfectious Causes of Odynophagia?*

Infectious esophagitis is an uncommon cause of odynophagia in immunocompetent patients. Rather the clinician should focus on noninfectious causes of odynophagia. These are listed in the following box.

Noninfectious Causes of Odynophagia
Acute radiation esophagitis
Behcet's disease
Corrosive esophagitis
Crohn's disease
Dermatologic conditions
Benign mucous membrane pemphigoid
Bullous pemphigoid
Epidermolysis bullosa dystrophica
Pemphigus vulgaris
Esophageal cancer
Gastroesophageal reflux disease
Graft-versus-host disease
Pill-induced esophagitis

Proceed to Step 12

> **STEP 12:** *Are There Any Clues in the Patient's Clinical Presentation That Point to the Etiology of the Odynophagia?*

Clues in the patient's history that may point to the etiology of the odynophagia are listed in the following table.

Historical Clue	Condition Suggested
Sudden onset of odynophagia following ingestion of a pill	Pill-induced esophagitis
Ingestion of pill while in bed Ingestion of pill with no or inadequate amounts of fluid	Risk factors for pill-induced esophagitis
Heartburn	Gastroesophageal reflux disease
Intentional ingestion of corrosive substance	Corrosive esophagitis
Undergoing radiation therapy for malignancy (ie, bronchogenic, lymphoma, esophageal, metastatic breast)	Acute radiation esophagitis
Skin rash	Pemphigus vulgaris Bullous pemphigoid Epidermolysis bullosa dystrophica Benign mucous membrane pemphigoid

One or more of the following:
  Achalasia
  Barrett's esophagus
  Heavy alcohol use
  Heavy tobacco use
  History of lye ingestion
  Plummer-Vinson syndrome
	Risk factors for esophageal cancer

History of Crohn's disease	Crohn's esophagitis

These conditions are described in further detail below.

Pill-Induced Esophagitis

Pill-induced esophagitis should be suspected when there is sudden onset of odynophagia following the ingestion of a pill. Quite often, patients feel that the pill "has become stuck" while in transit. Some patients report constant substernal chest pain while others describe pain only with swallowing. When constant, the history usually reveals that the pain is worsened by swallowing. This is a helpful feature in differentiating the pain of pill-induced esophagitis from cardiac pain. Sometimes, the pain awakens the patient from sleep.

Not uncommonly, patients will describe pill ingestion with little or no fluids prior to the onset of the symptoms. Others will report pill ingestion while lying supine. Other risk factors for the development of pill-induced esophagitis are listed in the following box.

Risk Factors for the Development of Pill-Induced Esophagitis
Swallowing pills in the recumbent position
Swallowing pills with little or no fluid
Increased age
Larger pill size
Increased stickiness of pill
Decreased amplitude of esophageal contractions
Slow-release formulation
Enlarged left atrium

Although many different types of medications may cause esophageal injury, the common offenders are listed in the following box.

Common Medicinal Causes of Esophageal Injury	
Antimicrobial / antiviral agents*	NSAIDs
Doxycycline	Quinidine
Tetracycline	Theophylline
Clindamycin	Alprenolol
Penicillin	Ferrous sulfate
Erythromycin	Alendronate
Zalcitabine	Pamidronate
Zidovudine	Potassium chloride
Aspirin	Ascorbic acid

*Doxycycline accounts for 50% of antibiotic-related cases

It is important to realize that there are atypical presentations of pill-induced esophagitis. In some patients, for example, the onset of symptoms may be delayed, occurring days to weeks after ingestion of the pill.

Gastroesophageal Reflux Disease

Heartburn and regurgitation are the typical symptoms of gastroesophageal reflux disease. Odynophagia may accompany these symptoms in patients who develop esophageal ulceration. Esophageal ulceration may develop in the stratified squamous epithelium that lines the esophagus. Alternatively, it may develop in the setting of Barrett's esophagus. Barrett's esophagus refers to the replacement of the normal stratified squamous epithelium with abnormal columnar epithelium. Ulcerations may develop in the columnar epithelium. In fact, one study noted esophageal ulceration in 66% of patients with Barrett's esophagus.

Esophageal Cancer

When symptomatic, patients with esophageal cancer usually complain of dysphagia. On occasion, other symptoms such as odynophagia, retrosternal discomfort, cough, hoarseness, or melena may be the predominant manifestation. In fact, 50% of patients with esophageal cancer report odynophagia.

Corrosive Esophagitis

Corrosive or caustic injury to the esophagus may be the result of alkali (drain openers, cleaning preparations) or acid (toilet bowl cleaners, battery fluids, swimming pool cleaners) ingestion. In adults, ingestion is usually intentional. Although the clinical presentation of corrosive esophagitis is varied, patients may complain of dysphagia, odynophagia, chest pain, abdominal pain, and hoarseness. Feared complications of corrosive esophagitis include esophageal perforation and upper airway obstruction.

Acute Radiation Esophagitis

Esophageal injury is not uncommon in patients receiving radiation for treatment of cancer of the esophagus or other organs that are near the esophagus. Symptoms of dysphagia, odynophagia, chest pain, or retrosternal burning may develop during the radiation therapy. In some patients, the symptoms of acute radiation esophagitis may not develop until shortly after the completion of the radiation therapy.

Behcet's Disease

Behcet's disease is a systemic illness having a predilection to affect individuals in the Mediterranean region and Japan. It is characterized by the following:

- Aphthous ulcerations of the mouth and genitalia
- Ocular inflammation (iridocyclitis, conjunctivitis)

In addition, patients may have disease affecting the skin, joints, and central nervous system. Superficial or deep vein thrombophlebitis is not uncommon in these patients.

The gastrointestinal system may be involved in Behcet's disease. Ulceration of the terminal ileum and right colon is the most common manifestation, often mimicking inflammatory bowel disease. Although rare, esophageal involvement may occur including ulceration, stricture, or perforation. With esophageal involvement, patients may report odynophagia.

Crohn's Disease

Esophageal involvement is rarely encountered in patients with Crohn's disease. In almost all cases, there is concomitant inflammation elsewhere in the gastrointestinal tract. Early in the course of Crohn's disease of the esophagus, ulcers and erosions may be noted. Odynophagia is a common complaint in many of these patients. With advancing disease, patients may develop strictures, sinus tracts, and even fistulas

Dermatologic Conditions

Dermatologic conditions that may involve the esophagus include the following:

- Pemphigus vulgaris
- Bullous pemphigoid
- Benign mucous membrane pemphigoid
- Epidermolysis bullosa dystrophica

Epidermolysis bullosa dystrophica is a hereditary condition characterized by the presence of cutaneous bullae. Both autosomal dominant and recessive inheritance of the disease have been described. Clinically significant esophageal involvement is more common in the autosomal recessive form of the disease. Ulceration of esophageal bullae may result in odynophagia. Healing of the lesions may result in scarring and stricture formation.

Graft-Versus-Host Disease

Graft-versus-host disease may be divided into acute and chronic forms. The acute phase of the disease is not characterized by esophageal involvement. In chronic graft-versus-host disease, however, the esophagus is often affected. Although most patients with chronic graft-versus-host disease have antecedent acute graft-versus-host disease, about 30% of patients with the chronic form will not have a history of acute graft-versus-host disease.

Esophageal involvement may take the form of diffuse desquamation, strictures, and web formation. Clinically, esophageal disease often manifests with dysphagia, odynophagia, and symptoms of gastroesophageal reflux. Because bone marrow transplant patients are also predisposed to the development of infectious esophagitis, the diagnosis is one of exclusion.

Proceed to Step 13

> **STEP 13:** *What is the Diagnostic Procedure of Choice in the Evaluation of Odynophagia?*

The diagnostic procedure of choice in the evaluation of odynophagia is endoscopy. While the accuracy of double-contrast barium radiography may approach that of endoscopy, in general, barium radiography is less sensitive and specific in the detection of disease involving the esophageal mucosa. While double-contrast barium radiography can detect ulcerative lesions of the esophagus, biopsy is necessary to establish the histologic diagnosis.

Barium radiography may be contraindicated in some diseases manifesting with odynophagia. For example, barium may be irritating in the setting of perforation complicating corrosive esophagitis. In addition, its use may prevent adequate endoscopic visualization of the esophageal mucosa.

Endoscopy is also necessary to establish the diagnosis of infectious esophagitis, should it occur in those who do not have an apparent predisposition to infection. For these reasons, then, endoscopy is favored over barium radiography in the evaluation of the patient with odynophagia. When infectious esophagitis is diagnosed in the apparently immunocompetent patient, a search should be undertaken for an underlying abnormality of immunoregulation.

Not all cases of odynophagia require endoscopy. When the presentation is classic for pill-induced esophagitis, endoscopy is not necessary. Indications for endoscopy in patients suspected of having pill-induced esophagitis are listed in the following box.

Indications for Endoscopy in Patients Suspected of Having Pill-Induced Esophagitis
Atypical presentation
Gradual onset of symptoms
Persistence of symptoms
Uncertainty regarding onset of symptoms in relation to ingestion of pill
Immunocompromised state
Prominent dysphagia

In addition, the clinician may elect to forego endoscopy in the patient presenting with classic symptoms of GERD (heartburn and regurgitation). However, lack of improvement with therapy for GERD warrants the performance of endoscopy.

REFERENCES

Clinical Practice of Gastroenterology, Brandt LJ (ed), Philadelphia, PA: Current Medicine, Inc, 1999.

Current Diagnosis and Treatment in Gastroenterology, Grendell JH, McQuaid KR, Friedman SL (eds), Stanford, CT: Appleton & Lange, 1996.

Laine L and Bonacini M, "Esophageal Disease in Human Immunodeficiency Virus Infection," *Arch Intern Med*, 1994, 154(14):1577-82.

Sutton FM, Graham DY, and Goodgame RW, "Infectious Esophagitis," *Gastrointest Endosc Clin N Am*, 1994, 4(4):713-29.

Wilcox CM and Karowe MW, "Esophageal Infections: Etiology, Diagnosis, and Management," *Gastroenterologist*, 1994, 2(3):188-206.

Yee J and Wall SD, "Infectious Esophagitis," *Radiol Clin North Am*, 1994, 32(6):1135-45.

ODYNOPHAGIA

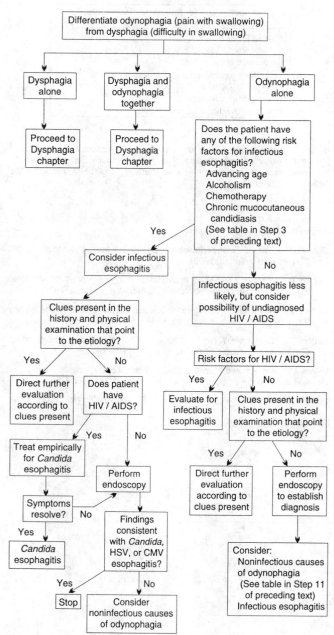

PALPITATIONS

STEP 1: *What are Palpitations?*

Palpitations are defined as an uncomfortable awareness of the heartbeat. Various surveys performed in the general medical outpatient setting have revealed that palpitations are among the ten most commonly reported symptoms. Any alteration of the heart rate, rhythm, or force of contractility may cause a patient to experience a disagreeable sensation of the heartbeat or palpitation. Patients with palpitations often use terms such as "pounding", "skipping", "fluttering", "racing", "stopping", or "jumping" to describe the sensation they are experiencing. Although most cases are due to a benign etiology, the clinician should realize that palpitations may be the manifestation of a potentially life-threatening arrhythmia.

Proceed to Step 2

STEP 2: *What are the Causes of Palpitations?*

The causes of palpitations are listed in the following box.

Causes of Palpitations	
Cardiac	Medications / drug use
Extrasystoles	Alcohol
Premature atrial beats	Aminophylline
Premature AV junctional (nodal) beats	Amphetamine abuse
Premature ventricular beats	β-agonists
Tachyarrhythmia	Caffeine
Atrial fibrillation	Cocaine abuse
Atrial flutter	Digoxin
Multifocal atrial tachycardia	Ephedrine
Sinus tachycardia	Nicotine
Supraventricular tachycardia	Sympathomimetic agents
Ventricular tachycardia	Thyroid hormone
Bradyarrhythmia	Psychiatric
Second degree AV block	Anxiety
Sinus bradycardia	Bereavement
Third degree AV block	Depression
Medical illness	Panic disorder
Anemia	Somatization disorder
Fever	
Hypercalcemia	
Hyperthyroidism	
Hypoglycemia	
Hypokalemia	
Hypomagnesemia	

Proceed to Step 3

> **STEP 3:** *Are There Any Clues in the Patient's History That Point to the Etiology of the Palpitations?*

Clues in the patient's history that point to the etiology of the palpitations are listed in the following table.

Historical Clue	Condition Suggested
History of chest pain or MI	Coronary artery disease (substrate for arrhythmia)
History of murmur	Valvular heart disease (substrate for arrhythmia)
History of rheumatic fever	Valvular heart disease (substrate for arrhythmia)
Leg swelling Orthopnea Paroxysmal nocturnal dyspnea (PND)	Congestive heart failure (substrate for arrhythmia)
History of heart disease	Cardiac cause of palpitations
History of depression, anxiety, panic disorder, or somatization disorder	Psychiatric cause of palpitations
Related to medication or drug use	Medication/drug use (see box in Step 2)
Palpitations begin and end abruptly	Supraventricular or ventricular tachycardia
Gradual onset and cessation of palpitations	Sinus tachycardia
Sudden relief of palpitations with vagal maneuvers: Breath-holding Induced gagging or vomiting Stooping	Paroxysmal supraventricular tachycardia
Associated symptoms of: Anxiety Dizziness Lump in throat Tingling in hands and face	Anxiety state characterized by sinus tachycardia and hyperventilation
Family history of similar symptoms or sudden death	Hypertrophic cardiomyopathy Long QT syndrome Wolff-Parkinson-White syndrome
"Skipped beats" or "flip-flopping sensation"	Extrasystoles
Fatigue Heat intolerance Increased appetite Increased sweating Nervousness Weakness Weight loss	Hyperthyroidism
Patient's description of pulse during palpitations*: Rapid and irregular	 Atrial fibrillation Atrial flutter with variable conduction Multifocal atrial tachycardia
Rapid and regular	Atrial flutter with fixed conduction Sinus tachycardia Supraventricular tachycardia Ventricular tachycardia
Following alcohol use	Alcohol†

(Continued)

(continued)

Historical Clue	Condition Suggested
Caffeine use	Exacerbation of supraventricular arrhythmias Extrasystoles
Tobacco use	Exacerbation of supraventricular arrhythmias Extrasystoles
Recent illicit drug use	Amphetamine abuse Cocaine abuse

Risk factors for atherosclerosis:
  Age
  Diabetes mellitus
  Family history
  Gender
  Hyperlipidemia
  Hypertension
  Smoking
	Coronary artery disease (substrate for arrhythmia)

Full sensation in the throat Neck pounding Sensation of palpitation in neck	AV nodal reentrant tachycardia Ventricular tachycardia (less often)
Polyuria following palpitations	Supraventricular tachycardia
Occurring during exercise	Exercise-induced arrhythmia

*Patients sometimes take their own pulse during an episode of palpitations. If so, the patient may be able to describe the rate and regularity of the rhythm. In those who do not take their pulse, it is useful to tap out various rhythms on the patient's chest or examination table. By doing so, the patient may be able to identify the rhythm that caused the palpitations. Alternatively, the clinician may elect to have the patient tap out the rate and rhythm. In one study, up to 33% of patients with palpitations were able to describe the rate and rhythm of the palpitations.

†Alcohol, even in small amounts, can precipitate arrhythmias (premature beats, atrial fibrillation) in patients with underlying heart disease. In large amounts (binge drinking), it can induce arrhythmias in individuals with structurally normal hearts.

Proceed to Step 4

> **STEP 4:** *Are There Any Clues in the Patient's Physical Examination That Point to the Etiology of the Palpitations?*

Most patients are free of symptoms at the time the physical examination is performed. In these cases, the goals of the physical examination include the following:

- Identification of signs consistent with underlying heart disease (substrate for arrhythmia)

- Identification of a systemic illness that may be causing the palpitations

Clues in the patient's physical examination that may point to the etiology of the palpitations are listed in the following table.

Physical Examination Finding	Condition Suggested
Fever	Sinus tachycardia

Hyper-reflexia
Ocular signs
  Infrequent blinking
  Lid lag
  Stare
Proptosis (Graves' disease)
Tremor
Warm, moist skin
	Hyperthyroidism

Arcus senilis Xanthomas	Coronary artery disease (substrate for arrhythmia)
Bilateral lower extremity edema Elevated jugular venous pressure Laterally displaced PMI S3	Congestive heart failure (substrate for arrhythmia)
Midsystolic click with or without heart murmur	Mitral valve prolapse
Heart murmur	Valvular heart disease (substrate for arrhythmia)
Harsh holosystolic murmur at left sternal border that increases with Valsalva	Hypertrophic cardiomyopathy

On occasion, the clinician may be fortunate to examine a patient during an episode of palpitations. Physical examination findings useful to note when the patient is symptomatic are listed in the following table.

Physical Examination Finding	Condition Suggested
Irregularly, irregular rhythm	Atrial fibrillation Atrial flutter with variable conduction Multifocal atrial tachycardia
Regular tachycardia (100-170 beats/minute) that transiently slows down with vagal maneuvers	Sinus tachycardia
Tachycardia with rate of 150 beats per minute (abruptly decreases with vagal maneuvers only to quickly return to 150 beats/minute)	Atrial flutter
Cannon a waves (with slow rhythm) in jugular venous waveform	Complete heart block
Cannon a waves (with fast rhythm) in jugular venous waveform	Ventricular tachycardia
Variable first heart sound	Ventricular tachycardia
Prominent a wave in jugular venous waveform	AV nodal re-entrant tachycardia
Bulging noted in the neck during episode of palpitations (positive frog sign)	AV nodal re-entrant tachycardia
Termination of tachycardia with vagal maneuvers	Supraventricular tachycardia

Of note, a normal heart rate and rhythm during an episode of palpitations strongly argues against a cardiac etiology.

Proceed to Step 5

STEP 5: *What are the Results of the EKG?*

An EKG is essential in every patient presenting with palpitations. An EKG performed during an episode of palpitations may identify an arrhythmia. Most often, however, the clinician will perform the EKG in an asymptomatic patient. Even when asymptomatic, the EKG may provide some valuable information. The clinician should focus on identifying any EKG abnormalities suggestive of the presence of structural heart disease. The table below describes the significance of abnormalities noted on inspection of the EKG in patients with palpitations.

EKG Finding	Significance of the EKG Finding
Left or right atrial enlargement	Increased risk of supraventricular arrhythmia
Delta wave Short PR interval	Wolff-Parkinson-White syndrome
Prolonged QT interval	Torsade de pointes Other forms of ventricular tachycardia
Q waves	Myocardial infarction (substrate for arrhythmia)
Sinus bradycardia	Nonspecific (consider possibility of sick sinus syndrome)
Bundle branch block	Possible heart block or ventricular tachycardia
Left or right ventricular hypertrophy	Presence of structural heart disease (substrate for arrhythmia)
Marked left ventricular hypertrophy with deep septal Q waves in leads I, avL, V4-V6	Hypertrophic cardiomyopathy
Normal or nonspecific	Does not rule out presence of organic heart disease

If the EKG captures a rhythm disturbance while a patient is experiencing palpitations, then the evaluation should proceed according to the rhythm disturbance identified.

Otherwise, *Proceed to Step 6.*

STEP 6: *What Laboratory Tests Should be Considered in the Patient Presenting With Palpitations?*

When indicated, the clinician may elect to perform the following laboratory tests:

- Hemoglobin
- Thyroid function tests
- Electrolytes (potassium, calcium)
- Blood glucose

The results of these tests may uncover anemia, hyperthyroidism, hypokalemia, hypercalcemia, and hypoglycemia. All of these conditions are associated with palpitations.

If laboratory testing reveals a systemic condition or medical illness that is causing the palpitations, *Stop Here.*

If laboratory testing does not reveal a systemic condition or medical illness that is causing the palpitations, *Proceed to Step 7.*

STEP 7: *Does the Patient Have Underlying Structural Heart Disease?*

It is said that up to 40% of patients with palpitations will have a diagnosis established after the history, physical examination, laboratory tests, and EKG. In the remainder, the clinician should ask the following questions:

- Does the patient have underlying heart disease that would predispose to an arrhythmic cause of the palpitations?

- Does the patient have severe or significant symptoms?

When the history, physical examination, or EKG provides evidence for structural heart disease, arrhythmia must be excluded by further evaluation. Although many patients complain of palpitations alone, others report accompanying chest pain, shortness of breath, light-headedness, dizziness, presyncope, or syncope. While the presence of these symptoms does not conclusively establish an arrhythmic cause, it does provide information regarding the effects of an arrhythmia, should one be present, on the cardiac output and blood pressure. In patients with significant symptoms, further evaluation to exclude an arrhythmic cause is necessary.

If the history, physical examination, and EKG findings are suggestive of an arrhythmia, *Proceed to Step 8.*

If the history, physical examination, and EKG findings suggest the presence of structural or organic heart disease (raising concern for arrhythmic cause), *Proceed to Step 8.*

If the history, physical examination, and EKG findings do not suggest that the patient is at risk for an arrhythmic cause of the palpitations and there is no evidence of structural heart disease, *Proceed to Step 14.*

STEP 8: *What Testing Should be Performed in the Patient Suspected of Having an Arrhythmic Cause of the Palpitations?*

Testing that is available to establish the etiology of the palpitations include the following:

- Ambulatory EKG monitoring (Holtor monitoring)
- Intermittent recorder (event, loop)
- Electrophysiologic study
- Exercise stress testing

    Exercise stress testing may be warranted in patients who develop palpitations during or after exercise.

Which test to perform is dependent on the patient's clinical presentation.

Proceed to Step 9

STEP 9: *Is Electrophysiologic Study Indicated?*

When palpitations are accompanied by life-threatening symptoms or those suggestive of hemodynamic compromise (syncope and presyncope), consideration should be given to performing an electrophysiologic study. Class I indications for electrophysiologic study in patients with palpitations are listed in the following box.

Class I Indications* for Electrophysiologic Study in Patients With Unexplained Palpitations

- Patients with rapid pulse rate documented by medical personnel and in whom EKG recordings fail to document the cause
- Patients with palpitations preceding a syncopal event

*Class I represents those conditions for which there is evidence and/or general agreement that a given procedure or treatment is useful and effective

Adapted from the "Guidelines for Clinical Intracardiac Electrophysiological and Catheter Ablation Procedures. A Report of the American College of Cardiology/American Heart Association Task Force on Practice Guidelines (Committee on Clinical Intracardiac Electrophysiologic and Catheter Ablation Procedures). Developed in Collaboration with the North American Society of Pacing and Electrophysiology," *Circulation*, 1995, 92(3):673-91.

If an electrophysiology study is indicated, *Stop Here*.

If an electrophysiology study is not indicated, *Proceed to Step 10.*

STEP 10: *How Frequent are the Palpitations?*

When an electrophysiologic study is not performed, the clinician should assess the frequency of palpitations to dictate further testing. Choices available to the clinician include ambulatory EKG monitoring and placement of an intermittent recorder. Either test seeks to record the EKG during a time when the patient is symptomatic. By capturing the rhythm during an episode of palpitations, the clinician can determine if the symptoms are related to an arrhythmia.

In patients with daily or frequent symptoms, it is reasonable to perform ambulatory EKG monitoring over a 24-hour period. Since the usefulness of 24-hour ambulatory EKG monitoring depends on a cardiac event occurring during a limited period of time, it may not be worthwhile in patients who have infrequent episodes of palpitations. In these cases, the clinician may elect to provide the patient with an intermittent recorder. The patient can activate the intermittent recorder when symptoms occur. The recorded EKG may then be viewed at a later time. The intermittent recorder does require the patient to have the cognitive ability to activate the recorder when symptoms develop.

If ambulatory EKG monitoring is chosen as the test of choice, *Proceed to Step 11.*

If an intermittent monitor is to be placed as the test of choice, *Proceed to Step 12.*

> **STEP 11:** *What are the Results of the Ambulatory EKG Monitoring?*

Ambulatory EKG monitoring involves the recording of the electrocardiographic signal over a certain time period. Most often, the clinician will elect to perform 24-hour monitoring. During the period of monitoring, the patient is free to pursue normal activities. At a later time, the recording can be played back. Rhythm abnormalities identified during review of the recording are correlated with symptoms recorded in the patient's diary. Of the four possible outcomes with ambulatory EKG monitoring, two are particularly revealing:

- An arrhythmia capable of producing the patient's symptoms is documented during an episode of palpitations

    With this finding, an arrhythmic cause of the palpitations is established. Further evaluation and management depends on the rhythm disturbance identified.

- No rhythm disturbance is documented during an episode of palpitations

    An arrhythmia is excluded in patients who have no rhythm disturbance documented during an episode of palpitations.

The other two outcomes, which are usually considered to be nondiagnostic, include the following:

- An arrhythmia is documented but patient is asymptomatic during the time when the rhythm disturbance is recorded

    In these cases, the recorded arrhythmia may or may not be related to the palpitations that prompted the study.

- No rhythm disturbance is documented in an asymptomatic patient

    This finding does not exclude an arrhythmia because the rhythm disturbance may not have occurred during the period of ambulatory EKG monitoring. Because of the spontaneous variability of cardiac arrhythmias, a symptomatic arrhythmia may not be identified during a single 24-hour ambulatory EKG.

If an arrhythmia capable of producing the patient's symptoms is documented during an episode of palpitations, then the evaluation should proceed according to the abnormal rhythm identified.

If no rhythm disturbance is documented during an episode of palpitations, then an arrhythmic cause has been excluded. The patient should be reassured that the palpitations are not due to a cardiac cause. ***Stop Here.***

If no rhythm disturbance is documented in an asymptomatic patient, then ***Proceed to Step 12.***

If an arrhythmia is documented but the patient is asymptomatic at the time of the abnormal rhythm, ***Proceed to Step 13.***

STEP 12: *What are the Results of the Intermittent Recorder?*

Placement of an intermittent recorder should be considered in patients who have infrequent palpitations. It should be reserved for patients who have the cognitive ability to use the device.

For patients who are unable to comply with the intermittent recorder, the clinician should perform ambulatory EKG monitoring. In these cases, several periods of ambulatory EKG monitoring may be required to establish the diagnosis.

The two basic types of intermittent recorders are loop and event recorders. It is possible to use either type over a prolonged period of time to identify arrhythmias occurring in patients with infrequent palpitations.

If the intermittent recorder reveals no rhythm disturbance during an episode of palpitations, then the patient does not have an arrhythmic cause of the palpitations. ***Stop Here.***

If the patient is not able to use the intermittent recorder, ***Proceed to Step 11.***

If the intermittent recorder captures a rhythm disturbance during an episode of palpitations, then the evaluation should proceed according to the abnormal rhythm identified.

If the etiology of the palpitations is not determined with the use of an intermittent recorder, consider cardiology consultation, especially if an arrhythmic cause remains a major consideration.

STEP 13: *What is the Significance of an Arrhythmia That is Detected During Ambulatory EKG Monitoring at a Time When the Patient is Asymptomatic?*

The detection of an asymptomatic rhythm abnormality does not imply that the rhythm disturbance is the cause of the palpitations. Premature ventricular and atrial contractions may have no specific meaning when detected in asymptomatic patients. Short runs of supraventricular or ventricular tachycardia are more concerning but, in the absence of symptoms, these rhythm disturbances should not be considered to be the cause of the patient's palpitations. These findings should prompt the clinician to pursue further evaluation. The documentation of sustained ventricular tachycardia (>30 seconds) is an ominous finding, even in an asymptomatic patient.

If there is any uncertainty about the significance of a rhythm disturbance detected in an asymptomatic patient, it is reasonable to seek the expertise of a cardiologist. Otherwise, these patients should be considered for either repeat ambulatory EKG monitoring or the placement of an intermittent recorder. In those who are considered to be at high risk for an arrhythmia, the clinician should discuss with cardiology the need for electrophysiology study when clinically significant arrhythmias are not detected by ambulatory monitoring.

End of Section.

STEP 14: *Should the Clinician Reassure the Patient or Recommend Ambulatory EKG Monitoring?*

When the history, physical examination, and EKG findings do not suggest a cardiac etiology of the palpitations, no further evaluation is necessary. In these cases, the patient should be reassured that the palpitations are not due to a serious cause. In those who remain overly concerned about their symptoms, the clinician may elect to perform ambulatory EKG monitoring to document the benign nature of the palpitations, especially if the palpitations are frequent. Alternatively, the clinician may place an intermittent recorder for the same purpose, particularly in patients who have infrequent symptoms.

In these patients, the clinician should revisit the history. In particular, a review of the medication history is warranted. It is also worthwhile to explore the patient's use of illicit drugs, tobacco, alcohol, and caffeine.

The clinician should also consider some of the psychiatric conditions associated with palpitations. Psychiatric conditions are common causes of palpitations. In many of these conditions, there is heightened awareness of the heartbeat. Appropriate treatment of a psychiatric condition, if present, may lead to the disappearance of the palpitations.

REFERENCES

Brugada P, Gursoy S, Brugada J, et al, "Investigation of Palpitations," *Lancet*, 1993, 341(8855):1254-8.

Burn S and Kaye G, "Identifying the Causes of Syncope and Palpitations," *Practitioner*, 1995, 239(1556):666-9.

"Guidelines for Clinical Intracardiac Electrophysiological and Catheter Ablation Procedures. A Report of the American College of Cardiology/American Heart Association Task Force on Practice Guidelines (Committee on Clinical Intracardiac Electrophysiologic and Catheter Ablation Procedures). Developed in Collaboration with the North American Society of Pacing and Electrophysiology," *Circulation*, 1995, 92(3):673-91.

Kopp DE and Wilber DJ, "Palpitations and Arrhythmias. Separating the Benign From the Dangerous," *Postgrad Med*, 1992, 91(1):241-4, 247-8, 251.

Murtagh J, "Palpitations," *Aust Fam Physician*, 1992, 21(4):475, 478-82.

Vohra JK, "Palpitations: Reassurance or More?" *Med J Aust*, 1999, 170(9):442-8.

Weitz HH and Weinstock PJ, "Approach to the Patient With Palpitations," *Med Clin North Am*, 1995, 79(2):449-56.

Zimetbaum P and Josephson ME, "Evaluation of Patients With Palpitations," *N Engl J Med*, 1998, 338(19):1369-73.

PALPITATIONS

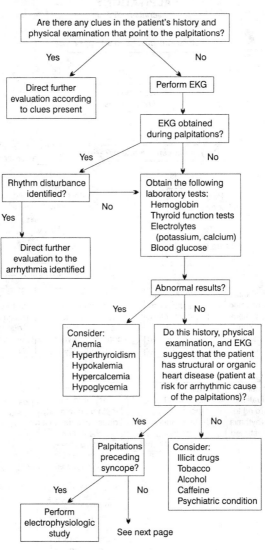

Are there any clues in the patient's history and physical examination that point to the palpitations?

Yes → Direct further evaluation according to clues present

No → Perform EKG

EKG obtained during palpitations?

Yes → Rhythm disturbance identified?

No → Obtain the following laboratory tests:
Hemoglobin
Thyroid function tests
Electrolytes (potassium, calcium)
Blood glucose

Yes → Direct further evaluation to the arrhythmia identified

Abnormal results?

Yes → Consider:
Anemia
Hyperthyroidism
Hypokalemia
Hypercalcemia
Hypoglycemia

No → Do this history, physical examination, and EKG suggest that the patient has structural or organic heart disease (patient at risk for arrhythmic cause of the palpitations)?

Yes → Palpitations preceding syncope?

No → Consider:
Illicit drugs
Tobacco
Alcohol
Caffeine
Psychiatric condition

Yes → Perform electrophysiologic study

No → See next page

PALPITATIONS
(continued)

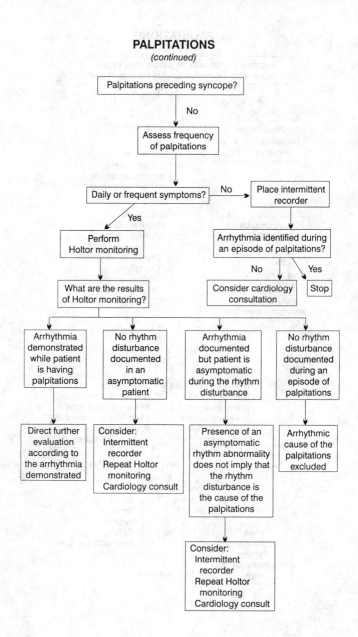

Palpitations preceding syncope?

No

Assess frequency of palpitations

Daily or frequent symptoms? — No → Place intermittent recorder

Yes

Perform Holtor monitoring

Arrhythmia identified during an episode of palpitations?

No   Yes

Consider cardiology consultation   Stop

What are the results of Holtor monitoring?

| Arrhythmia demonstrated while patient is having palpitations | No rhythm disturbance documented in an asymptomatic patient | Arrhythmia documented but patient is asymptomatic during the rhythm disturbance | No rhythm disturbance documented during an episode of palpitations |

Direct further evaluation according to the arrhythmia demonstrated

Consider: Intermittent recorder Repeat Holtor monitoring Cardiology consult

Presence of an asymptomatic rhythm abnormality does not imply that the rhythm disturbance is the cause of the palpitations

Arrhythmic cause of the palpitations excluded

Consider: Intermittent recorder Repeat Holtor monitoring Cardiology consult

PRURITUS (Generalized)

STEP 1: *What are the Causes of Pruritus?*

Pruritus is the most commonly encountered symptom in dermatology. Although generalized pruritus is often the result of a primary skin disease, in some cases, it may be a clue to the presence of an underlying systemic condition. The causes of generalized pruritus are listed in the following box.

Causes of Generalized Pruritus	
Diabetes mellitus	Polycythemia vera
Hyperthyroidism	Postmenopausal
Hypothyroidism	Pregnancy
Iron deficiency anemia	Primary skin disease
Liver disease	Psychologic
Medications	Uremia
Neoplasm	
Hodgkin's disease	
Leukemia	
Non-Hodgkin's lymphoma	
Solid tumors (pancreatic, stomach)	

Proceed to Step 2

STEP 2: *Are There Any Clues in the Patient's History That Point to the Etiology of the Generalized Pruritus?*

Clues in the patient's history that may point to the etiology of the generalized pruritus are listed in the following table.

Historical Clue	Condition Suggested
Skin rash	Primary skin disease
Associated with hot flashes	Postmenopausal
Fatigue Heat intolerance Increased appetite Increased sweating Nervousness Palpitation Weight loss	Hyperthyroidism
Cold skin Constipation Dry skin Hair loss Sensation of cold Weakness Weight gain	Hypothyroidism
Fever Night sweats Weight loss	Hodgkin's lymphoma Non-Hodgkin's lymphoma
History of venous or arterial thrombosis	Polycythemia vera

(continued)

(continued)

Historical Clue	Condition Suggested
Burning pain in feet or hands (erythromelalgia)	Polycythemia vera
Sensation of bugs crawling on the skin	Psychogenic
Antidepressants Aspirin Barbiturates Belladonna alkaloids CNS stimulants Estrogens Hepatotoxic drugs Opiates	Medication-induced

Proceed to Step 3

STEP 3: *Are There Any Clues in the Patient's Physical Examination That Point to the Etiology of the Generalized Pruritus?*

Clues in the patient's physical examination that point to the etiology of the generalized pruritus are listed in the following table.

Physical Examination Finding	Condition Suggested
Splenomegaly	Hodgkin's lymphoma Non-Hodgkin's lymphoma Polycythemia vera
Facial plethora	Polycythemia vera
Lymphadenopathy	Hodgkin's lymphoma Non-Hodgkin's lymphoma

Fine tremor of fingers and tongue
Hyper-reflexia
Ocular signs
  Infrequent blinking
  Lid lag
  Palmar erythema
Plummer's nail (onycholysis)
Pretibial myxedema (Grave's disease)
Proptosis (Grave's disease)
Stare
Thyroid acropachy
Warm, moist skin
	Hyperthyroidism

Deepening and hoarseness of voice Dry, cool skin Large tongue Periorbital puffiness Prolonged relaxation phase of deep tendon reflexes Rough and doughy skin Sparse hair	Hypothyroidism

Proceed to Step 4

STEP 4: *Does the Patient Have a Primary Skin Disease?*

The approach to the patient with generalized pruritus begins with a thorough skin examination. The presence of skin lesions does not conclusively establish that the pruritus is secondary to a primary skin disease. Excoriations are not uncommon in patients with pruritus. In addition, thickening with accentuation of the skin lines may occur. This is known as lichenification. Persistent rubbing of the skin may also lead to the development of papules, plaques, or nodules. These skin changes have a predilection for the scalp, extremities, and the posterior neck. It is essential that the clinician recognize that these manifestations are not the cause of the pruritus but represent the end result of scratching or rubbing. In general, however, the absence of a skin rash argues against pruritus that is the result of a primary skin disease.

If the pruritus is secondary to a primary skin disease, ***Stop Here.***

If the pruritus is not secondary to a primary skin disease, ***Proceed to Step 5.***

STEP 5: *What is the Response to Treatment?*

Once primary skin disease has been excluded as the cause of the generalized pruritus, the investigation should be tailored to the disease suggested by clinical clues from the history and physical examination. In the absence of clinical clues, it is appropriate to treat these patients symptomatically with oral antihistamines and topical nonsteroidal creams or lotions. Other useful recommendations include less frequent bathing, "pat" drying after a bath, and avoiding irritant fabrics such as wool. No further evaluation is necessary if there is improvement in the patient's symptoms after two weeks of symptomatic therapy.

If symptomatic therapy is successful and the pruritus does not return after discontinuation of symptomatic therapy, ***Stop Here.***

If symptomatic therapy is not successful and/or the pruritus returns after discontinuation of symptomatic therapy, ***Proceed to Step 6.***

STEP 6: *What Laboratory Tests Should be Obtained?*

Further evaluation is indicated in those who do not respond to symptomatic therapy. It is also recommended when pruritus returns after discontinuation of the symptomatic therapy. In these patients, the following laboratory tests are recommended.

- Hemoglobin / hematocrit
- Iron studies (serum iron, TIBC, ferritin)
- Serum BUN / creatinine
- Liver function tests (alkaline phosphatase, bilirubin, AST, ALT)
- Thyroid function tests (TSH, free thyroxine index or free T_4 level)
- Serum glucose level
- HIV test
- FSH level
- Stool for occult blood

The clinical significance of abnormalities in these laboratory tests are described in the following table.

Laboratory Test Abnormality	Condition Suggested
Decreased TSH Elevated free thyroxine index or free thyroxine level	Hyperthyroidism
Elevated TSH Decreased free thyroxine index or free thyroxine level	Hypothyroidism
Elevated serum glucose	Diabetes mellitus*
Elevated alkaline phosphatase	Cholestatic liver disease
Elevated hemoglobin / hematocrit	Polycythemia vera†
Elevated serum BUN / creatinine	Uremia
Microcytic or normocytic anemia Decreased serum iron Low ferritin Elevated TIBC Decreased transferrin saturation (<10% or 15%)	Iron deficiency anemia
Elevated urine / serum hCG	Pregnancy
Elevated FSH	Postmenopausal‡
Positive HIV test	HIV

* There is some debate about the association of generalized pruritus and diabetes mellitus. This association was first described in a case report in the 1920s. Since then, a controlled study found that generalized pruritus is no more common in diabetic patients than in individuals with normal glycemic control.

† The generalized pruritus of polycythemia vera is known as bath itch because it is typically water-induced. Occurring in about 50% of patients with polycythemia vera, in some cases, the pruritus precedes the development of the disease. It usually begins after the patient finishes bathing and may last up to one hour. Several recent reports have described similar complaints in patients with the hypereosinophilic syndrome or myelodysplasia.

‡ Although postmenopausal itch is often localized, in some patients, it may be generalized. When generalized pruritus is present, it is typically episodic, tending to coincide with other postmenopausal symptoms such as hot flashes.

If laboratory testing reveals the etiology of the pruritus, *Stop Here.*

If laboratory testing does not reveal the etiology of the pruritus, *Proceed to Step 7.*

STEP 7: *Is the Generalized Pruritus Due to a Malignancy?*

Less than 1% of patients referred to a dermatologist for generalized pruritus are found to have a malignancy. Since polycythemia vera has already been discussed above, it will not be considered here. Recall that pruritus is one manifestation of cholestatic liver disease. Malignancy is a major cause of extrahepatic cholestasis. In these patients, the laboratory tests described in Step 6 will suggest the diagnosis of cholestasis. As a result, cholestasis secondary to malignancy will also not be discussed here.

The major considerations are non-Hodgkin's and Hodgkin's lymphoma. Generalized pruritus occurs in less than 10% of patients with non-Hodgkin's lymphoma. In some of these patients, other systemic complaints including fever, weight loss, and night sweats may be present. Overall, approximately 40% of patients with non-Hodgkin's lymphoma present with these latter systemic complaints. Physical examination will reveal the presence of peripheral lymphadenopathy in more than 66% of patients.

Many patients with Hodgkin's disease experience generalized pruritus. In the majority, the pruritus occurs after the diagnosis has been made. In a minority, it may occur early in the disease course, even preceding the diagnosis by months or years. Systemic symptoms such as fever, night sweats, and weight loss are present in many individuals. Since mediastinal lymph nodes are involved in up to 60% of cases, it is reasonable to obtain a CXR even in the absence of systemic symptoms.

Generalized pruritus is the second most common dermatologic manifestation of leukemia (after purpura). Although it typically occurs late in the disease course, occasionally, it may be present early. An examination of the peripheral blood smear may be warranted.

Solid malignancies may also be associated with generalized pruritus but the decision to undertake an extensive evaluation should take into account the fact that generalized pruritus as the initial manifestation is rare and that testing can be quite expensive. Most authorities recommend a search for malignancy only in the presence of localized symptoms. Of the visceral malignancies, generalized pruritus most commonly occurs in patients with pancreatic or stomach cancer.

If the generalized pruritus is secondary to a malignancy, ***Stop Here.***

If the generalized pruritus is not secondary to a malignancy, ***Proceed to Step 8.***

STEP 8: *Has a Thorough Skin Examination Been Performed?*

The following primary skin diseases may result in generalized pruritus with minimal to no skin findings on physical examination:

- Aquagenic pruritus
- Fiberglass dermatitis
- Scabies
- Xerosis

Xerosis, also known as the winter itch, is a common cause of generalized pruritus in cooler climates. It should be suspected when the onset of the pruritus occurs during the winter months. Excessive dryness of the skin is usually apparent.

Infestation with scabies may result in subtle manifestations that may go unnoticed. Physical examination, however, may reveal burrows. If found, the burrow is pathognomonic for scabies. Microscopy of skin scrapings may demonstrate ova, mites, or feces.

An occupational history of contact with fiberglass should prompt consideration of fiberglass dermatitis, an irritant dermatitis that can also result in subtle skin manifestations. Fiberglass particles may be seen on microscopy of skin scrapings.

Itching that occurs after a bath or shower may be due to aquagenic pruritus, a condition that is usually associated with itching after the skin is wetted with water of any temperature. Aquagenic pruritus is not characterized by any skin findings and the itching usually abates within an hour. In 33% of patients, a positive family history may be elicited.

If one of the above subtle skin diseases is present, ***Stop Here.***

If one of the above subtle skin diseases is not present, ***Proceed to Step 9.***

STEP 9: *Is the Generalized Pruritus Medication-Induced?*

A thorough medication history is essential to exclude occult drug hypersensitivity. The following medications may be associated with generalized pruritus.

- Antidepressants
- Aspirin
- Barbiturates
- Belladonna alkaloids
- CNS stimulants
- Estrogens
- Hepatotoxic drugs
- Opiates

The resolution of the generalized pruritus after discontinuation of the medication supports the diagnosis.

If the patient has medication-induced generalized pruritus, *Stop Here.*

If the patient does not have medication-induced pruritus, *Proceed to Step 10.*

STEP 10: *Does the Patient Have Psychogenic Pruritus?*

Generalized pruritus may be due to anxiety or depression. The generalized pruritus of psychiatric disease should be a diagnosis of exclusion. Psychiatric consultation is often necessary in these cases.

If a psychiatric cause is not likely, then the patient should be treated symptomatically. Periodic follow-up is necessary to assess if the patient has developed signs and symptoms of an underlying disease.

End of Section.

REFERENCES

Greco PJ and Ende J, "Pruritus: A Practical Approach," *J Gen Intern Med*, 1992, 7(3):340-9.

Kantor GR, "Evaluation and Treatment of Generalized Pruritus," *Cleve Clin J Med*, 1990, 57(6):521-6.

Klecz RJ and Schwartz RA, "Pruritus," *Am Fam Phys*, 1992, 45(6):2681-6 (review).

Lober CW, "Should the Patient With Generalized Pruritus Be Evaluated for Malignancy?" *J Am Acad Dermatol*, 1988, 19(2 Pt 1):350-2 (review).

Sher TH, "Clinical Evaluation of Generalized Pruritus," *Compr Ther*, 1992, 18(9):14-9 (review).

Yosipovitch G and David M, "The Diagnostic and Therapeutic Approach to Idiopathic Generalized Pruritus," *Int J Dermatol*, 1999, 38(12):881-7 (review).

PRURITUS (GENERALIZED)

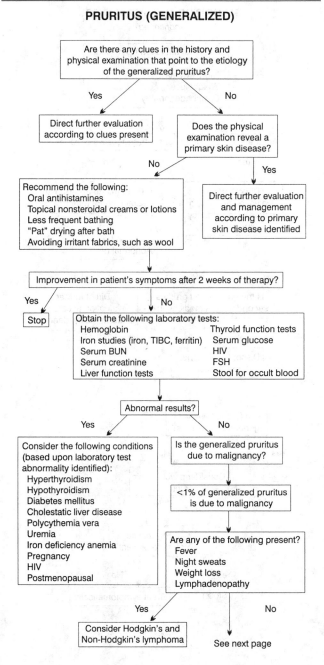

Are there any clues in the history and physical examination that point to the etiology of the generalized pruritus?

Yes → Direct further evaluation according to clues present

No → Does the physical examination reveal a primary skin disease?

Yes → Direct further evaluation and management according to primary skin disease identified

No → Recommend the following:
Oral antihistamines
Topical nonsteroidal creams or lotions
Less frequent bathing
"Pat" drying after bath
Avoiding irritant fabrics, such as wool

Improvement in patient's symptoms after 2 weeks of therapy?

Yes → Stop

No → Obtain the following laboratory tests:
Hemoglobin   Thyroid function tests
Iron studies (iron, TIBC, ferritin) Serum glucose
Serum BUN   HIV
Serum creatinine   FSH
Liver function tests   Stool for occult blood

Abnormal results?

Yes → Consider the following conditions (based upon laboratory test abnormality identified):
Hyperthyroidism
Hypothyroidism
Diabetes mellitus
Cholestatic liver disease
Polycythemia vera
Uremia
Iron deficiency anemia
Pregnancy
HIV
Postmenopausal

No → Is the generalized pruritus due to malignancy?

<1% of generalized pruritus is due to malignancy

Are any of the following present?
Fever
Night sweats
Weight loss
Lymphadenopathy

Yes → Consider Hodgkin's and Non-Hodgkin's lymphoma

No → See next page

PRURITUS (GENERALIZED)
(continued)

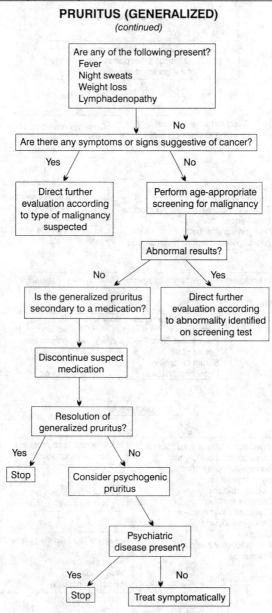

Are any of the following present?
Fever
Night sweats
Weight loss
Lymphadenopathy

↓ No

Are there any symptoms or signs suggestive of cancer?

Yes → Direct further evaluation according to type of malignancy suspected

No → Perform age-appropriate screening for malignancy

Abnormal results?

No → Is the generalized pruritus secondary to a medication?

Yes → Direct further evaluation according to abnormality identified on screening test

Discontinue suspect medication

↓

Resolution of generalized pruritus?

Yes → Stop

No → Consider psychogenic pruritus

↓

Psychiatric disease present?

Yes → Stop

No → Treat symptomatically

RED EYE

STEP 1: What are the Causes of Red Eye?

Red eye is commonly encountered in the primary care setting. In fact, it is the most common ocular disorder that primary care physicians encounter. As such, it behooves the clinician to become familiar with the causes of the red eye, most of which are benign. Since there are serious causes of red eye, the clinician must be able to recognize features in the patient's clinical presentation suggestive of these conditions. The common causes of red eye are listed in the following box.

Common Causes of Red Eye	
Acute angle-closure glaucoma	Corneal abrasion
Acute anterior uveitis	Corneal ulcer
Blepharitis	Episcleritis
Chalazion	Keratitis
Conjunctivitis	Orbital / preseptal cellulitis
Allergic	Pterygium
Bacterial	Scleritis
Chlamydial	Stye
Contact lens use	Subconjunctival hemorrhage
Dry eye	
Toxic or chemical reaction	
Viral	

Proceed to Step 2

STEP 2: Are There Any Clues in the Patient's History That Point to the Etiology of the Red Eye?

Clues in the patient's history that point to the etiology of the red eye are listed in the following table.

Historical Clue	Condition Suggested
Recent trauma	Acute anterior uveitis
	Corneal abrasion
	Corneal ulcer
	Subconjunctival hemorrhage
Pain in the eye	Acute angle-closure glaucoma
	Acute anterior uveitis
	Corneal abrasion
	Corneal foreign body
	Corneal ulcer
	Episcleritis
	Keratitis
	Scleritis
Absence of eye pain	Conjunctivitis*
	Subconjunctival hemorrhage

(continued)

(continued)

Historical Clue	Condition Suggested
Impaired vision	Acute angle-closure glaucoma
	Acute anterior uveitis
	Cavernous sinus thrombosis
	Corneal ulcer
	Keratitis
	Orbital cellulitis
	Orbital tumor
	Scleritis
Contact lens overwear	Corneal ulcer
	Keratitis

Recent exposure to any of the following:
  Chlorinated water
  Cosmetics
  Hairspray
  Industrial dust
  Smog
  Smoke
	Chemical conjunctivitis

Personal or family history of atopy	Allergic conjunctivitis
Abrupt onset of redness	Contact lens use
	Corneal foreign body
	Reaction to topical drops
	Subconjunctival hemorrhage
	Trauma
	Ultraviolet light exposure (sun lamp)
Recent removal of contact lens	Eye injury or irritation secondary to contact lens
Exposure to ultraviolet light (sun lamp or welding arc)	Eye injury or irritation secondary to ultraviolet light
Recently started topical medication	Eye injury or irritation secondary to topical medication
Recurrent episodes of red eye	Acute anterior uveitis
	Allergic conjunctivitis
	Episcleritis
	Scleritis
"Feels as though something is in my eye preventing me from keeping my eye open"	Corneal process
Antecedent or concurrent upper respiratory tract symptoms	Viral conjunctivitis
Vaginal or urethral discharge	Chlamydial conjunctivitis (inclusion type)
	Hyperacute bacterial conjunctivitis (gonococcal)
Rhinorrhea	Allergic conjunctivitis
	Viral conjunctivitis
Nausea / vomiting	Acute angle-closure glaucoma
Photophobia	Acute angle-closure glaucoma
	Acute anterior uveitis
	Keratitis
	Other corneal disease
Matting of the eyelashes on awakening	Conjunctivitis
Discharge	Conjunctivitis

*Patients with conjunctivitis may describe mild discomfort, using the terms "scratchiness" or "burning" to describe the sensation. Significant pain, however, is not typical of conjunctivitis.

Proceed to Step 3

STEP 3: *Are There Any Clues in the Patient's Physical Examination That Point to the Etiology of the Red Eye?*

Clues in the patient's physical examination that point to the etiology of the red eye are listed in the following table.

Physical Examination Finding	Condition Suggested
Impaired visual acuity	Acute angle-closure glaucoma Acute anterior uveitis Corneal ulcer Keratitis Scleritis
Circumcorneal injection	Acute angle-closure glaucoma Acute anterior uveitis Keratitis
Follicular changes of the palpebral conjunctiva (under the lids)	Viral or chlamydial conjunctivitis
Papillary (red bumps) changes of the palpebral conjunctiva (under the lids)	Allergic conjunctivitis
"Cobblestone" papillary changes of the palpebral conjunctiva (under the lids)	Eye irritation from contact lens Seasonal allergic conjunctivitis
Pupil moderately dilated (4-6 mm) and fixed	Acute angle-closure glaucoma
Preauricular lymphadenopathy	Allergic conjunctivitis Bacterial conjunctivitis Viral conjunctivitis
Increased intraocular pressure	Acute angle-closure glaucoma
Pupil small (1-2 mm) and poorly reactive to light	Acute anterior uveitis Corneal abrasion Keratitis
Fever Periorbital edema and erythema Toxic appearance	Orbital cellulitis

Proceed to Step 4

STEP 4: *Does the Patient Need to Be Referred to Ophthalmology?*

The clinician should refer the patient with red eye to an ophthalmologist when any of the features listed in the following box are present.

Alarming Clinical Features that Warrant Urgent Referral to Ophthalmology in the Patient with a Red Eye	
Impaired visual acuity	Proptosis
Perilimbal injection	Severe, deep pain
Photophobia	

If the patient does not have alarming clinical features that warrant urgent ophthalmology referral, *Proceed to Step 5.*

The presence of one or more alarming clinical features suggests that the patient may have a serious cause of red eye, one that may lead to irreversible loss of vision. Referral to ophthalmology is necessary in these cases. A full ophthalmological evaluation may reveal one of the diagnoses listed in the following box.

Causes of Red Eye That are Characterized By Alarming Clinical Features	
Acute angle closure glaucoma*	Episcleritis
Acute anterior uveitis	Keratitis
Corneal injury (abrasion, ulceration)†	Scleritis

*Individuals who have a shallow or narrow anterior chamber angle are predisposed to the development of acute angle closure glaucoma. An acute attack is usually the result of some stimulus associated with pupillary dilation. Examples include dim lighting, use of certain medications (anticholinergic, sympathomimetic), and emotional upset. An acute attack may also be precipitated in predisposed individuals whose pupils are dilated during an ophthalmological examination. Acute angle closure glaucoma typically presents with sudden onset of pain and blurred vision. Pain, however, is not invariably present. In some cases, nausea and vomiting may be the prominent symptoms.

†Trauma to the globe may result in corneal abrasion. Affected patients usually complain of eye pain and foreign body sensation. A corneal foreign body may or may not be present. Patients are often able to tell the clinician exactly when and how the abrasion occurred. In fact, this is so characteristic of corneal abrasion that the diagnosis should be doubted if a patient is vague about the how and when the abrasion occurred. A history typical for corneal abrasion in a patient who uses soft contact lenses should prompt concern for infectious keratitis and corneal ulceration. The symptoms of corneal ulceration are similar to those characteristic of corneal abrasion. Although trauma is a major cause of corneal ulceration, infection is also a concern. The use of cosmetic contact lenses, particularly when worn overnight, is the most common cause of infectious corneal ulceration.

The clinical features that allow these causes of red eye to be differentiated from one another are listed in the following table.

	Acute-Angle Closure Glaucoma	Acute Anterior Uveitis	Scleritis	Episcleritis	Keratitis
Pain	Yes	Yes	Yes	Yes	Yes
Visual Acuity	Decreased	Decreased	Normal	Normal	Decreased
Discharge	No	No	No	No	Usually some
Corneal Appearance	May be hazy	Normal	Normal	Normal	Corneal opacity
Redness	Around cornea	Around cornea	Localized of diffuse	Focal	Around cornea
Pupil	Mid-dilated and fixed	Small and poorly reactive to light	Normal	Normal	Normal
Cells or Flare in Anterior Chamber	None	Present	None	None	Occasional
Intraocular Pressure*	Elevated	Low or normal	Normal	Normal	Normal

*The intraocular pressure should not be measured if discharge or corneal ulceration are noted.

Although these cases are usually treated and managed by ophthalmology, on occasion, the ophthalmologist may need to consult the primary care provider regarding issues related to the following diagnoses.

Anterior Uveitis

Approximately 50% of anterior uveitis cases are idiopathic. The other causes are listed in the following box.

Causes of Anterior Uveitis	
Autoimmune disorders	Infection
Ankylosing spondylitis	Adenovirus
Crohn's disease	Herpes simplex virus
Juvenile rheumatoid arthritis	Herpes zoster
Psoriasis	Syphilis
Reiter's syndrome	Tuberculosis
Sarcoidosis	Malignancy
Ulcerative colitis	Large cell lymphoma
Idiopathic	Leukemia
	Malignant melanoma

Because 50% of cases are idiopathic, an extensive evaluation is not necessary in all patients with acute anterior uveitis. However, further evaluation is indicated in patients with recurrent, bilateral, or granulomatous disease. Patients who have signs and symptoms of a condition associated with anterior uveitis should have testing performed to confirm the diagnosis. When the etiology is not clear, many authorities recommend obtaining the tests listed in the following box.

Tests That May be Helpful in Determining the Etiology of Anterior Uveitis	
ANA	PPD
CBC	RPR/FTA-ABS
Chest radiograph	Other tests based upon the clinical
ESR	presentation (eg, HLA-B27, sacroiliac x-ray)

Scleritis / Episcleritis

The causes of scleritis and episcleritis are listed in the following box.

Causes of Episcleritis / Scleritis	
Connective tissue diseases	Infection
Ankylosing spondylitis	Aspergillus
Polyarteritis nodosa	Herpes simplex
Psoriatic arthropathy	Herpes zoster
Rheumatoid arthritis	Pseudomonas
Systemic lupus erythematosus	Pyogenic cocci
Wegener's granulomatosis	Toxoplasmosis
Granulomatous diseases	Metabolic conditions
Leprosy	Gout
Sarcoidosis	Thyrotoxicosis
Syphilis	
Tuberculosis	

Adapted from O'Connor GR, "Uveal Tract and Sclera," *General Ophthalmology*, 13th ed, Vaughn D, Asbury Y, Riordan-Eva P (eds), Norwalk, CN: Appleton & Lange, 1992, 150-68; also from Hara JH, "The Red Eye: Diagnosis and Treatment," *Am Fam Phys*, 1996, 54(8):2423-30 (review).

Although the preceding table lists the many causes of episcleritis and scleritis, the clinician should realize that the etiology of the great majority of episcleritis cases is unknown. This is in contrast to scleritis in which a systemic disease is frequently present. In these cases, an underlying cause should be identified.

End of Section.

STEP 5: *Does the Patient Have Conjunctivitis?*

Conjunctivitis is the most common cause of the red eye. Historical features supportive of conjunctivitis include the following:

- Red eye that is not painful

  Most patients with conjunctivitis do not describe pain. However, they may report a mild discomfort. "Scratchiness" or "burning" are some of the terms used to describe this sensation.

- Visual acuity is unchanged

  Visual impairment does not occur in conjunctivitis. However, some patients may complain of an intermittent blurring of vision. However, the blurry vision characteristically clears with a blink.

- Subacute onset

  Most patients with conjunctivitis present with symptoms that started over a course of a few days. An exception to this rule is in the patient with hyperacute bacterial conjunctivitis, which is usually due to the gonococcal organism. In these cases, the onset of the ocular symptoms may be abrupt.

- Discharge

  Discharge that accompanies the eye redness is strongly suggestive of conjunctivitis. Matting of the eyelashes on awakening is another characteristic feature.

- Absence of photophobia

  Photophobia is not a feature of uncomplicated conjunctivitis. It can, however, occur when there is concurrent inflammation of the cornea. When both the cornea and conjunctiva are inflamed, the patient is considered to have keratoconjunctivitis.

Physical examination typically reveals conjunctival injection that is more pronounced in the periphery. A discharge is often noted.

If the patient has a history and physical examination compatible with conjunctivitis, ***Proceed to Step 6.***

If the patient does not have a history and physical examination compatible with conjunctivitis, ***Proceed to Step 8.***

STEP 6: *What is the Etiology of the Conjunctivitis?*

The most common types of conjunctivitis include the following:

- Viral
- Bacterial
- Allergic
- Chlamydial

Clues in the history that point to the etiology of the conjunctivitis are listed in the following table.

Historical Clue	Condition Suggested
Recent upper respiratory tract infection	Infectious conjunctivitis (especially viral)
Urethral discharge	Gonococcal or chlamydial conjunctivitis
Unilateral followed by bilateral symptoms and signs	Infectious conjunctivitis
Purulent discharge	Bacterial conjunctivitis
Personal or family history of hay fever, allergic rhinitis, asthma, or atopic dermatitis	Allergic conjunctivitis
Copiously purulent discharge	Gonococcal conjunctivitis
Difficulty in opening eyes in the morning due to matting of eyelids	Suggestive of bacterial conjunctivitis
Itching	Allergic conjunctivitis
History of connective tissue disease Diuretic use Antidepressant medication	Risk factors for conjunctivitis secondary to dry eyes

Findings in the physical examination that point to the etiology of the conjunctivitis are listed in the following table.

Physical Examination Finding	Condition Suggested
Preauricular lymphadenopathy*	Viral conjunctivitis Chlamydial conjunctivitis Hyperacute conjunctivitis (N. gonorrhoeae)
Herpes labialis Shingles	Viral conjunctivitis (herpes simplex virus)
Urethral discharge (spontaneous or by urethral stripping)	Gonococcal or chlamydial conjunctivitis

*Preauricular lymphadenopathy is quite uncommon in bacterial conjunctivitis. It may be appreciated, however, in patients with hyperacute bacterial conjunctivitis or unusual bacterial causes of conjunctivitis such as cat-scratch fever or tularemia.

Proceed to Step 7

STEP 7: *What Laboratory Tests Should be Performed in the Patient With Conjunctivitis?*

Laboratory testing is not necessary in most cases of viral, allergic, or bacterial conjunctivitis. One exception to this rule is in the patient suspected of having hyperacute bacterial conjunctivitis, a type of infectious conjunctivitis that is characterized by a particularly abrupt onset and abundant purulent discharge. Not uncommonly, affected individuals will relate a history of rapid discharge accumulation, having to wipe the eye again almost immediately.

Because hyperacute bacterial conjunctivitis may progress to involve the cornea with resultant perforation, it is incumbent upon the clinician to recognize these cases. Examination may reveal only mild inflammation early in the course of the illness. The illness can quickly progress to manifest with marked swelling of the eye, redness of the eyelids, and severe chemosis.

In most cases, the gonococcal organism is implicated. As such, these patients tend to be sexually active adolescents or young adults. Not uncommonly, affected individuals may complain of symptoms suggestive of urethritis or vaginitis. If the gram stain of the exudate reveals many polymorphonuclear leukocytes along with intracellular gram-negative diplococci, an urgent ophthalmology consultation should be obtained. Culture is also recommended in these cases.

Laboratory tests are also indicated in patients suspected of having chlamydial conjunctivitis. In addition, whenever the diagnosis of gonococcal or chlamydial conjunctivitis is established, the clinician should assess the patient for other sexually transmitted diseases.

End of Section.

STEP 8: *What are Considerations in the Patient With Red Eye Who Does Not Have Signs and Symptoms Consistent With Conjunctivitis?*

When the clinical presentation is not consistent with conjunctivitis, the clinician should consider the following conditions:

- Subconjunctival hemorrhage

  Subconjunctival hemorrhage is a common cause of eye redness. Typically unilateral, subconjunctival hemorrhage is characterized by a localized and sharply circumscribed area of redness. The conjunctiva near this area is not inflamed. Patients do not complain of eye pain or change in vision. While many cases do not have an identifiable precipitant, other cases may be due to trauma, anticoagulant therapy, or bleeding disorders. Eye redness that follows vigorous coughing is particularly suggestive of subconjunctival hemorrhage.

- Stye

- Chalazion

- Blepharitis

REFERENCES

Bertolini J and Pelucio M, "The Red Eye," *Emerg Med Clin North Am*, 1995, 13(3):561-79.

Davey CC, "The Red Eye," *Br J Hosp Med*, 1996, 55(3):89-94.

Hara JH, "The Red Eye: Diagnosis and Treatment," *Am Fam Phys*, 1996, 54(8):2423-30.

Leibowitz HM, "The Red Eye," *N Engl J Med*, 2000, 343(5):345-51.

O'Connor GR, "Uveal Tract and Sclera," *General Ophthalmology*, Vaughn D, Asbury Y, Riordan-Eva P (eds), 13th ed, Norwalk, CN: Appleton & Lange, 1992, 150-68.

Morrow GL and Abbott RL, "Conjunctivitis," *Am Fam Phys*, 1998, 57(4):735-46.

Weber CM and Eichenbaum JW, "Acute Red Eye. Differentiating Viral Conjunctivitis From Other, Less Common Causes," *Postgrad Med*, 1997, 101(5):185-6, 189-92, 195-6.

RED EYE

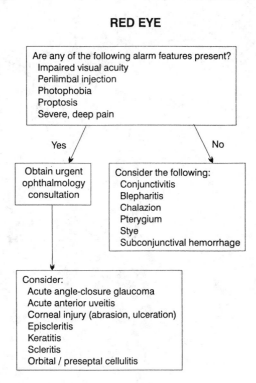

Are any of the following alarm features present?
  Impaired visual acuity
  Perilimbal injection
  Photophobia
  Proptosis
  Severe, deep pain

Yes

No

Obtain urgent
ophthalmology
consultation

Consider the following:
  Conjunctivitis
  Blepharitis
  Chalazion
  Pterygium
  Stye
  Subconjunctival hemorrhage

Consider:
  Acute angle-closure glaucoma
  Acute anterior uveitis
  Corneal injury (abrasion, ulceration)
  Episcleritis
  Keratitis
  Scleritis
  Orbital / preseptal cellulitis

SCROTAL PAIN (ACUTE)

STEP 1: What are the Causes of Acute Scrotal Pain?

Establishing the cause of acute scrotal pain can be difficult. The three most common causes of acute scrotal pain are epididymitis, testicular torsion, and torsion of a testicular appendage. Of the three, testicular torsion is the least common but, because of its seriousness, the patient with acute scrotal pain should be considered to have testicular torsion until proven otherwise. The causes of acute scrotal pain are listed in the following box.

Causes of Acute Scrotal Pain	
Abdominal aortic aneurysm	Orchitis*
Acute bacterial prostatitis	Pancreatitis
Acute peritonitis	Polyarteritis nodosa
Bites (venomous, tick)	Renal colic
Epididymitis*	Testicular cancer
Familial Mediterranean fever	Testicular torsion*
Fournier's gangrene	Testicular trauma*
Henoch-Schönlein purpura	Torsion of testicular appendage*

*Common cause

Proceed to Step 2

STEP 2: Are There Any Clues in the Patient's History That Point to the Etiology of the Acute Scrotal Pain?

Clues in the patient's history that point to the etiology of the acute scrotal pain are listed in the following table.

Historical Clue	Condition Suggested
Abrupt onset	Testicular torsion*
Age >30	Argues against testicular torsion
Bilateral	Acute bacterial prostatitis Acute seminal vesiculitis Epididymitis Fournier's gangrene Orchitis Polyarteritis nodosa
Dysuria	Epididymitis
Fever	Epididymitis Orchitis
Hematuria	Henoch-Schönlein purpura Polyarteritis nodosa Renal colic
History of previous episodes that resolved spontaneously	Testicular torsion
Nausea/vomiting	Orchitis Testicular torsion†
Skin rash	Henoch-Schönlein purpura Polyarteritis nodosa

(continued)

(continued)

Historical Clue	Condition Suggested
Systemic symptoms of fever, anorexia, weakness, weight loss, and malaise	Henoch-Schönlein purpura Polyarteritis nodosa
Urethral discharge	Epididymitis
Occurring with physical exertion	Testicular torsion‡
Begins at night, often waking the patient	Testicular torsion

* The onset is gradual, however, in up to 25% of patients with testicular torsion.

† Nausea and vomiting are not invariably present in patients with testicular torsion. Studies have shown that nausea and vomiting may be present in 30% to 80% of cases. These complaints are unusual in epididymitis and torsion of a testicular appendage.

‡ In 10% to 20% of cases, testicular torsion is associated with physical exertion.

Proceed to Step 3

> **STEP 3: *Are There Any Clues in the Physical Examination That Point to the Etiology of the Acute Scrotal Pain?***

The physical examination may be very enlightening in the patient presenting with acute scrotal pain, especially if performed early in the disease course. Clues in the patient's physical examination that point to the etiology of the acute scrotal pain are listed in the following table.

Physical Examination Finding	Condition Suggested
Blue dot sign	Torsion of testicular appendage
Erythema gives way to skin blackening and induration	Fournier's gangrene
Erythema of perineum, perianal area, penis, scrotum, lower abdomen, and buttocks	Fournier's gangrene
Patient appears comfortable	Epididymitis Torsion of testicular appendage
Patient appears uncomfortable	Testicular torsion
Petechial or purpuric rash	Henoch-Schönlein purpura Polyarteritis nodosa
Presence of cremasteric reflex*	Argues against testicular torsion
Swelling and tenderness of the preauricular area	Orchitis (mumps)
Urethral discharge	Epididymitis

*The reflex can be assessed by lightly stroking the inner thigh. When the ipsilateral testicle elevates 0.5 or more cm, the patient is said to have the cremasteric reflex. In almost all cases, the reflex is absent in patients with testicular torsion. However, in other causes of acute scrotal pain, the reflex may be absent as well. As such, only the presence of the reflex is useful in the patient presenting with acute scrotal pain, in that it argues against the diagnosis of testicular torsion.

The clinician should also try to elicit findings in the physical exam considered by some authorities to be pathognomonic of testicular torsion. These findings are listed in the following box.

Physical Examination Findings Considered to be Pathognomonic for Testicular Torsion
• Abnormal elevation of the affected testicle with a palpable twist in the spermatic cord*
• Abnormal axis of the affected testicle in the upright position†
• Abnormal position of the epididymis within the scrotum‡

* The testis is often high due to the shortening of the spermatic cord.

† Transverse orientation of the testis is often appreciated in testicular torsion.

‡The epididymis may assume a medial, lateral, or anterior position. The position of the epididymis is dependent on the degree of torsion.

If the history and physical examination provide clues to the etiology of the acute scrotal pain, the clinician should direct the evaluation accordingly.

If the etiology of the acute scrotal pain is not clear after a thorough history and physical examination, *Proceed to Step 4.*

STEP 4: *Is There a History of Scrotal Trauma?*

When a history of scrotal trauma is elicited, the clinician should consider the conditions in the following box.

Considerations in Patients Having a History of Scrotal Trauma	
Epididymal hematoma	Scrotal hematoma
Hematocele	Testicular hematoma
Hydrocele	Testicular rupture
Post-traumatic epididymitis	Testicular torsion
Pyocele	Torsion of testicular appendage
Retroperitoneal or intraperitoneal hemorrhage with a patent processus vaginalis	

Minor episodes of scrotal trauma are not uncommon in men. On occasion, however, a serious injury may result, often due to a direct blow to the groin. Because there are no features in the patient's clinical presentation that allow the clinician to reliably differentiate between the above possibilities, a color Doppler ultrasonography study should be obtained if the patient's pain is not significantly improved within one hour of the injury.

If the patient has one of the above conditions, *Stop Here.*

If the patient does not have one of the above conditions, *Proceed to Step 5*.

STEP 5: *Does Laboratory Testing Have Any Role in the Patient Presenting With Acute Scrotal Pain?*

In general, laboratory studies are not very helpful in the evaluation of the patient with acute scrotal pain. Nonetheless, a urinalysis and culture should be performed in almost all patients with acute scrotal pain. The finding of pyuria is suggestive of epididymitis. However, the presence of pyuria does not conclusively establish the presence of an infectious cause of the scrotal pain nor does it exclude testicular torsion.

The urinalysis may also be revealing in patients suspected of having Henoch-Schönlein purpura or polyarteritis nodosa. In these patients, an active urinary sediment may be noted.

A urethral swab should be obtained in patients who have a urethral discharge. The following studies should be performed:

- Gram's stain
- Testing for *Neisseria gonorrhoeae*
- Testing for *Chlamydia trachomatis*

A WBC count is not necessary in all patients. Leukocytosis is suggestive of epididymitis.

Proceed to Step 6

STEP 6: *Does the Patient Have Testicular Torsion?*

It is of the utmost importance that the clinician distinguish testicular torsion from all other causes of acute scrotal pain. Time is of the essence since salvage of testicular function is unlikely beyond 12 hours.

Testicular torsion is rare in those >35 years of age and most cases are described in individuals <20 years of age. An association with physical exertion or trauma has been described. The onset of testicular torsion is typically abrupt. A gradual onset should not exclude the diagnosis, however, since such an onset has been described in about 30% of patients. Not uncommonly, the pain of testicular torsion radiates to the inguinal or lower abdominal regions. In some cases, the pain may begin in the lower abdomen or groin. In many cases, nausea and vomiting accompany the unilateral testicular pain. Of note, some patients may describe a history of similar symptoms in the past. Interestingly, most patients relate that these prior episodes resolved spontaneously.

Early in the course of the disease, testicular swelling, which is sometimes marked, may be noted. The classic physical examination findings, which some authorities consider to be pathognomonic of testicular torsion, are listed in the following box.

Physical Examination Findings Considered to be Pathognomonic for Testicular Torsion
• Abnormal elevation of the affected testicle with a palpable twist in the spermatic cord*
• Abnormal axis of the affected testicle in the upright position†
• Abnormal position of the epididymis within the scrotum‡

* The testis is often high due to the shortening of the spermatic cord.

† Transverse orientation of the testis is often appreciated in testicular torsion.

‡ The epididymis may assume a medial, lateral, or anterior position. The position of the epididymis is dependent on the degree of torsion.

Examination later in the course of the illness may reveal the presence of a reactive hydrocele and overlying erythema of the scrotal wall. The cremasteric reflex is usually absent in testicular torsion. Its presence argues for another cause of acute scrotal pain.

Nearly 50% of patients have the classic presentation described above. However, the clinician should realize that many patients do not present classically. The presence of fever, dysuria, or urethral discharge argues against the diagnosis but does not exclude testicular torsion.

In patients who present classically, the clinician can send the patient directly for surgery without further evaluation. In those who are older (>30 years) or in younger patients with atypical presentations, it is preferable to perform color Doppler ultrasonography to confirm the diagnosis.

If the patient has a classic presentation for testicular torsion, proceed to surgery.

If the patient is >30 years of age or the presentation is not classic for testicular torsion, **Proceed to Step 7**.

STEP 7: *What are the Results of the Ultrasound?*

When testicular torsion is a consideration but the presentation is atypical, the clinician may elect to perform color Doppler ultrasonography. It should not be performed in the following patients:

- Clinical findings strongly suggestive of testicular torsion
- History of recurrent similar episodes of scrotal pain separated by pain-free intervals (>2 weeks)
- Definite clinical criteria for epididymitis (see Step 9)
- Study cannot be obtained quickly

In the former two, the clinician should plan for operative intervention because of the concern for testicular torsion. Patients who present with signs and symptoms meeting the clinical criteria for epididymitis do not require a study. When the study cannot be performed expeditiously in patients suspected of having testicular torsion, surgical exploration may be warranted.

The radiologic choices available to the clinician include 99m technetium pertechnetate radioisotope scanning and color Doppler ultrasonography. In both studies, the demonstration of decreased or absent perfusion to the affected testis when compared to the unaffected testis establishes the diagnosis of testicular torsion. The sensitivity and specificity of both tests are high but ultrasound has several advantages over radioisotope scanning. These advantages are considered in the following box.

Advantages of Color Doppler Ultrasonography Over Radioisotope Scanning
Can be performed in <30 minutes
No intravenous injection of radionuclide required
No radiation
Provides detailed anatomic information
Usually available at all hours of the day

In contrast, epididymitis is characterized by normal or increased flow. Normal to increased flow may also be seen in patients with torsion of a testicular appendage.

If the ultrasound is positive for testicular torsion, the patient should undergo operative intervention. *Stop Here.*

If the ultrasound is equivocal for testicular torsion, the clinician should consider surgical exploration.

If the ultrasound is negative for testicular torsion, *Proceed to Step 8.*

STEP 8: *Does the Patient Have Any Other Emergent Cause of Acute Scrotal Pain?*

The emergent causes of acute scrotal pain are considered in the following box.

Emergent Causes of Acute Scrotal Pain	
Abdominal aortic aneurysm	Testicular torsion
Fournier's gangrene	Peritonitis with patent processus
Testicular rupture	vaginalis

Of these possibilities, testicular torsion and rupture have already been considered and will not be discussed here. The remainder of this step will describe the other conditions in some detail.

Fournier's Gangrene

While Fournier's gangrene is rare, it is a potentially life-threatening cause of acute scrotal pain. It is characterized by a polymicrobial infection of the scrotum and its surrounding areas. While it has been reported in all age groups, it tends to have a predilection for older patients, particularly in those with underlying medical illnesses such as diabetes mellitus. Examination of the affected area usually reveals edema, erythema, skin necrosis, crepitus, and bullae formation.

Abdominal Aortic Aneurysm

Although most patients with an abdominal aortic aneurysm present with abdominal or back pain, there have been reports of isolated acute scrotal pain as the initial presentation. It should be more of a consideration in the older male with hypertension or atherosclerosis. Acute scrotal pain caused by an abdominal aortic aneurysm usually reflects a change in the aneurysm, either sudden expansion or small leak. The physical examination may reveal a pulsatile mass but the absence of this finding in no way excludes the diagnosis. If this is a consideration, the clinician can elect to perform an ultrasound of the abdomen along with the color Doppler ultrasound study of the testicles.

Peritonitis With Patent Processus Vaginalis

Acute scrotal pain secondary to acute peritonitis is rare. It can occur, however, when the processus vaginalis, which usually obliterates by the second year of life, remains patent. In fact, this patency has been described in up to 40% of men. This patency allows the free passage of purulent intra-abdominal fluid into the scrotum in patients with acute peritonitis.

If an emergent cause of acute scrotal pain is present, *Stop Here.*

If an emergent cause of acute scrotal pain is not present, *Proceed to Step 9.*

STEP 9: *Does the Patient Have Epididymitis or Orchitis?*

Epididymitis and orchitis are two common causes of acute scrotal pain that need to be differentiated from testicular torsion. Step 7 described the color Doppler ultrasonography findings that allow the clinician to make this distinction. In this step, the clinical features of epididymitis and orchitis will be described in further detail.

Epididymitis

Epididymitis is the most common cause of acute scrotal pain. It is the diagnosis in approximately 75% of postpubertal patients presenting with acute scrotal pain. Although epididymitis may be traumatic or reactive in etiology, most cases are infectious. The likely pathogens vary depending on the age and setting. In prepubertal boys, structural or functional abnormalities of the genitourinary tract are often present. These abnormalities predispose to infection with coliform bacteria.

Sexually transmitted pathogens, which include *Chlamydia trachomatis* and *Neisseria gonorrhoeae*, are the main considerations in sexually active men <35 years of age. Many of these patients have a concomitant urethritis but a urethral discharge is a complaint in only 50%. In this group of patients, coliform bacteria are rarely the cause of the epididymitis. One exception to this rule is in homosexual males who may develop infection due to coliform organisms.

In those >35 years of age, prostatic enlargement may predispose to the development of epididymitis. In this group of patients, coliform bacteria once again become the major consideration followed by sexually transmitted pathogens.

The clinician should realize that there are no pathognomonic features of acute epididymitis. It is usually characterized by a gradual onset of scrotal pain. Fever and dysuria are common. Early in the illness, the tenderness and swelling may be localized to the epididymis. With progression of the disease, the inflammation spreads. Although a urethral discharge is apparent in many patients, in others, the clinician may have to milk the urethra to note the discharge. Up to 50% of patients have leukocytosis. Pyuria is present in many patients as well.

Clinical criteria have been developed to aid the clinician in the diagnosis of epididymitis. These clinical criteria are listed in the following box.

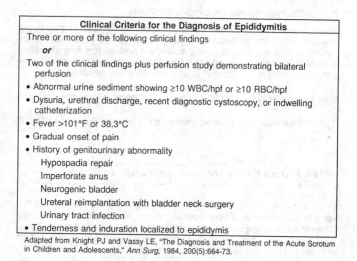

Clinical Criteria for the Diagnosis of Epididymitis
Three or more of the following clinical findings   *or*
Two of the clinical findings plus perfusion study demonstrating bilateral perfusion
• Abnormal urine sediment showing ≥10 WBC/hpf or ≥10 RBC/hpf
• Dysuria, urethral discharge, recent diagnostic cystoscopy, or indwelling catheterization
• Fever >101°F or 38.3°C
• Gradual onset of pain

• History of genitourinary abnormality
    Hypospadia repair
    Imperforate anus
    Neurogenic bladder
    Ureteral reimplantation with bladder neck surgery
    Urinary tract infection

• Tenderness and induration localized to epididymis

Adapted from Knight PJ and Vassy LE, "The Diagnosis and Treatment of the Acute Scrotum in Children and Adolescents," *Ann Surg*, 1984, 200(5):664-73.

The diagnosis of epididymitis is established when three or more of the above findings are present. Studies have shown that no diagnoses of testicular torsion were missed in patients having three or more of the above criteria. When two or fewer of the above findings were present, there was some overlap between testicular torsion and epididymitis.

Both color Doppler ultrasonography and nuclear scintigraphy can demonstrate the normal to increased blood flow that is typical of epididymitis. Ultrasound can also demonstrate the presence of an abscess, which is one complication of epididymitis.

Orchitis

Most cases of epididymitis are also characterized by inflammation of the testes, hence the term epididymo-orchitis. Isolated orchitis was more commonly encountered in the past but, with widespread mumps immunization, it is now rare. When isolated orchitis does occur, it is usually caused by a viral infection. The testicle is typically tender and enlarged. When due to the mumps virus, parotitis may also be present. In some patients, the orchitis follows the manifestations of parotitis.

If the patient has epididymitis or orchitis, ***Stop Here.***

If the patient does not have epididymitis or orchitis, ***Proceed to Step 10.***

STEP 10: *Does the Patient Have Torsion of a Testicular Appendage?*

Torsion of a testicular appendage is a common cause of acute scrotal pain. The pain is usually not as severe as that felt in testicular torsion. Unlike testicular torsion which often prompts the patient to present within hours after pain onset, the pain associated with torsion of a testicular appendage is often present for a few days prior to the patient's presentation. Nausea and vomiting are rare. Fever, dysuria, and urethral discharge are typically absent. The patient does not usually recall a history of similar episodes in the past.

Early in the course of the disease, the physical examination may be very revealing. Pathognomonic findings include the following:

- Palpable, tender nodule in the superior portion of the testicle
- Blue discoloration in the superior portion of the testicle (blue dot sign)

In some cases, transillumination may allow the clinician to view the torsed appendage through the scrotal wall. With progression of the disease, edema, and erythema may be appreciated. Color Doppler ultrasonography can demonstrate normal to increased testicular flow, a finding that torsion of a testicular appendage shares in common with epididymitis. The finding of a hypo- or hyperechoic area near the testis suggests a torsed appendage. Nonoperative management is recommended in patients with torsion of a testicular appendage.

If the patient has torsion of a testicular appendage, **Stop Here.**

If the patient does not have torsion of a testicular appendage, **Proceed to Step 11.**

> ### STEP 11: *What are Some of the More Uncommon Causes of Acute Scrotal Pain?*

After excluding the major causes of acute scrotal pain, the clinician can consider some of the more uncommon causes, which are detailed below.

Inguinal Hernia

Acute scrotal pain and swelling may be a manifestation of an inguinal hernia. In this condition, a loop of bowel or mesentery may push through a patent processus vaginalis. Fullness in the inguinal area is a clue to the diagnosis. Palpation of the testis is normal. If the hernia is incarcerated or strangulated, urgent operative intervention is necessary.

Henoch-Schönlein Purpura

Henoch-Schönlein purpura, a vasculitis having a predilection for children, usually presents with systemic symptoms, colicky abdominal pain, arthralgias/arthritis, and an active urinary sediment. A rash is often present. The acute scrotal pain that occurs is uncommon, reported in up to 10% of cases. Seldom does it occur in the absence of the other manifestations of this disease.

Testicular Neoplasm

Acute scrotal pain is not a common presentation of a testicular neoplasm but it certainly warrants consideration. Testicular cancer may present with acute scrotal pain when hemorrhage occurs within the tumor mass.

The other causes of acute scrotal pain listed in the box in Step 1 will not be discussed here. The reader is encouraged to consult appropriate resources for more information regarding these uncommon causes of acute scrotal pain should the etiology of the scrotal pain remain unclear.

REFERENCES

Barloon TJ, Weissman AM, and Kahn D, "Diagnostic Imaging of Patients with Acute Scrotal Pain," *Am Fam Phys*, 1996, 53(5):1734-50.

Burgher SW, "Acute Scrotal Pain," *Emerg Med Clin North Am*, 1998, 16(4):781-809.

Cuckow PM and Frank JD, "Torsion of the Testis," *BJU Int*, 2000, 86(3):349-53.

Galejs LE, "Diagnosis and Treatment of the Acute Scrotum," *Am Fam Phys*, 1999, 59(4):817-24.

Hawtrey CE, "Assessment of Acute Scrotal Symptoms and Findings. A Clinician's Dilemma," *Urol Clin North Am*, 1998, 25(4):715-23.

Horstman WG, "Scrotal Imaging," *Urol Clin North Am*, 1997, 24(3):653-71.

Knight PJ and Vassy LE, "The Diagnosis and Treatment of the Acute Scrotum in Children and Adolescents," *Ann Surg*, 1984, 200(5):664-73.

Lindsey D and Stanisic TH, "Diagnosis and Management of Testicular Torsion: Pitfalls and Perils," *Am J Emerg Med*, 1988, 6(1):42-6.

Sidhu PS, "Clinical and Imaging Features of Testicular Torsion: Role of Ultrasound," *Clin Radiol*, 1999, 54(6):343-52.

Siegel MJ, "The Acute Scrotum," *Radiol Clin North Am*, 1997, 35(4):959-76.

SCROTAL PAIN (ACUTE)

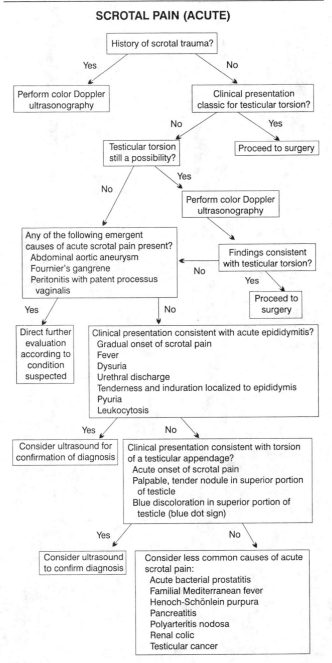

SHORTNESS OF BREATH (ACUTE)

STEP 1: *What is Dyspnea?*

Dyspnea or shortness of breath can be defined as the subjective sensation of breathing difficulty. It should be differentiated from the terms described in the box below.

Definitions	
Orthopnea:	Dyspnea in the recumbent position
Paroxysmal nocturnal dyspnea:	Dyspnea in the recumbent position that awakens the patient from sleep
Tachypnea:	Rapid breathing
Platypnea:	Dyspnea in the upright position
Trepopnea:	Dyspnea in one lateral position but not the other

Dyspnea may be acute or chronic. Acute dyspnea refers to the immediate or sudden onset of shortness of breath. Chronic dyspnea is defined as breathing difficulty that persists for at least one month. In this chapter, the approach to the patient presenting with acute dyspnea is considered.

Proceed to Step 2

STEP 2: *What are the Causes of Acute Dyspnea?*

The causes of acute dyspnea are listed in the following box.

Causes of Acute Dyspnea	
Acute myocardial infarction/ischemia	Metabolic acidosis
Asthma exacerbation	Noncardiogenic pulmonary edema
Cardiac tamponade	Pneumonia
Congestive heart failure/cardiogenic pulmonary edema	Pneumothorax
COPD exacerbation	Pulmonary embolism
Hyperventilation syndrome	Trauma
	Upper airway obstruction

Proceed to Step 3

STEP 3: *Does the Patient Have Acute Respiratory Failure?*

Acute shortness of breath may be the manifestation of a potentially life-threatening illness. As such, it should be evaluated as an urgent or emergent medical problem. Of utmost importance is an initial assessment of the patient focusing on the identification of imminent respiratory failure. In particular, the evaluation should focus on the following:

- Maintaining a patent airway
- Assisting ventilation (if indicated)

In cases where it is indicated, intubation should not be delayed in favor of obtaining a thorough history and physical examination. Once the ABCs (airway, breathing, circulation) have been addressed, the clinician can focus on the history, physical examination, and diagnostic studies. Diagnostic studies that are often obtained in the evaluation of the patient presenting with acute dyspnea are listed in the following box.

Diagnostic Studies That May be Indicated in the Patient With Acute Dyspnea	
Arterial blood gas	Neck radiograph and CT*
CBC	Peak expiratory flow rate (PEFR)
Chest radiograph	Pulse oximetry†
EKG	SMA 7
Nasopharyngolaryngoscopy*	

*These are considerations in patients suspected of having upper airway obstruction.

†The adequacy of oxygenation may be assessed by pulse oximetry. Unlike the arterial blood gas, it does not provide any information regarding ventilatory or acid-base status.

These diagnostic studies will be discussed in the steps that follow.

Proceed to Step 4

STEP 4: *Are There Any Clues in the Patient's History That Point to the Etiology of the Acute Dyspnea?*

Clues in the history that may point to the etiology of the acute shortness of breath are listed in the following table.

Historical Clue	Condition Suggested
History of asthma	Asthma exacerbation Complications of asthma: Pneumonia Pneumothorax
History of COPD	Acute COPD exacerbation Complications of COPD: Pneumonia Pneumothorax
History of chest wall trauma	Consider traumatic causes of acute dyspnea: Cardiac tamponade Diaphragmatic rupture Flail chest Hemothorax Pneumothorax Pulmonary contusion Spinal cord lesion
Risk factors for pulmonary embolism	Pulmonary embolism

(continued)

Historical Clue	Condition Suggested
Risk factors for pneumothorax	Pneumothorax
Leg pain or swelling	Pulmonary embolism
Dizziness Faintness Frequent sighing or yawning Numbness/tingling of toes, fingers, or perioral area	Hyperventilation syndrome
Recent procedure preceding acute dyspnea (ie, central line insertion, thoracentesis, needle biopsy of the lung, intercostal nerve block)	Iatrogenic pneumothorax
Chest pain	Acute myocardial infarction/ischemia Asthma Hyperventilation syndrome Pneumonia Pneumothorax Pulmonary embolism
Orthopnea Paroxysmal nocturnal dyspnea	Congestive heart failure
Risk factors for noncardiogenic pulmonary edema	Noncardiogenic pulmonary edema
History of congestive heart failure	Congestive heart failure (acute decompensation) Pneumonia Pulmonary embolism
Hemoptysis	Congestive heart failure/cardiogenic pulmonary edema Pneumonia Pulmonary embolism Pulmonary hemorrhage

The causes of acute dyspnea are discussed further in the remainder of this step.

Pneumonia

Pneumonia is the sixth leading cause of death in the United States. The symptoms that should prompt the clinician to consider pneumonia include shortness of breath, cough, sputum production, chest pain (often pleuritic), and fever. It is important to realize, however, that many patients with pneumonia also have nonrespiratory symptoms such as fatigue, headache, myalgias, nausea, and diaphoresis. Atypical presentations are not uncommon, especially in the elderly. In this age group, mental status change may be the most prominent manifestation of pneumonia.

The etiologic agents that commonly cause pneumonia in patients admitted to hospitals are listed in the following table.

Organism	Percentage of Cases (%)
Streptococcus pneumoniae	10-40
Viruses	5-20
H. influenzae	5-15
Mixed oral flora	3-15
Mycoplasma pneumoniae	2-18
Legionella species	2-14
Pneumocystis carinii	2-13
Chlamydia pneumoniae	2-10
Gram-negative bacilli	1-9
Staphylococcus aureus	1-8
Unknown	30-50

Adapted from *Medical Management of Pulmonary Diseases*, Davis GS (ed), New York, NY: Marcel Dekker, 1999, 295.

Clues present in the history that point to the etiologic organism are listed in the following table.

Historical Clue	Etiologic Organism Suggested
Cystic fibrosis	*Pseudomonas aeruginosa* *S. aureus*
Hospitalized patients	Enterobacteriaceae *Pseudomonas* *S. aureus*
Nursing home patient	*S. aureus* Tuberculosis Viral (RSV, adenovirus, influenza)
Alcohol use Loss of consciousness Recent dental work Sedative overdose Seizure	Risk factors for anaerobic infection due to oral aspiration

Hypogammaglobulinemia	Consider encapsulated organisms:
	   H. influenzae
	   S. pneumoniae

Severe neutropenia (<500 neutrophils/ μL)	*Aspergillus* Enterobacteriaceae *Pseudomonas aeruginosa* *S. aureus*
COPD or smoker	*H. influenzae* *M. catarrhalis* *S. pneumoniae*
Recent viral upper respiratory tract infection	Higher risk for secondary bacterial pneumonia (*S. pneumoniae, H. influenzae, S. aureus*)
Alcoholism	Anaerobes *Klebsiella pneumoniae* *S. aureus* *S. pneumoniae*

(continued)

Historical Clue	Etiologic Organism Suggested
Travel to or residence in Southwest United States	C. immitis Hantavirus Y. pestis
Travel to or residence in Southeast Asia	Melioidosis
Travel to or residence in Mississippi and Ohio River valley	Histoplasmosis
HIV	Consider the following: Bacterial organisms *Cryptococcus neoformans* *H. capsulatum* *M. tuberculosis* *Pneumocystis carinii*

Pneumothorax

Pneumothorax is defined as the presence of free air between the visceral and parietal pleura. The causes of pneumothorax can be categorized into spontaneous and iatrogenic types, as shown in the following box.

Causes of Pneumothorax	
Spontaneous	
Primary	
Secondary	
Asthma	Interstitial lung disease
Chronic obstructive pulmonary	Lymphangioleiomyomatosis
disease	Marfan syndrome
Cystic fibrosis	Pleural malignancy
Histiocytosis X	Sarcoidosis
Infection	Trauma
Bacterial	Tuberous sclerosis
Pneumocystis carinii pneumonia	
Tuberculosis	
Iatrogenic	
Chest compression	Positive pressure ventilation
Intercostal nerve block	Subclavian cannulation
Needle aspiration (lung biopsy)	Transbronchial biopsy

The typical patient who develops a primary spontaneous pneumothorax is a young male smoker between 20-40 years of age. Although not all patients are symptomatic, most describe the sudden onset of unilateral chest pain and shortness of breath. The symptoms of secondary spontaneous pneumothorax are essentially the same. In contrast to primary spontaneous pneumothorax, these patients can precipitously decline because the pneumothorax occurs in the setting of an existing pulmonary disease. This underlying pulmonary disease limits these patients' pulmonary reserve.

When mediastinal shift and compression of the contralateral lung occurs because of the progressive accumulation of air under pressure, a tension pneumothorax is said to be present. The symptoms of tension pneumothorax are similar to that encountered in uncomplicated spontaneous pneumothorax but may be exaggerated.

Pulmonary Embolism

Over 600,000 cases of pulmonary embolism occur every year in the United States. Because the symptoms and signs of pulmonary embolism are nonspecific, in many of these cases, the diagnosis is missed, only to be made at the time of autopsy.

Most often, pulmonary embolism develops when thrombi travel from the deep venous system to the pulmonary arterial tree, causing obstruction of blood flow. Approximately 70% of patients have a clot that can be demonstrated in the lower extremities by venography. Although most cases are due to thrombi originating in the deep venous system of the lower extremities, approximately 10% are thought to arise elsewhere. The majority of these originate in the upper extremity veins, especially in patients with indwelling central venous catheters.

In many cases, risk factors for venous thromboembolism are present. These risk factors are considered in the following box.

Risk Factors for Deep Venous Thrombosis and Pulmonary Embolism	
Acute myocardial infarction	Lupus anticoagulant
Antithrombin III deficiency	Malignancy
Behcet's disease	Obesity
Congestive heart failure	Oral contraceptive use
Dysfibrinogenemia	Polycythemia vera
Essential thrombocytosis	Postoperative
Estrogen replacement (high dose)	Postpartum
Hemolytic anemia	Pregnancy
Heparin-induced thrombocytopenia	Protein C deficiency
History of deep venous thrombosis	Protein S deficiency
History of pulmonary embolism	Resistance to activated protein C
Homocysteinuria	Trauma
Immobilization	Venography
Indwelling central venous catheters	Venous pacemakers

The classic triad of dyspnea, chest pain, and hemoptysis is seen in <20% of patients. No features of the chest pain are diagnostic for pulmonary embolism. While some patients present with pleuritic chest pain, others may manifest with a retrosternal heaviness that mimics what is considered classic for acute myocardial infarction. Symptoms encountered in patients proven to have pulmonary embolism by angiography are listed in the following table.

Symptom	Percent (%)
Dyspnea	93
Chest pain, pleuritic	74
Apprehension	59
Cough	53
Hemoptysis	30
Sweating	27
Chest pain, nonpleuritic	14
Syncope	13

Adapted from "The Urokinase Pulmonary Embolism Trial: A National Cooperative Study,"*Circulation*,1973, 47(2 Suppl):II1-108; also from "Urokinase-Streptokinase Embolism Trial: Phase II Results. A Cooperative Study," *JAMA*, 1974, 229(12):1606-13.

Because the signs and symptoms of pulmonary embolism are nonspecific, further evaluation is certainly indicated, especially in the setting of risk factors for venous thromboembolism. The clinician should realize, however, that not all patients have an apparent predisposition at the time of diagnosis.

COPD Exacerbation

Chronic obstructive pulmonary disease is the fourth leading cause of death in the United States. The American Thoracic Society defines COPD as the presence of chronic bronchitis and/or emphysema combined with airflow obstruction. Chronic bronchitis and emphysema are defined in the following box.

Definitions	
Chronic bronchitis:	Presence of productive cough for at least three months in each of two successive years
Emphysema:	Permanent airspace enlargement due to the destruction of alveolar walls

Symptoms of COPD should be separated from that of COPD exacerbation. Most patients with COPD usually present after the age of 50 with progressively worsening shortness of breath. Almost invariably, patients report a long history of smoking. Although a smoking history does not have to be present to establish the diagnosis, its absence should at least prompt the clinician to consider alternative causes of shortness of breath. In the nonsmoker, COPD may still occur secondary to passive smoke inhalation, α_1-antitrypsin deficiency, or occupational exposures.

Although most patients describe chronic shortness of breath, typically worsened by exertion, others present with a more abrupt illness. In these latter patients, the acute illness may be the initial manifestation of their COPD. Those who do report chronic symptoms consistent with COPD may also describe an acute worsening characterized by increased shortness of breath and cough productive of purulent sputum.

This periodic worsening of the COPD patient's pulmonary status is termed an acute exacerbation. Patients with acute exacerbation of COPD may also complain that the consistency of their sputum has become more tenacious, often making it difficult for them to expectorate their secretions. Many patients also notice increased wheezing. Not uncommonly, patients report increasing bronchodilator use. COPD exacerbation should clearly be a concern in patients who present with symptoms listed in the following box.

Symptoms Consistent With COPD Exacerbation	
Increasing cough	Increase in viscosity of secretions
Increase in purulence of secretions	Worsening dyspnea
Increasing sputum production	

Asthma Exacerbation

Asthma is a chronic condition characterized by episodic exacerbations. As such, most patients with asthma who have acute dyspnea secondary to an asthma exacerbation will relate a history of similar episodes. In a minority of patients, however, acute dyspnea may be the initial manifestation of asthma.

In between the episodic exacerbations, patients with asthma are usually free of symptoms.

Symptoms that should prompt the clinician to consider asthma exacerbation include the following:

- Dyspnea
- Chest tightness
- Wheezing
- Cough

The clinician should realize that wheezing is not specific for asthma and may be appreciated in many conditions. Some of these conditions include congestive heart failure, COPD, aspiration, pulmonary embolism, and upper airway obstruction.

Congestive Heart Failure / Cardiogenic Pulmonary Edema

Over 4 million people in the United States suffer from congestive heart failure. Many of these individuals have chronic symptoms consistent with congestive heart failure. These symptoms are described in the following table.

Type of Evidence	Highly Suggestive	Less Specific
Symptom	Orthopnea PND	Decreased exercise tolerance Discomfort when bending Nocturnal cough Fatigue Leg swelling

Adapted from Kannel WB and Belanger AJ, "Epidemiology of Heart Failure," *Am Heart J,* 1991, 121(3 Pt 1):951-7; also from *Primary Cardiology*, Goldman L and Braunwald E (eds), Philadelphia, PA: WB Saunders Co, 1998, 311.

It is not uncommon for patients with congestive heart failure to have clinical decompensation. Acute dyspnea is the hallmark of these congestive heart failure exacerbations. In some cases, transmission of the increased left-sided heart pressures to the pulmonary circulation may result in the flow of fluid into the alveoli. When this occurs, cardiogenic pulmonary edema is said to be present. In addition to acute dyspnea, patients with cardiogenic pulmonary edema may report a cough productive of pink, frothy sputum.

Although most patients with congestive heart failure exacerbation have a known history of congestive heart failure, in other cases, patients may present with an illness compatible with congestive heart failure in the absence of known history of cardiac disease.

Noncardiogenic Pulmonary Edema

The major type of noncardiogenic pulmonary edema is the acute respiratory distress syndrome (ARDS). Approximately 100,000 cases of ARDS are described in the United States each year. In ARDS, hypoxemic respiratory failure is the end result of a process that increases alveolar capillary permeability. Conditions associated with ARDS are listed in the following box.

Conditions Associated With ARDS	
Aspiration	Poisonous snakebite
Cardiopulmonary bypass (pump lung)	Pneumonia
Disseminated intravascular congestion	Prolonged hypotension
Drug ingestion	Sepsis
Fat embolism	Toxic inhalation
Multiple blood transfusions	Corrosive
administered emergently	Gases
Near-drowning	Smoke
Pancreatitis	Trauma

Eighty percent of cases are due to systemic or pulmonary infection, severe trauma, or aspiration of gastric contents. After the patient suffers an insult known to be associated with ARDS, hours to days may pass before the patient becomes symptomatic. In most cases, the inciting event is quite apparent. Acute dyspnea is invariably present in patients with ARDS. Although the dyspnea may initially be exertional, there is rapid progression to severe dyspnea at rest.

Acute Myocardial Infarction / Ischemia

Most patients with acute myocardial infarction or ischemia complain of chest pain. It is not uncommon, however, for shortness of breath to accompany the chest pain. The clinician should realize, however, that some patients with acute myocardial infarction or ischemia may present with acute shortness of breath alone. In these cases, the shortness of breath may represent an anginal or ischemic equivalent. For further information regarding the clinical presentation of acute myocardial infarction or ischemia, proceed to the chapter on Chest Pain (Acute) *on page 53*.

Upper Airway Obstruction

Mechanical obstruction of the upper airway may present with acute dyspnea. If the obstruction is not relieved, asphyxiation may occur. Causes of acute upper airway obstruction are listed in the following box.

Causes of Acute Upper Airway Obstruction		
Angioedema	Ingestion or inhalation	Neoplasm
Diphtheria	of caustic agents	Oropharyngeal abscess
Epiglottitis	Acids	Peritonsillar
Foreign body aspiration*	Alkalis	Retropharyngeal
Granulomatous disease	Heat (intense)	Trauma
Hemorrhage†	Smoke	Blunt
Infectious mononucleosis	Steam	Penetrating
		Vocal cord paralysis

*In adults, foreign body aspiration usually occurs in the setting of alcohol use, dentures, or poor chewing habits. It typically occurs during a meal when a food bolus becomes trapped in the hypopharynx or upper larynx, resulting in either partial or complete obstruction. The panic-stricken patient may be unable to breathe or talk and may be noted to place one or both hands over the front of the neck.

†In the absence of trauma, hemorrhage should be a consideration primarily in patients who are receiving anticoagulation therapy. On occasion, blood dyscrasias such as hemophilia may present with acute upper airway obstruction secondary to spontaneous hemorrhage.

The clinical presentation of upper airway obstruction varies depending upon the underlying etiology. Historical clues that should prompt consideration of upper airway obstruction include facial or neck trauma, eating prior to the development of symptoms, smoke or gas inhalation, fever or other signs of infection (recent upper respiratory tract infection, pharyngeal pain), and exposure to potential allergen (medication, food, insect strings).

Hyperventilation Syndrome

That an association exists between emotional illness or factors and hyperventilation is well recognized. When a patient presents with signs and symptoms of hyperventilation due to emotional factors, the hyperventilation syndrome, also known as psychogenic dyspnea, is said to be present. This syndrome has a predilection for women, usually occurring in the third or fourth decades of life.

Recurrent episodes characterized by symptoms such as dizziness, faintness, and visual disturbances are quite common. Shortness of breath has been reported in up to 90% of patients. Chest pain is also a commonly encountered complaint. When it is present, the pain usually has no relation to exertion, a feature that is important in distinguishing hyperventilation syndrome from myocardial ischemia. Patients may also describe numbness or tingling of the fingers, toes, and perioral area. Clues in the history that should prompt the clinician to consider the hyperventilation syndrome are listed in the following box.

Historical Clues That Should Prompt Consideration of the Hyperventilation Syndrome
Concern about a life-threatening illness
Feels nervous
Female 20-40 years of age
Has visited numerous physicians
Many vague and unrelated minor complaints
Nervousness runs in family
Shortness of breath and chest pain are not related to exertion

Adapted from Brashear RE, "Hyperventilation Syndrome," *Lung*, 1983, 161(5):257-73.

Proceed to Step 5

STEP 5: *Are There Any Clues in the Physical Examination That Point to the Etiology of the Patient's Acute Shortness of Breath?*

Clues present in the patient's physical examination that may point to the etiology of the acute dyspnea are discussed in remainder of this step.

Pneumonia

Physical examination findings in patients with pneumonia along with their clinical significance are listed in the following table.

Physical Examination Finding	Clinical Significance
Fever	Often present
	May be absent in immunocompromised patient or in patient with significant comorbidities (eg, uremia)
	May be absent in overwhelming infection
Hypotension	Suggests pneumonia complicated by sepsis
Pulse temperature deficit (relative bradycardia for amount of fever)	Consider the following organisms: *Chlamydia* *Legionella* *Mycoplasma pneumoniae* Tularemia Viral
Herpes labialis	Seen in up to 40% of pneumonia cases due to *S. pneumoniae*
Bullous myringitis	Seen infrequently in pneumonia due to *Mycoplasma pneumoniae*
Erythema nodosum	*Mycoplasma pneumoniae*
Erythema multiforme	*Mycoplasma pneumoniae*
Cerebellar ataxia	*Legionella pneumophilia* *Mycoplasma pneumoniae*
Poor dentition	Mixed infection due to aspiration of anaerobes and aerobes that colonize oropharynx
Edentulous	Argues against aspiration (anaerobic infection)
Evidence of consolidation (dullness to percussion, e to a changes, bronchial breath sounds)*	Highly suggestive of bacterial pneumonia

*Dullness to percussion and reduced breath sounds should prompt the clinician to consider a parapneumonic effusion or empyema.

Pneumothorax

Physical examination findings consistent with primary spontaneous pneumothorax include hyper-resonance to percussion and decreased breath sounds. The signs of secondary spontaneous pneumothorax are the same. In some of these patients, however, the underlying lung disease (eg, COPD) may mask some of the physical examination findings of pneumothorax (ie, breath sounds may be reduced in both pneumothorax and COPD).

Patients with tension pneumothorax usually appear quite ill and may be noted to be in severe cardiovascular and respiratory distress. These patients are often agitated, restless, and cyanotic. Vital signs may reveal tachycardia, tachypnea, and hypotension. The hallmarks of tension pneumothorax include jugular venous distention, absent breath sounds on the ipsilateral side, and hyper-resonance to percussion. It is important to realize that hypotension is not invariably present, especially in those who are presenting early in the disease course.

Pulmonary Embolism

Signs present in those proven to have pulmonary embolism by angiography are listed in the following table.

Sign	Percent (%)
Tachypnea >16/minute	92
Rales	58
Accentuated second heart sound	53
Tachycardia >100/minute	44
Fever >37.8°C	43
Diaphoresis	36
S3 or S4 gallop	34
Thrombophlebitis	32
Lower extremity edema	24
Cardiac murmur	23
Cyanosis	19

Adapted from "The Urokinase Pulmonary Embolism Trial: A National Cooperative Study," *Circulation*, 1973, 47(2 Suppl):II1-108; also from "Urokinase-Streptokinase Embolism Trial: Phase II Results. A Cooperative Study," *JAMA*, 1974, 229(12):1606-13.

COPD Exacerbation

The physical examination finding that is considered the hallmark of COPD is a prolonged expiratory phase. Early in the disease course, the clinician may only be able to detect this finding with forced expiration. Later in the disease course, it is evident even with normal breathing. Expiratory wheezes may or may not be present. Hyper-resonance to percussion, distant breath sounds, and an increase in the anteroposterior diameter of the chest are all findings consistent with hyperinflation. With the development of pulmonary hypertension and right heart failure, the clinician may note jugular venous distention, hepatojugular reflux, peripheral edema, and accentuation of the pulmonic component of the second heart sound. The clinician should realize, however, that the findings of pulmonary hypertension and right heart failure are not specific to COPD but can accompany any disease process (ie, left heart failure) that results in pulmonary hypertension and right heart failure.

In patients with acute exacerbation of COPD, the physical examination findings are similar. Many of these patients, however, present in respiratory distress due to limited pulmonary reserve. The clinician may note the following findings:

- Use of accessory muscles of respiration
- Pursed lip breathing
- Wheezing
- Tachypnea
- Tachycardia
- Findings of hypercapnia (warm, flushed skin/papilledema/strong peripheral pulses)
- Fever (only if pneumonia is present)
- Coarse rhonchi or rales (reflect presence of secretions in the large airways)

Asthma

Between asthma exacerbations, patients may have a completely normal physical examination. Physical examination findings consistent with an asthma exacerbation include the following:

- Tachypnea

- Tachycardia

- Wheezing (inspiratory and/or expiratory)

- Prolonged expiratory phase

- Increased anteroposterior diameter of the thorax

- Hyper-resonance to percussion

Suggestive of severe asthma are respiratory rate >30/minute, pulsus paradoxus, silent chest, cyanosis, agitation, confusion, somnolence, heart rate >120 beats/minute, and the inability to complete sentences.

Congestive Heart Failure / Cardiogenic Pulmonary Edema

Physical examination findings found in patients with congestive heart failure are listed in the following box.

Type of Evidence	Highly Suggestive	Less Specific
Signs	Displaced left ventricular impulse Jugular venous distention Narrow pulse pressure Pulsatile hepatomegaly Rales S3 gallop	Ascites Hypotension Peripheral edema Tachycardia

Adapted from Kannel WB and Belanger AJ, "Epidemiology of Heart Failure," *Am Heart J*, 1991, 121(3 Pt 1):951-7; also from *Primary Cardiology*, Goldman L and Braunwald E (eds), Philadelphia, PA: WB Saunders Co, 1998, 311.

Noncardiogenic Pulmonary Edema

Early in the course of the illness, the physical examination may be unremarkable except for an increase in the respiratory rate and a few fine inspiratory crackles. With illness progression, the patient may become anxious, agitated, and markedly tachypneic. Crackles can be appreciated throughout both lung fields. Cyanosis is not uncommon. Clinical deterioration can occur over a period of several hours, often requiring intubation and mechanical ventilation.

Upper Airway Obstruction

Signs of upper airway obstruction are listed in the following box.

Signs of Upper Airway Obstruction	
Anxiety	Lack of air movement
Cyanosis	Lack of phonation
Gagging	Salivation
Inspiratory stridor	Snoring respirations
Intercostal indrawing	Use of accessory muscles of respiration

The physical examination may also reveal findings suggestive of the etiology of upper airway obstruction. Singed eyebrows and nasal vibrissae suggests smoke inhalation. Mucous membrane erythema and soot deposition/blistering are signs of noxious inhalation. Unilateral pharyngeal swelling, trismus, and deviation of the uvula should prompt consideration of peritonsillar abscess.

Hyperventilation Syndrome

The hyperventilation syndrome should be considered a diagnosis of exclusion. Many experts advocate the performance of the hyperventilation provocative test. In this test, the patient is instructed to breathe deeply and rapidly for 2-3 minutes. The reproduction of the typical symptoms provides support for the diagnosis.

Proceed to Step 6

STEP 6: *Are There Any Radiographic Findings That Point to the Etiology of the Acute Shortness of Breath?*

In some patients with acute dyspnea, the chest radiograph may be diagnostic (ie, pneumothorax, pulmonary edema). In other cases, interpretation of the chest radiographic findings in the context of the patient's clinical presentation provides support for a particular diagnosis. It is important to realize that a normal chest radiograph does not exclude a serious cause of the acute dyspnea. Causes of acute dyspnea that may present with a normal chest radiograph include acute myocardial infarction/ischemia, pulmonary embolism, cardiac tamponade, metabolic acidosis, and upper airway obstruction. Chest radiographic findings that point to the etiology of the acute shortness of breath are described in the remainder of this step.

Pneumonia

In most cases, the chest radiographic findings do not allow the clinician to determine the etiologic organism. Sometimes, however, characteristics of the pulmonary infiltrate may provide clues to the pathogen, as shown in the following table.

Chest Radiographic Finding	Etiologic Organism Suggested
Lobar or segmental consolidation	Pyogenic bacterial organism
Bilateral diffuse alveolar or interstitial infiltrates	*Legionella* *Mycoplasma pneumoniae* *Pneumocystis carinii* Viral
Nodular shadows	Fungi *Legionella* Mycobacteria *Nocardia*
Cavitation	Anaerobes *S. aureus* Gram-negative bacilli Hemolytic streptococci *Rhodococcus equi* Mycobacteria *Nocardia* Fungi *Legionella* (in immunocompromised patients)
Hilar adenopathy	Suggests associated malignancy *Mycoplasma pneumoniae* *Chlamydia pneumoniae* Tuberculosis (primary infection) Histoplasmosis Coccidioidomycosis Tularemia Pertussis Plague Measles Toxoplasmosis

Pleural effusion	Suggestive of bacterial infection
	 Argues against the following pathogens:
	   Chlamydia pneumoniae
	   Mycoplasma pneumoniae
	   Viral

Involvement of superior or basilar segment of either lower lobe or posterior segment of upper lobe	Consider aspiration pneumonia (oral anaerobes)

Chest radiography is also useful in differentiating pneumonia from other causes of acute dyspnea. Radiographic findings may also be used to gauge the severity of the illness (ie, multilobar involvement is suggestive of severe illness). The chest radiograph may reveal the presence of a pleural effusion in up to 40% of adult patients with pneumonia. These effusions are termed parapneumonic effusions. Pleural effusions that are less than 1 cm thick on lateral decubitus films are likely to resolve with appropriate treatment. Thoracentesis should be considered in patients who have effusions that exceed 1 cm in thickness. In these cases, the major concern is empyema, which can be readily excluded by analysis of the pleural fluid.

It is not necessary to obtain follow up chest radiographs in patients with pneumonia who are improving clinically. The clinician should, however, obtain another chest radiograph if the patient has persistent fever, lack of improvement with therapy, or a deterioration in the clinical status. One possibility in these cases is the development of a pleural effusion. If present, consideration should be given to performing a thoracentesis to differentiate an uncomplicated from a complicated effusion (including empyema).

In patients who are clinically improving, there is no need to repeat the chest radiograph until at least 8 weeks have passed. If the radiographic abnormalities have not resolved at this time, then the clinician should consider bronchial obstruction (foreign body or malignancy) or an alternative diagnosis. The clinician should realize, however, that there are factors that may delay resolution of the parenchymal infiltrate. These factors include older age, underlying pulmonary disease (especially COPD), and type of organism. Further evaluation of a persistent pulmonary infiltrate may include spiral CT scan of the chest or bronchoscopy.

Pneumothorax

In patients with primary spontaneous pneumothorax, the chest radiograph usually confirms the diagnosis. On occasion, the chest radiograph may be unrevealing in the patient suspected of having pneumothorax. In these cases, the clinician may wish to obtain a chest radiograph in complete expiration. This film will make the pneumothorax more apparent.

Secondary spontaneous pneumothorax can also be confirmed by chest radiography. In patients with tension pneumothorax, the acuity of the presentation does not usually allow the clinician to confirm the diagnosis by obtaining a chest film. In these cases, the clinician often has to treat the patient presumptively because a delay in treatment may adversely affect the patient's outcome. If obtained, the chest radiograph will reveal complete lung collapse along with mediastinal shift.

Pulmonary Embolism

Chest radiographic abnormalities are commonly encountered in patients with pulmonary embolism. Unfortunately, the findings are nonspecific. These findings are listed in the following box.

Chest Radiographic Findings Suggestive of Pulmonary Embolism	
Normal*	Atelectasis
Focal infiltrates	Pleural effusion
Elevated hemidiaphragm†	

*At the time of presentation, normal chest radiographs are noted in approximately 30% of patients.

†Nearly 50% of all patients will have an elevated hemidiaphragm at the time of presentation.

There are several radiographic findings that, although rare, are considered classic for pulmonary embolism. Westermark's sign refers to focal pulmonary oligemia. Hampton's hump, a finding suggestive of pulmonary infarction, is said to be present when a triangular, pleural-based density (with apex pointing to the hilum) is appreciated next to the diaphragm.

COPD Exacerbation

There are no chest radiographic findings that establish the diagnosis of COPD exacerbation but, in many patients, the characteristic findings of COPD will be present. These radiographic findings are listed in the following box.

Chest Radiographic Findings Suggestive of COPD	
Bullae	Hyperlucency of the lungs
Hyperinflation	Long, narrow heart shadow
Flattening or inversion of the hemidiaphragmatic domes	Rapid tapering of vascular markings (peripheral oligemia)
Increased retrosternal airspace	

Many of the above chest radiographic findings, particularly the combination of hyperinflation and peripheral oligemia, are fairly specific for COPD. However, these findings are relatively insensitive. A considerable number of patients with early COPD may not have any of the findings described above. While the radiographic findings of COPD are more common in advanced disease, the absence of these findings does not exclude the presence of severe disease. In patients suspected of having COPD exacerbation, the chest radiograph is also important in excluding pneumothorax and pneumonia.

Asthma Exacerbation

A chest radiograph is not indicated in all patients suspected of having an asthma exacerbation. It should, however, be performed if any of the following hold true:

- Clinical presentation consistent with pneumothorax or pneumomediastinum

- Failure to respond to appropriate therapy

- Fever (suggestive of pneumonia) or other manifestations suggestive of infection

- Signs and symptoms (eg, wheezing) consistent with asthma in a patient without a history of asthma

If obtained, the chest radiograph in uncomplicated asthma exacerbation may reveal findings consistent with hyperinflation (flattened hemidiaphragms, increased anteroposterior diameter of the chest). Scattered atelectasis may also be appreciated. With resolution of the acute episode, the radiographic findings consistent with air trapping disappear.

Congestive Heart Failure / Cardiogenic Pulmonary Edema

Chest radiographic findings consistent with congestive heart failure are listed in the following box.

Chest Radiographic Findings Consistent With Congestive Heart Failure	
Cardiomegaly*	Increased interstitial markings
Cephalization of pulmonary venous vessels†	Pleural effusion
Diffuse alveolar densities‡	

*Cardiomegaly is considered to be a fairly specific indicator of an increased left ventricular end-diastolic volume. It is, however, a relatively insensitive finding.

†Cephalization refers to the dilation and constriction of vessels supplying the upper and lower lobes of the lung, respectively.

‡The alveolar densities of cardiogenic pulmonary edema are usually confined to the inner 2/3 of the lungs. This is often described as a "butterfly" or "bat-wing" appearance.

Noncardiogenic Pulmonary Edema

The pulmonary parenchymal changes that occur in noncardiogenic pulmonary edema are similar to those observed in congestive heart failure/cardiogenic pulmonary edema. However, cardiomegaly, cephalization, and pleural effusions are quite uncommon.

It can be particularly difficult to differentiate cardiogenic from noncardiogenic pulmonary edema based upon chest radiographic findings. Some investigators maintain that the radiographic findings listed in the following table are useful in making this distinction.

	Cardiogenic Pulmonary Edema	Noncardiogenic Pulmonary Edema
Heart Size	Enlarged (usually)	Normal (usually)
Width of Pulmonary Vascular Pedicle	Widened	Normal or reduced in size
Interstitial Thickening	Septal lines	No septal lines
Regional Distribution of the Pulmonary Edema	Diffuse distribution (initially perihilar or basilar)	Peripheral rather than central pattern
Pleural Effusions	Often occurs early in the course of the illness	May rarely occur late in the course of the illness

Upper Airway Obstruction

In some cases of upper airway obstruction, the lateral neck radiograph may be particularly revealing. In patients with epiglottitis, the lateral radiograph may demonstrate findings consistent with edema and inflammation of the epiglottis and aryepiglottic folds. The hallmark radiographic finding is the thumb sign.

In patients with retropharyngeal abscess, a lateral neck radiograph should be obtained with the neck extended. An increase in the width of the soft tissue anterior to the vertebrae is consistent with the diagnosis. In adults, the width of the soft tissue should not exceed 7 and 22 mm at C2 and C6, respectively. On occasion, the clinician may note an air-fluid level which reflects the presence of gas in the abscess.

Confirming the diagnosis of foreign body aspiration often requires chest radiography. In some cases, the foreign body may be visualized within the tracheal or bronchial air column. When a foreign body is not visualized in patients suspected of having foreign body aspiration, the clinician should consider obtaining films in inspiration and expiration which may facilitate the diagnosis. The clinician should realize that radiographic studies are not indicated in patients who present with complete obstruction due to a foreign body. In these cases, emergent intervention is required to relieve the obstruction.

Also useful in the evaluation of upper airway obstruction is fiberoptic rhinopharyngolaryngoscopy or CT scan of the neck.

If the patient has a pneumothorax, **Stop Here**.

If the patient has upper airway obstruction, **Stop Here**.

If the patient has hyperventilation syndrome, **Stop Here**.

If the initial evaluation is consistent with pneumonia, **Proceed to Step 7**.

If the initial evaluation is consistent with pulmonary embolism, **Proceed to Step 8**.

If the initial evaluation is consistent with COPD exacerbation, **Proceed to Step 9**.

If the initial evaluation is consistent with asthma exacerbation, **Proceed to Step 10**.

If the initial evaluation is consistent with congestive heart failure / cardiogenic pulmonary edema, **Proceed to Step 11**.

If the initial evaluation is consistent with noncardiogenic pulmonary edema, **Proceed to Step 12**.

> ### STEP 7: *What Tests are Available in Establishing the Etiologic Pathogen of Pneumonia?*

Testing that is available in establishing the etiologic organism of the pneumonia is discussed in the remainder of this step. It is important to realize, however, that a microbial pathogen may not be identified in up to 50% of cases despite extensive testing.

Routine Laboratory Testing

Routine laboratory tests include CBC, electrolytes, liver function tests, BUN, and creatinine. These tests are not indicated in all patients with pneumonia because, in most cases, they provide very little information as to the etiologic agent. If obtained, leukocytosis may be noted. It is, however, a nonspecific finding. Furthermore, the absence of leukocytosis does not exclude pneumonia. A low white blood cell count in the patient with pneumonia is a poor prognostic sign. Abnormal liver function tests are not uncommon but do not have enough reliability in predicting the pathogen. Laboratory test abnormalities associated with a poor outcome are listed in the following box.

Laboratory Test Abnormalities Associated With Poor Outcome	
WBC count <4 X 10^9 cells/L	Serum BUN >7 mmol/L
WBC count >30 X 10^9 cells/L	PaO_2 <8 kPa

Gram Stain of Expectorated Sputum

Approximately 60% of patients with pneumonia produce sputum. Although the gross appearance of the sputum produced is not very reliable in identifying the etiologic organism, it may point to a particular etiologic organism, as shown in the following table.

Gross Appearance of Sputum Produced	Etiologic Organism Suggested
Mucopurulent*	Bacterial organism
Watery or scant	Atypical pathogen
Rusty	S. pneumoniae
Dark, red, mucoid ("currant jelly")	Klebsiella pneumoniae
Foul-smelling	Mixed anaerobic infection secondary to aspiration

*A mucopurulent sputum has also been described in up to 50% of mycoplasma and adenoviral pneumonia.

Although there continues to be debate regarding the usefulness of the sputum Gram stain in the evaluation of the patient with pneumonia, it still plays a prominent role in the laboratory evaluation of these patients. Proponents of the sputum Gram stain maintain that it is simple, quick, and inexpensive. Furthermore, a properly prepared Gram stain that is not contaminated by oropharyngeal flora may help guide initial antibiotic therapy.

Not all sputum specimens should be examined. Those that do not meet the following criteria should be discarded:

- >25 PMNs per low powered field
- <10 epithelial cells per low powered field

When these criteria are not met, the sputum sample can be considered to be contaminated with oral secretions. In these cases, a repeat sputum specimen should be submitted for Gram staining.

Findings on the Gram stain that point to the etiologic organism are listed in the following table.

Finding on Gram Stain	Etiologic Organism Suggested
Gram-positive lancet-shaped diplococci	S. pneumoniae
Small Gram-negative coccobacillary organisms	H. influenzae
Gram-positive in tetrads or grape-like clusters	S. aureus
Few bacteria	Legionella Mycoplasma Viral

Acid-fast staining of the sputum should be performed in patients suspected of having tuberculosis. Acid-fast smears can also detect weakly acid-fast organisms such as Legionella, Nocardia, and Rhodococcus equi. Giemsa staining of expectorated material is useful in the diagnosis of Pneumocystis carinii pneumonia in AIDS patients.

Also available to the clinician are direct fluorescent antibody testing (DFA) for Legionella and Pneumocystis carinii. The sensitivity and specificity of DFA testing in the diagnosis of these two causes of pneumonia are listed in the following table.

	Sensitivity (%)	Specificity (%)
Legionella	25-75	>90
Pneumocystis carinii	80	90

Sputum Culture

Some of the pneumonia pathogens may colonize the upper respiratory tract without causing disease. As a result, contamination of the sputum specimen is not uncommon, reducing the specificity of sputum culture. The sensitivity of sputum culture also suffers because of the following factors:

- Overgrowth of nonpathogenic organisms

- Loss of fastidious organisms due to delays in processing of the specimen

- Many of the common pulmonary pathogens are not able to be cultured by routine techniques (*Mycoplasma, Chlamydiae, Legionella, Pneumocystis carinii*, mycobacteria, and fungi)

- The administration of even a single dose of antibiotic can lower the yield of the sputum culture

The yield of the sputum culture can be improved if the laboratory screens the specimen prior to culture. Specimens that do not meet the following criteria should not be cultured:

- >25 PMNs per low powered field

- <10 epithelial cells per low powered field

Although sputum culture has its limitations, the isolation of an organism that is not part of the normal respiratory flora should prompt the clinician to consider the possibility that the organism is the etiologic agent.

Blood Culture

Blood cultures are not indicated in all patients with pneumonia. Cultures should be obtained, however, in all hospitalized patients. If possible, cultures should be obtained prior to the start of antimicrobial therapy. The yield of blood cultures is significantly lower when cultures are obtained after the institution of antibiotic therapy. Blood cultures are usually positive in <25% of patients with pneumonia. Isolation of an organism known to cause pneumonia should prompt the clinician to strongly consider the organism to be the etiologic agent of the pneumonia.

Invasive Procedures

Invasive procedures available in the diagnosis of pneumonia include transtracheal aspiration, needle aspiration of the lung, bronchoscopy, and bronchoalveolar lavage. These invasive procedures are not performed in most patients with pneumonia. These procedures do deserve consideration, however, in patients who are severely ill or immunocompromised. Failure to respond to empiric therapy also warrants consideration of an invasive procedure. When indicated, it is preferable to perform bronchoscopy (with protected brush catheter) or bronchoalveolar lavage because these techniques carry less risk than needle aspiration of the lung or transtracheal aspiration.

Thoracentesis

Pleural effusions are common in patients with pneumonia, occurring in up to 40% of cases. Of utmost importance is the exclusion of empyema. Although the definitive diagnosis of empyema can only be based upon inspection and analysis of the pleural fluid, studies have shown that most effusions that are less than 1 cm in thickness on lateral decubitus chest films resolve with appropriate treatment. When the effusion exceeds 1 cm in thickness, thoracentesis is required to exclude empyema.

Serologic Studies

On occasion, serologic testing may be helpful in establishing the etiologic organism. Serologic methods are particularly useful in the diagnosis of viral, *Legionella*, and other atypical infections. In many cases, however, the results of the testing do not return at a time when the clinician has to begin therapy. This is because many of the serologic tests require paired sera (ie, convalescent titers) to demonstrate a fourfold or greater increase in antibody titer. Less sensitive and specific in the diagnosis of pneumonia caused by *L. pneumophilia*, *M. pneumoniae*, and *C. pneumoniae* is the demonstration of increased levels of IgM antibody in a single serum specimen.

A urinary antigen test to detect *Legionella pneumophilia* is available. It is important to realize that this test only detects the antigen of *L. pneumophilia* serogroup 1, which accounts for >70% of *L. pneumophilia* infection. The yield of urinary antigen testing is increased if the laboratory concentrates the urine. Although antigenuria may persist for several months after infection onset, most patients have disappearance of the urinary antigen within 6 weeks.

End of Section.

STEP 8: *Does the Patient Have Pulmonary Embolism?*

Signs, symptoms, and chest radiographic findings are not sufficiently sensitive or specific to establish the diagnosis of pulmonary embolism. The remainder of this step describes other tests that are available in the diagnosis of pulmonary embolism.

EKG

EKG abnormalities are present in 87% of patients with pulmonary embolism. The EKG abnormalities may be suggestive but are never diagnostic of pulmonary embolism. Tachycardia and nonspecific EKG findings are the most common abnormalities noted. Other findings that may be appreciated are listed in the following table.

EKG Abnormalities Noted in Pulmonary Embolism	
Atrial fibrillation	Right axis deviation
Nonspecific ST-T wave abnormalities	Right bundle branch block
Normal	SIQIIITIII pattern*
P. pulmonale	Tachycardia

*Refers to deep S wave in lead I and Q wave and T wave inversion in lead III

Laboratory Testing

Laboratory test abnormalities that have been appreciated in patients with pulmonary embolism are listed in the following box.

Laboratory Test Abnormalities Noted in Pulmonary Embolism	
Arterial hypocapnia*	Polycythemia‡
Arterial hypoxemia*	Positive (+) plasma D-dimer#
Elevated liver function tests	Thrombocytopenia/thrombocytosis§
Leukocytosis†	

*In the past, arterial blood gas analysis revealing arterial hypoxemia and hypocapnia were considered hallmarks of pulmonary embolism. The PIOPED study showed that many patients with pulmonary embolism have normal PaO_2 and $PaCO_2$ levels. The alveolar-arterial oxygen difference also has limited utility in the diagnosis of pulmonary embolism.

†The white blood cell count may be elevated to as high as 20×10^9 cells/L. A normal white blood cell count, however, is not uncommon.

‡Pulmonary embolism does not lead to an increase in the hemoglobin/hematocrit. Polycythemia is, however, a well recognized risk factor for venous thromboembolism.

#A positive D-dimer test is present in most patients with pulmonary embolism. However, the test is not specific, with positive test results being appreciated in many different conditions including acute myocardial infarction, pneumonia, and other systemic diseases. Therefore, a positive result provides very little diagnostic information in the diagnosis of pulmonary embolism. The test does, however, have an excellent negative predictive value (99%). A negative test result performed by ELISA argues strongly against the diagnosis of pulmonary embolism. Latex agglutination based D-dimer testing is also available but is less reliable.

§Most patients with pulmonary embolism have normal platelet counts. Thrombocytosis is a risk factor for pulmonary embolism (ie, essential thrombocytosis). Thrombocytopenia should raise concern for the possibility of heparin-induced thrombosis.

Ultrasonographic Examination of the Lower Extremities

The premise behind performing ultrasound of the lower extremities in patients with pulmonary embolism is that most emboli originate within the deep venous system of the lower extremities. When a patient with suspected pulmonary embolism is found to have a deep venous thrombosis, further evaluation is unnecessary as the patient can be considered to have pulmonary embolism. It is reasonable to perform testing for deep venous thrombosis even when symptoms and signs of deep venous thrombosis are lacking.

It is important to realize, however, that ultrasonographic examination of the lower extremities may be unremarkable in up to 66% of all patients with pulmonary embolism. One possible reason for this is that the entire thrombus may have embolized. Although venography studies are positive in nearly 70% of patients with pulmonary embolism, the invasiveness of the procedure and need for intravenous contrast limits its performance on a more widespread basis.

Ventilation-Perfusion Scanning of the Lungs (V/Q Scan)

Ventilation-perfusion scanning of the lungs should be performed in patients suspected of having pulmonary embolism, particularly when no other diagnosis for the patient's chest pain has been found. The PIOPED trial classified the results of ventilation-perfusion scanning into four possible groups:

- High probability
- Intermediate probability
- Low probability
- Normal

Intermediate and low probability scans are considered nondiagnostic. Unfortunately, most patients with pulmonary embolism have nondiagnostic scans, as shown in the following table.

Ventilation-Perfusion Results of PIOPED Study

V/Q Classification of Patients Who Had Angiography	Likelihood of Positive Angiogram (%)	Percent of All PE Cases With This Pattern (%)
High probability	88	41
Nondiagnostic	26	57
(formerly intermediate)	30	41
(formerly low)	16	16
Normal perfusion*	9	2

*Based on this data, a normal perfusion scan will miss about 2% of PE cases. Therefore, a normal ventilation-perfusion scan does not definitively exclude pulmonary embolism, but, in the absence of high clinical suspicion, provides a strong argument against the diagnosis. Many clinicians choose not to pursue further evaluation in patients with normal ventilation-perfusion scans.

The clinician should recognize several pitfalls in the use of the ventilation-perfusion scan. Although universal criteria for the interpretation of ventilation-perfusion scans have been proposed, not all radiologists agree upon these proposed criteria. In addition, errors in interpretation may occur with radiologists who are not experienced in the reading of these scans.

It is also important to realize that the results of the ventilation-perfusion scan should always be interpreted in light of the clinical suspicion for pulmonary embolism. It is this combination that should be used to guide further evaluation. When the clinical likelihood for pulmonary embolism is high, a high probability scan provides strong evidence for the diagnosis, often obviating the need for a more definitive test such as pulmonary angiography. When the clinical likelihood for pulmonary embolism is low, a normal scan strongly argues against the diagnosis of pulmonary embolism. Angiography, if performed in this group, will be negative in 95% of patients. Although a normal scan does not exclude the diagnosis, in the presence of a low clinical likelihood for pulmonary embolism, it should prompt the clinician to consider other possibilities for the patient's symptoms.

CT Scan

Spiral CT scan has been shown to have moderate to high sensitivity in the detection of emboli in the main, lobar, or segmental vessels. Furthermore, it is quite specific in the diagnosis. Subsegmental emboli, however, may not be visualized with spiral CT scan.

Transthoracic Echocardiography

In the patient presenting with signs and symptoms compatible with pulmonary embolism, echocardiographic findings of right ventricular hypokinesis and/or dilatation provides support for the diagnosis of pulmonary embolism, particularly when these findings cannot be explained by another disease process. These findings are more typical of massive pulmonary embolism and may be absent in minor events. The clinician should realize, however, that other conditions such as acute COPD exacerbations may present with similar findings.

Although an uncommon finding, echocardiographic demonstration of thrombus in the right atrium, ventricle, or proximal pulmonary artery argues strongly for the diagnosis of pulmonary embolism.

Pulmonary Angiography

Although it is an invasive test, pulmonary angiography remains the most reliable test for the diagnosis of pulmonary embolism. Findings consistent with pulmonary embolism include the following:

- Intraluminal filling defect
- Blockage of flow (dye cut-off)

The absence of these findings should prompt the clinician to determine if the procedure was performed properly. It is important to ensure that the entire pulmonary arterial tree was well visualized. Even an adequately performed pulmonary angiogram, however, may miss emboli present in very small arteries.

Pulmonary embolism is diagnosed with almost 100% certainty when the angiogram reveals one or both of the findings listed above. When the angiogram is negative, pulmonary embolism can be excluded with over 90% certainty.

The following table summarizes the advantages and disadvantages of the imaging methods currently used in the diagnosis of pulmonary embolism.

Feature	Transthoracic Echocardiography	V/Q Scan	Pulmonary Angiography	Spiral CT Scan
Widely available	+++	+++	++	++
Noninvasive	+++	++	−	++
Low interobserver variability	++	++	++	++
Well tolerated	+++	++	+	++
Detects massive PE	+++	++	+++	+++
Detects peripheral PE	−	+	+++	++
Low cost	+++	++	+	+

+++ = very good; ++ = satisfactory; + = poor; − = does not apply

Adapted from *Cardiology*, Crawford MH and DiMarco JP (eds), St Louis, MO: Mosby, 2001, 5.18.7.

End of Section.

STEP 9: *What is the Precipitant of the COPD Exacerbation?*

When a diagnosis of COPD exacerbation has been established, it behooves the clinician to search for a precipitant. Common precipitants of COPD exacerbation are listed in the following box.

Common Precipitants of COPD Exacerbation	
Infection	Left ventricular dysfunction*
Pneumonia	Pneumothorax†
Tracheobronchitis	Pulmonary embolism‡
Inflammation / bronchoconstriction	Sedative or narcotic use

*Left ventricular dysfunction or congestive heart failure can also cause an acute exacerbation of COPD. Because CHF and COPD share many of the same signs and symptoms, it can be difficult to distinguish the combination of COPD and CHF from COPD alone. Although orthopnea and paroxysmal nocturnal dyspnea are classic features of CHF, COPD patients, who have no underlying heart disease, may also present with these symptoms. Careful probing of the history may allow the clinician to make the distinction. The paroxysmal nocturnal dyspnea of CHF does not clear immediately after a patient rises or sits. In contrast, COPD patients classically have rapid resolution of their symptoms after sitting up and coughing. An EKG is always indicated in patients with COPD exacerbation to exclude arrhythmias and myocardial ischemia. In those who have a clinical presentation suggestive of left ventricular dysfunction, a transthoracic echocardiogram should be obtained. Echocardiography should also be considered in patients who fail to improve with standard therapy for COPD. In especially difficult cases, a therapeutic trial of diuretic medication or even heart catheterization may be needed to define the role of left ventricular dysfunction in the patient's acute dyspnea.

†Pneumothorax should be considered in every COPD patient who develops an acute exacerbation, particularly when there is sudden onset of shortness of breath and unilateral chest pain.

‡Pulmonary embolism is thought to be underdiagnosed as a cause of acute COPD exacerbation. The diagnosis of pulmonary embolism can be difficult to establish in COPD patients. The signs and symptoms of pulmonary embolism are nonspecific and many patients with COPD have these same clinical manifestations in the absence of pulmonary embolism. Pulmonary embolism should clearly be considered in patients with pleuritic chest pain (if no other etiology is present) or marked dyspnea without evidence of worsening bronchospasm or infection (no change in sputum, cough, or wheezing). Although the ventilation-perfusion scan is more likely to be nondiagnostic in COPD patients, it still remains the initial test of choice in COPD patients suspected to have pulmonary embolism.

Although most patients with COPD exacerbation present with a known history of COPD, on occasion, a patient may present with signs and symptoms of COPD exacerbation in the absence of documented COPD. In these cases, a diagnosis of COPD should be confirmed by performing pulmonary function tests. These should be performed, however, when the patient has recovered from the acute illness and is at baseline.

A decreased forced expiratory volume in 1 second (FEV_1) is commonly appreciated in COPD patients. Because COPD shares this finding in common with restrictive lung diseases, it is also necessary to determine the forced vital capacity (FVC). A reduced FEV_1 to FVC ratio is consistent with airflow limitation. It is important to realize that a reduced ratio is not entirely specific for COPD and may be noted in patients with asthma, cystic fibrosis, bronchiolitis, and upper airway abnormalities. Nearly 30% of COPD patients will show at least a 20% increase in FEV_1 after bronchodilator administration. Lung volume measurements consistent with COPD include increases in the functional residual capacity (FRC), residual volume (RV), and total lung capacity (TLC). Lung volumes may be normal, however, in early COPD. The carbon monoxide diffusion capacity is low in patients with emphysema. Normal levels may be seen, however, in patients with mild emphysema.

End of Section.

STEP 10: *Does the Patient Have an Asthma Exacerbation?*

Testing that may be indicated in the patient presenting with an asthma exacerbation are discussed further in the remainder of this step.

EKG

It is not necessary to obtain an EKG in all patients with asthma exacerbation. If obtained, the EKG is usually normal with the exception of sinus tachycardia. In those with severe disease, however, other EKG abnormalities may be noted. Right axis deviation, right bundle branch block, *P. pulmonale*, and nonspecific ST-T wave abnormalities have all been described. An EKG should also be obtained if the clinician suspects arrhythmia or myocardial ischemia.

Laboratory Testing

Routine laboratory tests (ie, CBC, electrolytes) are not necessary in most cases. The clinician should consider obtaining a white blood cell count in asthma patients suspected of having pneumonia. It is preferable to draw the blood for determination of the white blood cell count prior to the administration of corticosteroids since leukocytosis can occur due to corticosteroid-induced demargination of white blood cells. The differential count may reveal a mild eosinophilia. An eosinophil percentage exceeding 25% of the total white blood cell count should prompt consideration of an alternative diagnosis.

Significant hypokalemia can occur in patients given high doses of β-agonist therapy. In patients who are on theophylline, it is reasonable to obtain a theophylline level to identify those that have subtherapeutic or supratherapeutic levels.

Arterial Blood Gas

Arterial blood gas analysis is not indicated in all patients with asthma exacerbation. It should be obtained, however, if the exacerbation is of sufficient severity that a prolonged period of observation or hospital admission is required. In most cases, arterial blood gas analysis will reveal hypoxemia and hypocapnia. A normal $PaCO_2$ level should not always be considered reassuring, especially in patients with moderate to severe asthma. In these cases, a normal level may herald respiratory failure.

Pulmonary Function Testing

Assessment of pulmonary function by determining either the forced expiratory volume in 1 second (FEV_1) or the peak expiratory flow rate (PEFR) is important for the following reasons:

- Provides a rapid measure of disease severity
- Can be used to monitor the response to therapy
- Form the basis for guidelines used in admitting patients

During acute bronchospasm, spirometric findings consistent with asthma include a decreased FEV_1. The FEV_1 to FVC ratio is also reduced. With more severe obstruction, elevations in the residual volume and functional residual capacity may be noted. These latter findings are reflective of hyperinflation.

The hallmark finding is partial or complete reversal of airflow obstruction after bronchodilator administration.

Although the PEFR is less sensitive than spirometry, it is easier to perform at the bedside. It is important to realize that PEFR measurements are easily influenced by patient cooperation and effort. Therefore, management decisions should be based upon the average of three measurements. Normal PEFR in men and women range between 500-700 L/minute and 380-550 L/minute, respectively. A gradual improvement in the PEFR with treatment suggests that the patient is responding appropriately. The PEFR or FEV_1 may be used as measures of asthma severity, as shown in the following table.

Event or Measurement	Mild Asthma (%)	Moderate Asthma (%)	Severe Asthma (%)
FEV_1 or PEFR; % of predicted	>80	60-80	<60

Adapted from Boulet LP, Becker A, Berube d, et al, "Canadian Asthma Consensus Report," *CMAJ*, 1999, 161(11 Suppl):S1-61 (review).

Precipitating Factors in Asthma Exacerbation

Factors that may precipitate an asthma exacerbation are listed in the following box.

Factors That May Precipitate an Asthma Exacerbation	
Allergens	Medications
Change in weather	β-blockers (oral or ophthalmic)
Exercise	NSAIDs
Infection	Occupational
	Pollution
	Smoking

Every effort should be taken to identify the precipitant. Treatment or correction of the precipitating factor can play a large role in the prevention of future asthma exacerbations.

End of Section.

STEP 11: *What are the Underlying and Precipitating Causes of the Congestive Heart Failure / Cardiogenic Pulmonary Edema?*

Of major importance in the patient with an exacerbation of congestive heart failure / cardiogenic pulmonary edema is the determination of the following:

- Underlying cause of the congestive heart failure
- Precipitating cause of the congestive heart failure

The common underlying causes of congestive heart failure are listed in the following box.

Common Underlying Causes of Congestive Heart Failure	
Alcohol	Infiltrative cardiomyopathy
Coronary artery disease	Myocarditis
Dilated cardiomyopathy	Thyroid disorders
Hypertension	Valvular heart disease
Hypertrophic cardiomyopathy	

Identification of the underlying cause is important because appropriate treatment may prevent further congestive heart failure exacerbations.

Underlying causes of congestive heart failure should be separated from precipitating causes. Although acute dyspnea may be the result of progressively worsening heart failure alone, in many cases, a precipitating cause that is superimposed on the underlying cause is present. Every effort should be taken to identify the precipitating cause since appropriate treatment can lead to the resolution of the patient's acute dyspnea. In addition, avoidance of the precipitating causes of congestive heart failure may help prevent future exacerbations. Common precipitating causes are listed in the following box.

Common Precipitating Causes of Congestive Heart Failure	
Acute myocardial ischemia	Infection
Arrhythmia	Medication noncompliance
Dietary indiscretion	Negative inotropic medications
Emotional stress	β-blocker
Excessive alcohol use	Calcium channel blockers
Hyperthyroidism	NSAIDs
Hypothyroidism	Uncontrolled hypertension
Inadequate therapy	

The remainder of this section will discuss tests that the clinician may wish to obtain in an effort to identify both the underlying and precipitating causes of the congestive heart failure.

Laboratory Testing

Laboratory test abnormalities that should be considered in the evaluation of the congestive heart failure patient presenting with acute dyspnea are listed in the following table.

Laboratory Test Abnormality	Clinical Significance
Anemia	Anemia is a cause of high output CHF
	Anemia alone can be the cause of acute dyspnea
Elevated serum BUN/ creatinine	The clinical presentation of renal failure may closely resemble CHF exacerbation
	Abnormal serum BUN and creatinine levels may also reflect kidney hypoperfusion due to CHF

(continued)

483

(continued)

Laboratory Test Abnormality	Clinical Significance
Abnormal liver function tests	The clinical presentation of cirrhosis can mimic that of CHF exacerbation
	Abnormal liver function tests may also reflect congestive hepatopathy in patients with right-sided heart failure
Thyroid function tests	Acute dyspnea may be the manifestation of hypothyroidism or hyperthyroidism
Electrolytes	Hyponatremia is a poor prognostic finding
	Hypokalemia may be the result of diuretic therapy

EKG

Although EKG abnormalities are often nonspecific in patients with congestive heart failure, at times, the findings may provide clues to the cause of the congestive heart failure.

EKG Finding	Cause of CHF Suggested
Q waves ST-T wave abnormalities	Ischemic heart disease
Left ventricular hypertrophy	Hypertension
Low voltage	Hypothyroidism
	Pericardial effusion
	Infiltrative cardiomyopathy
Right ventricular hypertrophy	Pulmonary hypertension
Bundle branch block or intraventricular conduction delay	Common findings in congestive heart failure

Echocardiography

It is essential to assess left ventricular function in all patients who have a clinical presentation consistent with congestive heart failure. The two methods that are most commonly used to evaluate left ventricular function include the following:

- Echocardiography
- Radionuclide angiography

Of the two methods, echocardiography is more widely used. Two-dimensional echocardiography can provide information regarding ventricular function, chamber size, and wall motion abnormalities. It can help identify many of the underlying causes of congestive heart failure. Echocardiography with Doppler should be performed if valvular heart disease is suspected.

Wall motion abnormalities are suggestive of an ischemic etiology but may occur in dilated cardiomyopathy (nonischemic). The absence of wall motion abnormalities does not exclude ischemic heart disease. In fact, patients with severe ischemic heart disease may present with global hypokinesis.

It is important to realize that a normal ejection fraction in a patient who presents with signs and symptoms compatible with congestive heart failure does not exclude the diagnosis. Although most patients with congestive heart failure will have a depressed ejection fraction consistent with systolic dysfunction, approximately 40% of patients have diastolic dysfunction characterized by a normal ejection fraction. Diastolic dysfunction is just one consideration in patients who have a normal ejection fraction. Other considerations are listed in the following box.

Causes of Normal Ejection Fraction in Patients Presenting With Congestive Heart Failure
Inaccurate measurement of ejection fraction
Atrial fibrillation
Technical problems
Resolved systolic dysfunction
Prior ischemia
Prior tachyarrhythmia
Other cause of transient depression (ie, alcohol)
Ejection fraction unrepresentative of systolic function
Mitral regurgitation with underlying systolic dysfunction
Severe hypertension
Causes of heart failure unrelated to left ventricular dysfunction
High output heart failure
Isolated right heart failure
Primary valvular heart disease (ie, mitral stenosis)
Pericardial constriction or tamponade
Diastolic dysfunction

Adapted from *Cardiology*, Crawford MH and DiMarco JP (eds), St Louis, MO: Mosby, 2001, 5.6.2.

Therefore, a normal ejection fraction in a patient with congestive heart failure is not synonymous with diastolic dysfunction. Doppler echocardiography may, however, reveal other findings consistent with diastolic dysfunction such as alterations in the E to A ratio. Causes of diastolic dysfunction are listed in the following box.

Causes of Diastolic Dysfunction	
Acute myocardial ischemia	Infiltrative cardiomyopathy
Aortic stenosis	Amyloidosis
Chronic coronary artery disease	Hemochromatosis
Diabetes mellitus	Metabolic storage diseases
Hypertension	Sarcoidosis
Hypertrophic cardiomyopathy	Restrictive cardiomyopathy

End of Section.

STEP 12: *Does the Patient Have Noncardiogenic Pulmonary Edema?*

Adult respiratory distress syndrome (ARDS), the major type of noncardiogenic pulmonary edema, is defined by the following:

- Severe hypoxemia not responsive to the administration of supplemental oxygen ($PaO_2/FIO_2 < 200$)

- Widespread pulmonary infiltrates (involvement of three of six lung regions) not explained by cardiovascular disease or volume overload

It can be difficult, at times, to differentiate noncardiogenic from cardiogenic pulmonary edema. The following table describes some of the differences between these two conditions.

Adult Respiratory Distress Syndrome	Cardiogenic Pulmonary Edema / Volume Overload

Prior history
  Younger
  No history of heart disease
  Appropriate fluid balance
	Prior history
	  Older
	  Prior history of heart disease
	  Hypertension
	  Chest pain
	  New onset palpitations
	  Positive fluid balance

Physical examination
  Flat neck veins
  Hyperdynamic pulses
  Absence of edema
	Physical examination
	  Elevated neck veins
	  Left ventricular enlargement, life,
	    heave
	  S3
	  S4
	  Edema

EKG
  Sinus tachycardia
  Nonspecific ST-T wave abnormalities
	EKG
	  Evidence of prior or on going ischemia
	  Supraventricular tachycardia
	  Left ventricular hypertrophy

CXR
  Normal heart size
  Peripheral distribution of infiltrate
  Air bronchogram (80%)
	CXR
	  Cardiomegaly
	  Central or basilar infiltrate; peri-
	    bronchial and vascular congestion
	  Septal lines (Kerley's lines)
	  Air bronchograms (25%)
	  Pleural effusions

Hemodynamic measurements
  Pulmonary artery pressure <15 mm Hg
  Cardiac index >3.5 L/min/m^2
	Hemodynamic measurements
	  Pulmonary capillary wedge
	    pressure >18 mm Hg
	  Cardiac index <3.5 L/min/m^2 with
	    ischemia
	  Cardiac index >3.5 L/min/m^2 with
	    volume overload

Adapted from *Cecil Textbook of Medicine*, Goldman L and Bennett JC (eds), 21st ed, 2000, Philadelphia, PA: WB Saunders, 469.

REFERENCES

Bartlett JG, Breiman RF, Mandell LA, et al, "Community-Acquired Pneumonia in Adults: Guidelines for Management. The Infectious Diseases Society of America," *Clin Infect Dis*, 1998, 26(4):811-38.

Barton ED, "Tension Pneumothorax," *Curr Opin Pulm Med*, 1999, 5(4):269-74.

Boulet LP, Becker A, Berube D, et al, "Canadian Asthma Consensus Report," *CMAJ*, 1999, 161(11 Suppl):S1-61 (review).

Brashear RE, "Hyperventilation Syndrome," *Lung*, 1983, 161(5):257-73.

Cardiology, Crawford MH and DiMarco JP (eds), St Louis, MO: Mosby, 2001, 5.18.7.

Colice GL, Curtis A, Deslauriers J, et al, "Medical and Surgical Treatment of Parapneumonic Effusions: An Evidence-Based Guideline," *Chest*, 2000, 118(4):1158-71.

Cunha BA, "Community-Acquired Pneumonia. Diagnostic and Therapeutic Approach," *Med Clin North Am*, 2001, 85(1):43-77.

"Dyspnea. Mechanisms, Assessment and management: A Consensus Statement. American Thoracic Society," *Am J Respir Crit Care Med*, 1999, 159(1):321-40.

Garcia MJ, "Diastolic Dysfunction and Heart Failure: Causes and Treatment Options," *Cleve Clin J Med*, 2000, 67(10):727-9, 733-8.

Goodman PC, "Radiographic Findings in Patients With Acute Respiratory Distress Syndrome," *Clin Chest Med*, 2000, 21(3):419-33.

Kabbani SS and LeWinter MM, "Diastolic Heart Failure. Constrictive, Restrictive, and Pericardial," *Cardiol Clin*, 2000, 18(3):501-9.

Kannel WB and Belanger AJ, "Epidemiology of Heart Failure," *Am Heart J*, 1991, 121(3 Pt 1):951-7; also from *Primary Cardiology*, Goldman L and Braunwald E (eds), Philadelphia, PA: WB Saunders Co, 1998, 311.

Kline JA, Johns KL, Colucciello SA, et al, "New Diagnostic Tests for Pulmonary Embolism," *Ann Emerg Med*, 2000, 35(2):168-80.

Li JT, Pearlman DS, Nicklas RA, et al, "Algorithm for the Diagnosis and Management of Asthma: A Practice Parameter Update: Joint Task Force on Practice Parameters, Representing the American Academy of Allergy, Asthma and Immunology, the American College of Allergy, Asthma and Immunology, and the Joint Council of Allergy, Asthma and Immunology," *Ann Allergy Asthma Immunol*, 1998, 81(5 Pt 1):415-20.

Medical Management of Pulmonary Diseases, Davis GS (ed), New York, NY: Marcel Dekker, 1999, 295.

Michelson E and Hollrah S, "Evaluation of the Patient With Shortness of Breath: An Evidence Based Approach," *Emerg Med Clin North Am*, 1999, 17(1):221-37.

Morgan WC and Hodge HL, "Diagnostic Evaluation of Dyspnea," *Am Fam Phys*, 1998, 57(4):711-6.

Richardson C and Baldwin D, "Diagnosing Acute Shortness of Breath in Adult Patients," *Practitioner*, 2000, 244(1610):478-82.

Riedel M, "Acute Pulmonary Embolism 1: Pathophysiology, Clinical Presentation, and Diagnosis," *Heart*, 2001, 85(2):229-40.

Sahn SA and Heffner JE, "Spontaneous Pneumothorax," *N Engl J Med*, 2000, 342(12):868-74.

Seamens CM and Wrenn K, "Breathlessness, Strategies Aimed at Identifying and Treating the Cause of Dyspnea," *Postgrad Med*, 1995, 98(4):215-6, 219-22, 225-7.

Shamsham F and Mitchell J, "Essentials of the Diagnosis of Heart Failure," *Am Fam Phys*, 2000, 61(5):1319-28.

Skerrett SJ, "Diagnostic Testing for Community-Acquired Pneumonia," *Clin Chest Med*, 1999, 20(3):531-48.

Steinberg KP and Hudson LD, "Acute Lung Injury and Acute Respiratory Distress Syndrome. The Clinical Syndrome," *Clin Chest Med*, 2000, 21(3):401-17.

"The Urokinase Pulmonary Embolism Trial: A National Cooperative Study,"*Circulation*,1973, 47(2 Suppl):II1-108

Tresch DD, "Clinical Manifestations, Diagnostic Assessment, and Etiology of Heart Failure in Elderly Patients," *Clin Geriatr Med*, 2000, 16(3):445-56.

"Urokinase-Streptokinase Embolism Trial: Phase II Results. A Cooperative Study," *JAMA*, 1974, 229(12):1606-13.

Voelkel NF and Tuder R, "COPD: Exacerbation," *Chest*, 2000, 17(5 Suppl 2):376S-9S.

Ware LB and Matthay MA, "The Acute Respiratory Distress Syndrome," *N Engl J Med*, 2000, 342(18):1334-49.

SORE THROAT

STEP 1: *What are the Causes of Acute Sore Throat?*

Acute sore throat is a commonly encountered problem in primary care. While infectious pharyngitis is a major consideration in the patient presenting with acute sore throat, the clinician should realize that there are other causes of sore throat, some of which may be severe or life-threatening. The causes of acute sore throat are listed in the following box.

Causes of Acute Sore Throat	
Infectious pharyngitis	Head and neck disorders
Systemic disease	Allergy
Acute leukemia	Dental infection
Agranulocytosis	Foreign body
Still's disease	Neoplasm
Temporal arteritis	Otitis
Toxic shock syndrome	Salivary gland infection
Viral hepatitis	Sinusitis
Mediastinal disorders	Thyroiditis
Aortic dissection	Trauma
Aortitis	
Esophageal rupture	
Esophagitis	
Mediastinitis	
Myocardial infarction / angina pectoris	
Pneumomediastinum	

While there are many causes of the acute sore throat, most cases are due to infectious pharyngitis. The other conditions listed above are usually apparent on history and physical examination. These conditions will not be discussed here in this chapter. The remainder of this chapter will focus on the patient with infectious pharyngitis.

Proceed to Step 2

STEP 2: *Does the Patient Have Infectious Pharyngitis?*

As mentioned in Step 1, acute sore throat is not synonymous with infectious pharyngitis. Most patients with infectious pharyngitis report discomfort in the posterior pharynx, often accompanied by painful swallowing. Physical examination usually reveals erythema of the posterior pharynx. When the history and physical examination are atypical for infectious pharyngitis, the clinician should consider other causes of acute sore throat (listed in the box in Step 1).

Of importance in the patient presenting with infectious pharyngitis is the identification of the patient with group A β-hemolytic streptococcal pharyngitis. Recognition of group A β-hemolytic streptococcal pharyngitis followed by appropriate therapy will prevent the development of rheumatic fever and acute glomerulonephritis. In addition, the clinician should recognize the manifestations of the less common but potentially serious causes of infectious pharyngitis.

If the patient does not have typical features of infectious pharyngitis, consider other causes of acute sore throat.

If the patient has typical features of infectious pharyngitis, **Proceed to Step 3.**

STEP 3: *Does the Patient Have a Serious Illness?*

While most cases of infectious pharyngitis are benign and self-limited, occasionally, a patient may present with serious or even life-threatening illness. The causes of complicated sore throat are listed in the following box.

Causes of Complicated Sore Throat	
Diphtheria	Peritonsillar abscess
Epiglottitis	Retropharyngeal abscess
Infectious mononucleosis	

Clues to the presence of a complicated sore throat include the following:

- Trismus (difficulty opening the mouth because of tightening of the facial and jaw muscles)

- Asymmetric tonsillar swelling

- Associated respiratory symptoms (shortness of breath, wheezing, stridor)

The presence of one or more of these features should prompt consideration of the causes of complicated sore throat. Because these conditions are heterogeneous in their clinical presentation, the absence of all of these features does not exclude the causes of a complicated sore throat. These causes will be described in further detail below.

Epiglottitis

Although typically considered to be an infection of children, epiglottitis can occur in adults. Although epiglottitis is usually caused by *H. influenzae*, many other etiologic organisms have been described. Epiglottitis is characterized by cellulitis of the epiglottis and surrounding structures that can lead to complete airway obstruction. Because of this feared complication, the clinician should consider this possibility in any patient with sore throat. Typical symptoms include sore throat, odynophagia, fever, and dysphonia. Signs and symptoms of upper airway obstruction including wheezing, stridor, and orthopnea may be present. These as well as other signs and symptoms of epiglottitis are listed in the following box.

Signs and Symptoms of Epiglottitis	
Symptoms	**Signs**
Severe sore throat (100%)	Lymphadenopathy
Painful dysphagia (76%)	Drooling
Fever (88%)	Respiratory distress
Shortness of breath (78%)	
Anterior neck tenderness	
Hoarseness	
Muffling of the voice	

On physical examination, the patient may have difficulty opening the mouth. Occasionally, the clinician may be able to visualize the red and swollen epiglottis. In most cases, the examination is unrevealing. Laboratory testing is usually not helpful but may show nonspecific findings of leukocytosis with a left shift. Blood cultures should be sent in all suspected cases of epiglottitis. *H. influenzae* can be isolated from the blood in up to 25% of adults with epiglottitis.

When the physical exam is unimpressive, the diagnosis rests with visualization of the epiglottis by indirect or direct laryngoscopy. The role of radiography in the patient suspected of having epiglottitis is debated. While radiographs of the lateral neck may reveal epiglottic swelling, the sensitivity of the test is variable. In addition, false-positive rates as high as 30% have been described. Because patients with epiglottitis are at risk for airway compromise, obtaining films may result in a delay in securing the airway. If radiographs are obtained, a negative result should prompt the clinician to visualize the epiglottis directly, especially when epiglottitis is suspected.

Peritonsillar Abscess

Peritonsillar abscess, also known as quinsy, may complicate acute pharyngo-tonsillitis. With the development of an abscess, swallowing becomes difficult and painful. Opening the mouth may be difficult for some patients if the abscess encroaches upon the mastication muscles. Turning of the head may cause increased pain. Dribbling of saliva may be noted along with fetid breath. Physical examination typically reveals redness and swelling of the peritonsillar area with medial displacement of the tonsil. The findings are usually unilateral although bilateral involvement has been described. Although anaerobic bacteria is the major cause, group A β-hemolytic strepto-cocci, other streptococci, and *Staphylococcus aureus* have been isolated. If left untreated, the illness may resolve within 5-10 days if there is spontaneous discharge of the pus from the abscess. Major concerns in the patient with peritonsillar abscess are upper airway obstruction, mediastinitis, sepsis, and lateral extension resulting in involvement of the large vessels of the neck.

Retropharyngeal Abscess

In adults, retropharyngeal abscess tends to present with symptoms of sore throat, dysphagia, or neck pain. Although a small proportion of patients present with symptoms of airway compromise, most of these patients will relate a history of throat pain. Other signs and symptoms include nuchal rigidity, fever, cervical lymphadenopathy, drooling, and stridor.

A predisposing factor can be identified in most adult patients with retropha-ryngeal abscess. These factors include trauma, intraoral procedures, endo-tracheal intubation, and hypopharyngeal foreign bodies.

Although physical examination may reveal swelling of the posterior pharynx, an unremarkable exam does not exclude the diagnosis. A lateral neck x-ray is very helpful in establishing the diagnosis. In the majority of patients, the lateral radiograph will reveal retropharyngeal swelling. A retropharyngeal diameter exceeding 7 and 22 mm at C2 and C6, respectively, strongly argue for the diagnosis of retropharyngeal abscess. A CT scan may help establish the diagnosis when there is uncertainty. Although group A β-hemolytic strep-tococci and *S. aureus* are the major etiologic organisms, many others have been identified.

Diphtheria

Diphtheria is uncommon in the United States but may occur in unvaccinated individuals. The illness is characterized by a slow onset. Although common, fever is usually low-grade. The pharyngeal discomfort of diphtheria is not impressive. Examination usually reveals the firmly adherent tonsillar or pharyngeal membrane, the color of which may vary from light to dark gray. If suspected, a throat swab should be sent for culture using Loffler's medium.

If the patient has a complicated case of infectious pharyngitis, **Stop Here.**

If the patient does not have a complicated case of infectious pharyngitis, **Proceed to Step 4**.

STEP 4: *What are the Causes of Infectious Pharyngitis?*

Once the serious causes of infectious pharyngitis have been excluded, the clinician can then focus efforts on identifying the etiologic organism. In most cases, the etiologic organism will not be identified. Of particular importance is the identification of group A β-hemolytic streptococcal pharyngitis, the acute retroviral syndrome, and infectious mononucleosis.

The etiologic organisms of infectious pharyngitis are listed in the following box.

Causes of Infectious Pharyngitis	
Bacterial	
Group A β-hemolytic streptococci*	*Arcanobacterium hemolyticum*
	Corynebacterium diphtheriae
Group C streptococci*	*Neisseria gonorrhoeae*
Group G streptococci*	*Yersinia enterocolitica*
Anaerobic (Vincent's angina)	
Viral	
Adenovirus*	Influenza*
Coronavirus	Measles
Coxsackievirus	Parainfluenza*
Cytomegalovirus	Respiratory synctial virus
Enterovirus	Rhinovirus
Epstein-Barr virus*	Rubella
Herpes simplex virus	Varicella
HIV (acute retroviral syndrome)	
Other organisms	
Candida	*Mycoplasma pneumoniae*
Chlamydia pneumoniae	

*Common causes of infectious pharyngitis

Proceed to Step 5

STEP 5: *Are There Any Historical Clues That Point to the Etiology of the Infectious Pharyngitis?*

Historical clues that may point to the etiology of the infectious pharyngitis are listed in the following table.

Historical Clue	Etiologic Organism Suggested
Exposure to rabbits History of deer hunting	*Francisella tularensis*
Recent orogenital sexual activity	Acute retroviral syndrome Herpes simplex virus *Neisseria gonorrhoeae* Treponema pallidum
Rash	Acute retroviral syndrome *Arcanobacterium hemolyticum* Group A β-hemolytic streptococci Infectious mononucleosis (EBV)
History of swimming pool exposure	Adenovirus (pharyngoconjunctival fever)
Urethral or vaginal discharge	*Neisseria gonorrhoeae*
Family member with conjunctivitis	Adenovirus (pharyngoconjunctival fever)

Clues in the physical examination that may point to the etiology are listed in the following table.

Physical Examination Clue	Etiologic Organism Suggested
White plaque-like lesions (thrush)	Acute retroviral syndrome *Candida albicans*
Ulcerative lesions of oropharynx	Acute retroviral syndrome Coxsackievirus Herpes simplex virus Vincent's angina
Palatal petechiae	Epstein-Barr virus Group A β-hemolytic streptococci Rubella
Conjunctivitis	Adenovirus (pharyngoconjunctival fever)
Hepatomegaly	Epstein-Barr virus
Splenomegaly	Epstein-Barr virus
Pharyngeal exudate*	Adenovirus Anaerobic pharyngitis *Arcanobacterium hemolyticum* *Corynebacterium diphtheriae* Epstein-Barr virus Group A β-hemolytic streptococci Group C streptococci Group G streptococci Herpes simplex virus *Yersinia enterocolitica*

*Exudate is not always present in infectious pharyngitis due to these organisms. Therefore, the absence of an exudate does not exclude these possibilities. The pharyngitis that is associated with the common cold and influenza is not characterized by the presence of an exudate.

In most cases, the historical and physical examination findings do not allow the clinician to distinguish between the etiologic organisms. On occasion, however, the information obtained may be very suggestive of a particular organism.

If the patient has a rash, *Proceed to Step 6.*

If the patient has ulcerative lesions of the oropharynx, *Proceed to Step 7*.

If the patient has conjunctivitis, *Proceed to Step 8*.

If the patient has splenomegaly, *Proceed to Step 9*.

Otherwise, *Proceed to Step 10*.

> **STEP 6: *What are the Considerations in the Patient With Infectious Pharyngitis Who Has a Rash?***

When rash accompanies infectious pharyngitis, the clinician should consider the following possibilities:

- Group A β-hemolytic streptococci

  The scarlatiniform rash of scarlet fever may be appreciated in infections caused by a strain carrying the erythrogenic toxin. The rash characteristically begins on the trunk only to spread centrifugally. This sandpapery rash tends to blanch with pressure. One week after the onset of the rash, desquamation, particularly of the skin over the palms and soles, occurs.

- *Arcanobacterium hemolyticum*

  Arcanobacterium hemolyticum should be suspected when the infectious pharyngitis patient presents with rash. The rash is typically described as a diffuse, maculopapular rash on the trunk and extremities. Throat culture on sheep blood agar is preferred when this organism is suspected. Hemolysis is usually evident at 48-72 hours.

- Acute retroviral syndrome

  Various types of rash have been described during primary HIV infection including maculopapular, roseola-like, and diffuse urticaria.

- Infectious mononucleosis (EBV)

  A rash is present in about 5% of patients. The rash may be macular, petechial, urticarial, scarlatiniform, or erythema-multiforme-like. With the administration of ampicillin, >90% of patients will develop a pruritic, maculopapular eruption.

For more information regarding the acute retroviral syndrome, *Proceed to Step 10*.

For more information regarding infectious mononucleosis, *Proceed to Step 10*.

For more information regarding group A β-hemolytic streptococci, *Proceed to Step 11*.

STEP 7: *What are the Considerations in the Patient With Infectious Pharyngitis Who Has Oropharyngeal Ulcerations?*

Possibilities in the patient with infectious pharyngitis who has oropharyngeal ulcerations include the following:

- Primary herpes simplex virus infection

  Fever, headache, sore throat, and lymphadenopathy are all features of primary herpes simplex virus infection. Inflammation of the gingiva is apparent on exam along with vesicles. The vesicles commonly involve the palate and pharynx. Rupture of the vesicles occur several days later, resulting in painful ulcers. One to two weeks are usually required before the ulcers heal.

- Herpangina

  Multiple small ulcerations are also a feature of coxsackievirus infection of the oral mucosa and pharynx. As with primary herpes simplex virus infection, symptoms and signs include fever, headache, and lymphadenopathy. As a result, it may be difficult to distinguish primary herpes simplex infection from herpangina on clinical features alone. In contrast to primary herpes simplex infection, however, herpangina tends to occur during the summer months. In addition, the duration of the illness is usually shorter.

- Vincent's angina

  Vincent's angina, also known as necrotizing ulcerative gingivostomatitis, is caused by the organism, *Fusobacterium nucleatum*. This illness begins as a gingivitis, characterized by inflamed gingiva with ulcerations. The ulcers may be covered by a foul smelling, grayish exudate. With time, the infection involves the oral mucosa or posterior pharynx, producing similar ulcerations. Fever, tender lymphadenopathy, tonsillitis, and foul breath often accompany the illness. A crystal-violet stained smear of the exudate usually reveals the presence of many fusobacteria and spirochetes.

- Acute retroviral syndrome

  The acute retroviral syndrome is discussed in further detail in Step 10.

End of Section.

STEP 8: *What are Considerations in the Patient With Infectious Pharyngitis Having Conjunctivitis?*

Pharyngoconjunctival fever is the term used to describe conjunctivitis accompanying infectious pharyngitis. The etiologic organism is adenovirus. The illness is characterized by malaise, headache, and chills. Patients may complain of a severe sore throat. On exam, pharyngeal edema, as well as an exudate, may be noted. The conjunctivitis occurs in 33% to 50% of all cases of adenoviral pharyngitis. When present, it is bilateral in 25% of patients. On occasion, enterovirus may cause a similar picture.

End of Section.

STEP 9: *What Etiologic Organisms Should be Considered in the Infectious Pharyngitis Patient Presenting With Splenomegaly?*

The detection of splenomegaly in the patient with infectious pharyngitis should prompt consideration of infectious mononucleosis (EBV). Sixty percent of patients with infectious mononucleosis will have splenomegaly. The only other consideration is the acute retroviral syndrome, in which hepatosplenomegaly has been described in about 10% of patients.

Proceed to Step 10

STEP 10: *Does the Patient Have the Acute Retroviral Syndrome or Infectious Mononucleosis?*

Infectious mononucleosis (EBV) and the acute retroviral syndrome are diagnoses that may be missed if the clinician does not take the time to carefully consider these possibilities. This step will begin with a description of these two illnesses followed by a discussion of the features that may help differentiate the two.

Acute Retroviral Syndrome

Approximately 60% of patients with HIV infection experience an acute retroviral syndrome 3-6 weeks after primary infection. A high index of clinical suspicion and familiarity with the features of this syndrome are important in establishing the diagnosis. Recognition and diagnosis of this illness is important in preventing the further spread of the virus.

The illness is typically acute in onset, lasting 1-2 weeks. Sore throat is common and physical examination may reveal pharyngeal edema, usually without exudate.

Clinical Findings in the Acute Retroviral Syndrome	
General	**Dermatologic**
Anorexia	Alopecia
Arthralgias / myalgias (53%)	Diffuse urticaria
Cough	Erythematous maculopapular
Diarrhea (32%)	Mucocutaneous ulceration
Fever (97%)	Rash (70%)
Headache / retro-orbital pain (32%)	Roseola-like rash
Lymphadenopathy (77%)	
Nausea / vomiting (27%)	**Neurologic**
Pharyngitis (73%)	Encephalitis
Weight loss	Guillain-Barre syndrome
	Meningitis
	Myelopathy
	Peripheral neuropathy

Laboratory test abnormalities are generally nonspecific and do not allow differentiation of the acute retroviral syndrome from other acute viral illness. Leukopenia is common although, on occasion, leukocytosis may be appreciated. The differential count often reveals lymphopenia. Thrombocytopenia has been described in 45% of patients. An elevation in the transaminase levels has been noted in about 20% of patients. If CD4 and CD8 counts are obtained, an increase in the CD8 count along with an inversion in the CD4 to CD8 ratio may be noted.

Confirming the diagnosis requires determination of the serum p24 antigen levels or plasma HIV RNA. Seventy-five percent of patients with the acute retroviral syndrome will have detectable p24 antigenemia within the first two weeks after exposure. Determination of the plasma HIV RNA is more sensitive in the diagnosis of the acute retroviral syndrome. Assays for the HIV antibody (usually ELISA) should also be performed but may initially be negative. Follow-up to detect the appearance of the antibody is recommended.

Infectious Mononucleosis (EBV)

The Epstein-Barr virus is the major cause of infectious mononucleosis. Primarily affecting teenagers and young adults, infectious mononucleosis is an acute febrile illness. Most often, patients seek medical attention after about a week of nonspecific symptoms including headache, anorexia, and fever. At about this time in the course of the illness, adenopathy, splenomegaly, and pharyngitis may be noted. Pharyngitis, which is present in approximately 85% of patients, is often exudative and foul smelling. Almost all patients have posterior cervical lymphadenopathy. Some even have generalized lymphadenopathy.

Symptoms and Signs of Infectious Mononucleosis	
Symptoms	**Signs**
Malaise (100%)	Adenopathy (100%)
Sore throat (85%)	Fever (90%)
Warmth, chilliness (70%)	Pharyngitis (85%)
Anorexia (70%)	Splenomegaly (60%)
Headache (50%)	Bradycardia (40%)
Cough (40%)	Periorbital edema (25%)
Myalgia (25%)	Palatal enanthem (25%)
Arthralgia (5%)	Jaundice (10%)
Skin rash (5%)	
Diarrhea (5%)	
Photophobia (5%)	

A leukocytosis is commonly appreciated in patients with infectious mononucleosis, typically reaching a zenith during the second or third week of the illness. Early in the course of the illness, neutropenia may be noted. The differential count usually reveals an absolute lymphocytosis with marked atypical lymphocytes. The platelet count may be normal or depressed. The hemoglobin level is typically normal although, in a minority of cases, hemolytic anemia may be noted. A mild transaminitis is commonly encountered in the patient with infectious mononucleosis.

A positive monospot test corroborates the diagnosis. However, 5% to 10% of patients will have a negative test result. In these patients, the monospot test may be repeated. Alternatively, the clinician may elect to obtain Epstein-Barr viral serology.

Distinguishing the Acute Retroviral Syndrome from Infectious Mononucleosis

It can be difficult to distinguish infectious mononucleosis from the acute retroviral syndrome. In fact, the acute retroviral syndrome has classically been described as "mononucleosis-like." The clinical features that are helpful in differentiating the acute retroviral syndrome from infectious mononucleosis are listed in the following table.

	Acute Retroviral Syndrome	Infectious Mononucleosis (EBV)
Onset	Acute	Insidious
Tonsillar Hypertrophy	Little to none	Marked
Exudative Pharyngitis	Uncommon	Common
Mucocutaneous Ulceration	Common	Rare
Rash	Common	Rare (in the absence of ampicillin)
Diarrhea	In some	Does not occur
Jaundice	Rare	Reported in 8%
Enanthem	On hard palate	On border of hard and soft palate

Adapted from Gaines H, von Sydow M, Pehrson PO, et al, "Clinical Picture of Primary HIV Infection Presenting as a Glandular-Fever-Like Illness," *BMJ*, 1988, 297(6660):1363-8. Also adapted from Sande MA and Volberding PA (eds), *The Medical Management of AIDS*, 5th ed, Philadelphia, PA: WB Saunders Co, 1997, 95.

Because the pharyngitis of the acute retroviral syndrome and infectious mononucleosis may closely resemble streptococcal pharyngitis, all patients should be evaluated for group A β-hemolytic streptococcal pharyngitis.

For more information on group A β-hemolytic streptococcal pharyngitis, **Proceed to Step 11.**

STEP 11: *Does the Patient Have Group A β-Hemolytic Streptococcal Pharyngitis?*

Group A β-hemolytic streptococcal pharyngitis more commonly occurs during the winter and spring months. Following an incubation period of 2-4 days, individuals may complain of the abrupt onset of sore throat, fever, headache, and malaise. The classic features of group A β-hemolytic streptococcal pharyngitis are listed in the following box.

Classic Features of Group A β-Hemolytic Streptococcal Pharyngitis
Creamy white tonsillar exudate
Fever
Tender lymphadenopathy at the angle of the mandible

It is important to realize that <10% of patients will have all the classic features described in the previous box. Furthermore, some of these classic features may be noted in infectious pharyngitis due to other organisms. Symptoms that argue against group A β-hemolytic streptococcal pharyngitis include cough, hoarseness, conjunctivitis, coryza, ulcerative lesions, diarrhea, and rhinorrhea. The scarlatiniform rash of scarlet fever may be appreciated in infections caused by a strain carrying the erythrogenic toxin. The rash characteristically begins on the trunk only to spread centrifugally. This sandpapery rash tends to blanch with pressure. One week after the onset of the rash, desquamation, particularly of the skin over the palms and soles, occurs.

In general, the signs and symptoms of group A β-hemolytic streptococcal pharyngitis are not sufficiently specific to allow for diagnosis. A study performed recently allowed the separation of patients presenting with sore throat into three groups based on the following clinical features:

- Tonsillar exudate
- Tender anterior cervical adenopathy
- Fever (>100°F)

The percentage of patients having group A β-hemolytic streptococcal pharyngitis was then determined using throat culture as the gold standard.

Group	Clinical Features	% Having Positive Strep Cultures
1	Tonsillar exudate and Tender anterior cervical adenopathy and Temperature >100°F	42.1
2	Tonsillar exudate or Tender adenopathy or Temperature >100°F	13.5
3	None of the above findings	3.4

Deciding whether to perform laboratory testing for group A β-hemolytic streptococcal pharyngitis depends upon the presence of clinical and epidemiological findings that support the diagnosis. When clinical (as shown in the above table) and epidemiological findings (ie, close contact with well-documented case of streptococcal pharyngitis, high prevalence of group A β-hemolytic streptococcal pharyngitis in the community) supportive of the diagnosis are not present, laboratory testing is not necessary.

If clinical and epidemiological findings supportive of group A β-hemolytic streptococcal pharyngitis are not present, *Proceed to Step 12*.

The gold standard for the diagnosis is throat culture. However, the clinician should realize that false-negative cultures can occur, especially if the manner in which the culture was obtained was not appropriate. One disadvantage of the throat culture is that the results are often not available for 24-48 hours. To address this limitation of the throat culture, rapid antigen detection tests were developed.

Rapid antigen tests detect a carbohydrate antigen specific to the group A β-hemolytic streptococcus. Although the specificity of the test exceeds 95%, the sensitivity of the rapid antigen detection test varies from 60% to 95%, lower than that of culture. A positive result can be considered to represent infection. In these patients, treatment should be instituted with the following goals:

- Eradication of infection to prevent transmission
- Symptomatic relief
- Prevention of suppurative and nonsuppurative complications

When group A β-hemolytic streptococcal pharyngitis remains a consideration despite a negative rapid antigen test, the negative result should be confirmed with a throat culture.

If the patient has group A β-hemolytic streptococcal pharyngitis, *Stop Here.*

If the patient does not have group A β-hemolytic streptococcal pharyngitis, *Proceed to Step 12.*

STEP 12: *Does the Patient Have a Cause of Infectious Pharyngitis That Needs Further Evaluation or Treatment?*

Most cases not due to streptococcal pharyngitis, infectious mononucleosis, or the acute retroviral syndrome do not require further evaluation or treatment. One exception to this rule is in the patient with gonococcal pharyngitis. Most patients with gonococcal pharyngitis are completely asymptomatic. On occasion, however, symptoms may be severe. Gonococcal pharyngitis should be a consideration when homosexual males or women practicing fellatio present with infectious pharyngitis. Establishing the diagnosis requires culture with Thayer-Martin medium.

REFERENCES

Bisno AL, Gerber MA, Gwaltney JM, et al, "Diagnosis and Management of Group A Streptococcal Pharyngitis: A Practice Guideline. Infectious Diseases Society of America," *Clin Infect Dis*, 1997, 25(3):574-83.

Gaines H, von Sydow M, Pehrson PO, et al, "Clinical Picture of Primary HIV Infection Presenting as a Glandular-Fever-Like Illness," *BMJ*, 1988, 297(6660):1363-8.

Perkins A, "An Approach to Diagnosing the Acute Sore Throat," *Am Fam Phys*, 1997, 55(1):131-8, 141-2.

Perlmutter BL, Glaser JB, and Oyugi SO, "How to Recognize and Treat Acute HIV Syndrome," *Am Fam Phys*, 1999, 60(2):535-42, 545-6.

Peterson LR and Thomson RB, "Use of the Clinical Microbiology Laboratory for the Diagnosis and Management of Infectious Diseases Related to the Oral Cavity," *Infect Dis Clin North Am*, 1999, 13(4):775-95.

Pichichero ME, "Sore Throat After Sore Throat After Sore Throat. Are You Asking the Critical Questions?" *Postgrad Med*, 1997, 101(1):205-6, 209-12, 215-8.

Richardson MA, "Sore throat, Tonsillitis, and Adenoiditis," *Med Clin North Am*, 1999, 83(1):75-83.

The Medical Management of AIDS, 5th ed, Sande MA and Volberding PA (eds), Philadelphia, PA: WB Saunders Co, 1997, 95.

SYNCOPE

Syncope is defined as a transient loss of consciousness characterized by a loss of postural tone. It is typically sudden in onset with spontaneous recovery being the rule. Regardless of the etiology, syncope is the result of a decrease in or cessation of cerebral blood flow. While syncope is certainly an alarming symptom, in most cases, the etiology is benign. The challenge rests in identifying the patient with a serious cause. Prior to embarking on extensive evaluation to elucidate the etiology of the syncope, it is essential to differentiate syncope from dizziness, drop attacks, vertigo, coma, and seizures.

Proceed to Step 2

STEP 2: *Does the Patient Truly Have Syncope?*

It is usually not difficult to distinguish syncope from dizziness, drop attacks, vertigo, and coma based on the patient's clinical presentation. Loss of consciousness does not occur in patients with dizziness or vertigo. Drop attacks result in a fall with preservation of consciousness. Coma refers to a prolonged (rather than transient) loss of consciousness.

Differentiating syncope from seizure, however, is often more difficult. Clues that allow the clinician to differentiate between the two are listed in the following table.

	Syncope	Seizure
Facial Color	Pale	Blue
Frothing at Mouth	Absent	Present
Tongue Biting	Absent	Present
Disorientation After Event	Absent	Present
Sleepiness After Event	Absent	Present
Duration of Episode	Usually <5 minutes	Often >5 minutes
Aura	Absent	Sometimes present
Onset	More gradual	More sudden
Injury From Falling	More frequent	Less frequent
Upturning of the Eyes	Common	Uncommon
Urinary Incontinence	Uncommon	Common
Creatine Kinase Elevation	Uncommon	Common
Jerks	Rare	Frequent

If the patient has not had syncope, **Stop Here.**

If the patient has had syncope, **Proceed to Step 3.**

STEP 3: *What are the Causes of Syncope?*

The causes of syncope are listed in the following box.

Causes of Syncope	
Cardiac	Bradyarrhythmias
Organic heart disease	Sinus node disease
Myocardial infarction	AV block (2nd or 3rd)
Aortic stenosis	Pacemaker malfunction
Hypertrophic cardiomyopathy	Orthostatic hypotension
Pulmonary hypertension	Neurally-mediated syncope
Atrial myxoma	Vasovagal syncope
Pulmonary embolism	Situational syncope
Aortic dissection	Cough
Cardiac tamponade	Defecation
Mitral stenosis	Micturition
Arrhythmia	Swallow
Tachyarrhythmias	Carotid sinus syncope
Supraventricular tachycardia	Neurologic
Ventricular tachycardia	TIA/CVA
Torsade de pointes	Migraine
	Subclavian steal syndrome
	Psychiatric

Proceed to Step 4

STEP 4: *What are the Common Causes of Syncope?*

The information in the following table is pooled from the results of five studies performed in the 1980s, which looked at the common causes of syncope.

Cause	Mean Prevalence (%)
Neurally-mediated syncope	
Vasovagal attack	18
Situational syncope	5
Carotid-sinus syncope	1
Psychiatric disorders	2
Orthostatic hypotension	8
Medications	3
Neurologic disease	10
Cardiac syncope	
Organic heart disease*	4
Arrhythmias	14
Unknown	34

*Organic heart disease refers to structural heart disease that causes syncope, such as aortic stenosis, pulmonary hypertension, pulmonary embolism, or myocardial infarction.

Adapted from Linzer M, Yang EH, Estes NA, et al, "Diagnosing Syncope. Part 1: Value of History, Physical Examination, and Electrocardiography. Clinical Efficacy Assessment Project of the American College of Physicians," *Ann Intern Med*, 1997, 126(12):989-96 (review); also from Kapoor WN, "Syncope," *N Engl J Med*, 2000, 343(25):1856-62 (review).

Proceed to Step 5

> **STEP 5:** *Does the History and Physical Examination Readily Identify the Cause of the Syncope?*

It is said that the history and physical examination identify the cause of syncope in nearly 50% of cases. Neurally mediated syncope (vasovagal, situational, carotid sinus syncope) and orthostatic hypotension account for most of these cases. Clues in the history and physical examination that point to these conditions are listed in the following table.

Historical or Physical Examination Clue	Condition Suggested
Syncope following fear, anxiety, pain, etc	Vasovagal syncope
On standing/arising	Orthostatic hypotension
Occurring during or immediately after urination, swallowing, defecation	Situational syncope
Prolonged standing at attention	Vasovagal syncope
Prodrome of warmth, nausea, sweating, and light-headedness	Vasovagal syncope
Occurring with shaving, tight collar, sudden turn of the head	Carotid sinus syncope
Orthostatic change in blood pressure and heart rate	Orthostatic hypotension

The remainder of this step will consider these conditions in further detail.

Neurally-Mediated Syncope

It is important to differentiate neurally mediated from cardiac causes of syncope because the former is a benign condition, which has an excellent prognosis. A large number of patients with syncope will have a neurally mediated cause. The causes of neurally mediated syncope are listed in the box below.

Causes of Neurally-Mediated Syncope
Carotid sinus syncope
Situational
Cough
Defecation
Micturition
Swallow
Vasovagal

Vasovagal syncope, the common faint, is the most common cause of neurally mediated syncope. It typically has a precipitant. Common precipitants include prolonged standing, pain, and emotional upset. Not uncommonly, patients complain of prodromal symptoms such as nausea, weakness, and diaphoresis. Vasovagal syncope may, however, occur without any identifiable precipitants.

In carotid sinus syncope, episodes may be provoked when pressure is placed on the carotid sinus. As such, syncope may be precipitated by a tight collar, shaving, or sudden turning. Unfortunately, this classic history is elicited in only 25% of patients. Carotid sinus syncope is a fairly common cause of unexplained syncope in older individuals, particularly those >50 years of age, Carotid sinus syncope is discussed further in Step 12.

Orthostatic Hypotension

Patients with orthostatic hypotension classically complain of light-headedness or dizziness when moving from a supine to upright position. Some patients, however, may describe a weakness or even a blurring or loss of vision with the change in position. Yet others may have a syncopal event. The history often reveals the symptoms to be worse when the patient arises in the morning. The two most common causes of orthostatic hypotension include decreased intravascular volume and medications. The causes of orthostatic hypotension are listed in the following box.

Causes of Orthostatic Hypotension	
Medications	Alcoholism
Antidepressants	Adrenal insufficiency
Tricyclic	Aging
Monoamine oxidase inhibitors	Spinal cord lesions
Antihypertensive agents	Central brain lesions
Prazosin	Multiple system atrophy (Shy-Drager)
Hydralazine	Tabes dorsalis
Calcium channel blockers	Syringomyelia
ACE-inhibitors	Multiple sclerosis
Guanethidine	Mastocytosis
Methyldopa	Carcinoid syndrome
Clonidine	Volume depletion
α-adrenergic blockers	Blood loss
Tranquilizers	Prolonged bed rest
Phenothiazines	Prolonged standing
Barbiturates	Dehydration
Diabetes mellitus	Amyloidosis

To establish the diagnosis of orthostatic hypotension, the blood pressure and heart rate should be measured in both the supine and standing positions. After the supine values are obtained, values should be measured immediately upon standing and several minutes later. An orthostatic decrease in the systolic blood pressure of at least 20 mm Hg and/or diastolic blood pressure of at least 10 mm Hg is considered to be significant. A lowering of the systolic and/or diastolic blood pressure that is unaccompanied by an increase in the heart rate suggests autonomic neuropathy as the cause of the orthostatic hypotension.

If the patient has neurally mediated syncope or orthostatic hypotension, *Stop Here.*

If the patient does not have neurally mediated syncope or orthostatic hypotension, *Proceed to Step 6.*

STEP 6: *Do the History and Physical Examination Suggest the Etiology of the Syncope?*

Step 5 considered the causes of syncope that are readily identified by history and physical examination. In many cases, however, the history and physical examination are suggestive but not diagnostic of the etiology of the syncope. These conditions are listed in the following box.

Conditions in Which History and Physical Examination are Suggestive but Not Diagnostic of the Etiology of the Syncope	
Aortic dissection	Pulmonary embolism
Atrial myxoma	Pulmonary hypertension
Cardiac tamponade	Valvular heart disease
Myocardial infarction	Aortic stenosis
Neurologic disease	Hypertrophic obstructive
Migraine	cardiomyopathy
Subclavian steal syndrome	Mitral stenosis
TIA/CVA	

The remainder of this step will consider these causes of syncope in further detail.

Neurologic Causes of Syncope

Clues in the history and physical examination that point to a neurologic cause of syncope are listed in the following table.

Historical or Physical Examination Clue	Condition Suggested
Associated with vertigo, dysarthria, diplopia, and other motor or sensory findings localized to brainstem	Vertebrobasilar TIA/CVA Basilar artery migraine Subclavian steal syndrome
After upper extremity exercise	Subclavian steal syndrome
Focal neurologic deficits	Neurologic cause of syncope
Significant difference in systolic blood pressure between one arm and the other*	Subclavian steal syndrome

*Systolic blood pressure difference exceeding 20 mm Hg (between one arm and the other) carries a 90% association with subclavian steal syndrome. Such a difference may also be appreciated in patients with aortic dissection.

Neurologic causes of syncope are listed in the following box.

Neurologic Causes of Syncope	
TIA/CVA*	Migraine‡
Subclavian steal syndrome†	Seizure#

*Only 5% of transient ischemic attacks or cerebrovascular accidents are accompanied by syncope. Syncope is more common in those suffering vertebrobasilar TIA or CVA. In these patients, other neurological symptoms are always present, some of which include vertigo, dysarthria, diplopia, and paresthesias. Syncope is rarely appreciated in patients with carotid artery disease even when severe.

†When exercise of an arm leads to symptoms of basilar insufficiency including syncope, the clinician should consider the subclavian steal syndrome. In this syndrome, blockage of the subclavian artery proximal to the vertebral artery may lead to a reversal in blood flow, with blood flowing from the vertebrobasilar system into the arm. Other symptoms include transient weakness of the arm with exercise. Claudication of the arm with exercise is another feature of this syndrome. A greater than 20 mm Hg difference in the blood pressure between the two arms supports the diagnosis.

‡While close to 20% of patients with migraine report a faint sensation, syncope is uncommon. It does tend to occur, however, in patients with basilar artery migraine. This rare disorder, which typically begins in adolescence, is usually accompanied by other symptoms and signs of brainstem ischemia. All patients with migraine are susceptible to a vasovagal syncopal event from pain.

#The first step in the approach of the patient presenting with syncope is the differentiation of syncope from seizure. While the history often permits the clinician to do so, some types of seizures are nonconvulsive. An example is temporal lobe epilepsy. In this form of epilepsy, a sudden fall may occur, followed by a brief period of unconsciousness. There may be some degree of confusion after the loss of consciousness. An interictal EEG may show temporal lobe epileptic abnormalities.

Valvular Heart Disease

Syncope due to valvular heart disease deserves consideration when auscultation reveals the presence of a murmur. The types of valvular heart disease associated with syncope are listed in the following box.

Causes of Syncope Due to Valvular Heart Disease	
Aortic stenosis*	Hypertrophic obstructive cardiomyopathy‡
Mitral stenosis†	

*While dyspnea on exertion and chest pain are the two most common symptoms that prompt patients with aortic stenosis to seek medical care, syncope may be the initial manifestation in a small percentage of patients (15% to 30%). Classically, the syncope is exercise related, usually occurring during or after exercise. This is thought to be due to vasodilatation in the exercising muscles in the setting of a fixed cardiac output. Arrhythmia is another cause of syncope in aortic stenosis. Syncope is a poor prognostic factor in patients with aortic stenosis. Most patients will succumb to their disease within two to three years if valve replacement is not performed.

†Mitral stenosis is a rare cause of syncope. In these patients, exertional syncope is the result of the obstruction to left ventricular filling. With exertion, a higher cardiac output is needed and the obstruction to left ventricular filling prevents this from occurring. As a result, cerebral perfusion falls, leading to syncope.

‡A family history of syncope should prompt concern for hypertrophic obstructive cardiomyopathy. The absence of a family history does not exclude the diagnosis since sporadic cases are not uncommon. Common symptoms of this condition include shortness of breath, palpitations, exertional chest pain, near-syncope, and syncope. Syncope is reported in up to 30% of patients. Any factor (ie, Valsalva, coughing) that worsens left ventricular outflow obstruction can cause syncope. Predictors of syncope include age <30, nonsustained ventricular tachycardia, and left ventricular end diastolic volume index <60 mL/m^2.

The physical examination findings of these different types of valvular heart disease are considered in the following box.

Physical Examination Finding	Condition Suggested
Pulsus parvus et tardus	
Diminished pulse pressure	
Accentuated a wave in jugular venous pulse	
Lateral displacement of apical impulse	
Systolic thrill at base of heart	
Systolic murmur	
Loudest at base	
Harsh	Aortic stenosis
Crescendo-decrescendo murmur	
Low-pitched	
Best heard over aortic area	
Radiation to the carotid area	
Paradoxical splitting of second heart sound (or single soft S2)	
Fourth heart sound	
Opening snap	
Loud S1	Mitral stenosis
Rumbling diastolic murmur	
Bisferiens pulse	
Murmur	
Systolic ejection	
Best heard at left lower border radiating to apex	Hypertrophic obstructive cardiomyopathy
Prominent a wave in jugular venous pulse	
S4	

EKG findings noted in these conditions are listed in the following table.

Condition	EKG Findings
Mitral stenosis	Left atrial abnormality (50%)
	Atrial fibrillation (50%)
	Vertical or rightward mean QRS axis*
	Right ventricular hypertrophy*
Aortic stenosis	Left ventricular hypertrophy (90%)
	ST segment depression and T-wave inversion in lead I and left precordial leads
	Left atrial abnormality (80%)
	Atrial fibrillation (late finding)
Hypertrophic obstructive cardiomyopathy	Left ventricular hypertrophy
	ST-T wave changes
	Left atrial abnormality
	Abnormal Q waves (pseudoinfarct pattern)

*These findings suggest the development of pulmonary hypertension.

Chest radiographic findings that may be noted in these types of valvular heart disease are listed in the following table.

Condition	Chest Radiographic Finding
Mitral stenosis	Left atrial enlargement
	Pulmonary venous hypertension
	Enlargement of pulmonary arteries*
	Right ventricular enlargement*
Aortic stenosis	Heart size usually normal
	Apex can become prominent with rounding of left heart border
	Poststenotic dilatation of the aorta
	Calcification of aortic valve
Hypertrophic obstructive cardiomyopathy	Mild to moderate cardiomegaly (can be normal)
	Enlarged left atrial shadow

*These findings suggest the development of pulmonary hypertension.

Echocardiography can confirm the diagnosis of valvular heart disease.

Atrial Myxoma

Atrial myxoma is the most common intracavitary tumor of the heart, occurring more commonly on the left than the right. Systemic symptoms and signs include fever, cachexia, malaise, rash, arthralgias, clubbing, and Raynaud's phenomenon. Most often, patients will present with signs and symptoms of mitral valve obstruction. Systemic emboli are a real concern in atrial myxoma patients, most of which travel to the central nervous system. Not uncommonly, however, the initial presentation may be peripheral emboli of unclear etiology. The mechanism of syncope in atrial myxoma is similar to that of mitral stenosis. In addition to exertional syncope, patients with atrial myxoma may also develop syncope with postural changes. In some, syncope may occur with simply rolling over in bed. Physical examination findings consistent with atrial myxoma include tumor plop and diastolic rumble. Variability of the physical exam findings with changes in body position may also be noted. Echocardiography is useful in establishing the diagnosis.

Myocardial Infarction

5% to 12% of elderly patients may present with syncope as the presenting symptom of a myocardial infarction. Syncope may be the result of pump failure if sufficient amounts of myocardium have been jeopardized. Alternatively, a myocardial infarction may result in a bradyarrhythmia or tachyarrhythmia. In younger patients, myocardial infarction is a rare cause of syncope. The history, physical examination, EKG, and cardiac enzymes will help exclude myocardial infarction.

Pulmonary Embolism

Syncope due to pulmonary embolism should be a consideration, particularly in those who have a risk factor for venous thromboembolism. These risk factors are listed in the following box.

Risk Factors for Venous Thromboembolism	
Advancing age	Congestive heart failure
Hypercoagulable state	Obesity
Activated protein C resistance	Trauma
Antithrombin III deficiency	Pregnancy
Protein C deficiency	Oral contraceptives
Protein S deficiency	Malignancy
Dysfibrinogenemia	Nephrotic syndrome
Hyperhomocysteinemia	Paroxysmal nocturnal hemoglobinuria
Prothrombin gene mutation	Polycythemia vera
Antiphospholipid antibody syndrome	Essential thrombocytosis
Surgery	Immobilization

Syncope has been reported in up to 15% of patients with pulmonary embolism. Accompanying symptoms include sudden shortness of breath and central chest pain. When present, these symptoms suggest the presence of large emboli in the main or lobular pulmonary arteries (massive pulmonary embolism). Although CXR may be normal in some patients, in others focal oligemia (Westermark's sign), enlarged right descending pulmonary artery, or peripheral wedge-shaped density (Hampton's hump) may be appreciated. The principal test used to establish the diagnosis is ventilation/perfusion scan.

Aortic Dissection

Aortic dissection most commonly occurs between the fifth and seventh decades of life. It tends to have a predilection for men. Risk factors for aortic dissection include hypertension, Marfan's syndrome, Turner's syndrome, and pregnancy. An increased frequency of aortic dissection has been noted among individuals having coarctation of the aorta or bicuspid aortic valve. Dissection may also be iatrogenic, complicating cardiac catheterization, coronary artery bypass grafting, and intra-aortic balloon counterpulsation.

Most patients with dissection present with chest pain, often described as "ripping," "cutting," or "tearing." Although most describe chest pain, pain may be appreciated in the interscapular, lumbar, or epigastric regions. Particularly characteristic of the pain is its sudden onset and maximal intensity from the onset.

In a minority of patients, the aortic dissection is painless. Many of these patients present with a sudden neurological event with syncope being the most common manifestation. The syncope is almost always due to the rupture of the ascending aorta into the pericardial space, resulting in cardiac tamponade. Syncope occurs in 5% of patients with aortic dissection.

Physical examination findings vary depending on the location of the dissection. The following table makes a distinction between dissection of the ascending and descending aorta.

	Proximal Dissection	Distal Dissection
Murmur of Aortic Regurgitation	Approximately 50%	Rare
Pulse Deficit	Approximately 50%	15% to 20%
Neither AR Murmur Nor Pulse Deficit	15% to 20%	75%
Hypotension	20%	Rare
Severe Hypertension	Unusual	Frequent

Adapted from *Hurst's The Heart, Arteries and Veins*, 9th ed, Alexander RW, Schlant RC, and Fuster V (eds), New York, NY: McGraw-Hill, 1998, 2473.

Chest radiography may reveal dilatation of the ascending aorta in patients having proximal aortic dissection. Dilatation of the aortic knob and descending aorta may be appreciated with distal dissection. Confirmation of the diagnosis requires transesophageal echocardiography or CT scan.

Pulmonary Hypertension

Common symptoms of pulmonary hypertension include shortness of breath, chest pain, fatigue, edema, and syncope. Syncope may be exertional. In these cases, it is due the inability to increase right ventricular output with exercise. The chest pain of pulmonary hypertension may also be exertional, closely resembling angina. Physical examination findings consistent with pulmonary hypertension are listed in the following box.

Physical Examination Findings of Pulmonary Hypertension	
Abnormal c and v waves	Right-sided S3
Jugular venous distention	Right-sided S4
Prominent and delayed P2	Right ventricular heave
Prominent a wave	

EKG findings supportive of pulmonary hypertension include the following:

- Right atrial abnormality
- Right bundle branch block or right ventricular conduction delay
- S wave in lead I
- Tall, initial R wave in V1

Cardiac catheterization is the gold standard in the diagnosis of pulmonary hypertension. However, since it is an invasive test that may carry an increased risk of death in patients with severe pulmonary hypertension, the clinician may elect to perform noninvasive testing such as echocardiography to establish the diagnosis. Once the presence of pulmonary hypertension has been confirmed, the clinician should identify the etiology of the pulmonary hypertension. The causes are listed in the following box.

Causes of Pulmonary Hypertension	
α_1-antitrypsin deficiency	Cystic fibrosis
Alveolar hypoventilation	Hepatopulmonary syndrome
Central nervous system dysfunction	Interstitial lung disease
Chest wall dysfunction	Medications
Neuromuscular disease	Primary pulmonary hypertension
Obesity	Residence at high altitude
Sleep apnea	Thromboembolic disease
Chronic obstructive pulmonary disease	Veno-occlusive disease
Connective tissue disease	

Cardiac Tamponade

Cardiac tamponade is characterized by the development of increased pressure in the pericardial sac due to accumulation of fluid. If the pressure is sufficiently elevated, filling of the heart may be compromised, resulting in hypotension. There are many causes of cardiac tamponade. Most often, tamponade is due to viral or idiopathic pericarditis, malignancy, uremia, or trauma. Dyspnea is a commonly encountered complaint. Pleuritic chest pain may or may not be present.

Physical examination may reveal tachypnea, tachycardia, elevated jugular venous pressure, and pulsus paradoxus. Hypotension is not invariably present. In most cases, it is a late manifestation of tamponade. It is also important to realize that pulsus paradoxus is not specific for tamponade. Asthma and chronic obstructive pulmonary disease are two conditions in which pulsus paradoxus has been noted.

Beat to beat variation in the height of the EKG (electrical alternans) is an infrequent finding in patients with cardiac tamponade. Although a chest radiograph should be obtained, not all patients will have an enlarged cardiac silhouette. In cases characterized by the rapid accumulation of pericardial fluid, the silhouette may be normal.

Echocardiography is very useful in providing support for the diagnosis of tamponade. Echocardiographic findings consistent with tamponade include right and/or left atrial diastolic collapse and right ventricular diastolic collapse. It is important to realize that the echocardiographic findings are not 100% sensitive and specific in the diagnosis of cardiac tamponade. If there is any uncertainty, the clinician may wish to perform right heart catheterization.

If the etiology of the syncope is identified, **Stop Here.**

If the etiology of the syncope is not identified, **Proceed to Step 7.**

STEP 7: *Does the Patient Have Heart Disease?*

When the etiology of the syncope remains unclear after a thorough history and physical examination, the clinician should ascertain whether the patient has structural or organic heart disease. In some patients, a history of heart disease is known at the time of their presentation. In others, it is suspected from the history and physical examination findings. There is, however, a subset of patients in which heart disease is not suspected but is detected only with testing. It is important to identify the patient with structural or organic heart disease since syncope may be the manifestation of a potentially life-threatening arrhythmia.

An EKG should be obtained in most patients with syncope, particularly when the cause is not evident from the history and physical examination. While the yield of an EKG is low, the test is relatively inexpensive and noninvasive. The initial EKG identifies the cause of the syncope in only 5% of patients. It may, however, suggest an etiology in a fair number of patients. In fact, 25% to 50% of patients will have abnormalities that are nondiagnostic but suggestive of a particular etiology. The clinical significance of abnormalities identified on the EKG in patients with syncope are listed in the following table.

EKG Finding	Cause of Syncope Suggested
Normal or nonspecific	Does not rule out serious cause of syncope
Delta waves	WPW (possible supraventricular tachycardia)
Sinus bradycardia	Nonspecific (may indicate sick sinus syndrome)
Myocardial infarction	Arrhythmia Hemodynamic problem
Bundle branch block	Heart block Ventricular tachycardia
QT prolongation	Torsade de pointes
Paced rhythm	Consider pacemaker malfunction
First degree heart block	No obvious significance in most cases
Epsilon waves	Right ventricular dysplasia
Atrial fibrillation	Underlying structural heart disease Arrhythmic cause
Complete heart block	Complete heart block
Supraventricular tachycardia	Supraventricular tachycardia
Ventricular tachycardia	Ventricular tachycardia

Adapted from Grubb BP and Olshansky B, *Syncope: Mechanisms and Management*, Armonk, NY: Futura Publishing Co, 1997, 43.

The likelihood of an arrhythmia as the cause of the syncope is low when the EKG is normal. These patients have a low risk for sudden death. In summary, the EKG can provide important diagnostic and prognostic information in patients presenting with syncope.

If the history, physical examination, and EKG findings support the presence of structural or organic heart disease, *Proceed to Step 8*.

If heart disease cannot be excluded based on the history, physical examination, and EKG findings, *Proceed to Step 8*.

If heart disease can be excluded based on the history, physical examination, and EKG findings, *Proceed to Step 12*.

STEP 8: *Does the Patient Need an Echocardiogram and / or Exercise Stress Test?*

The clinician may wish to perform echocardiography in the following patients:

- Presence or absence of heart disease cannot be determined based on the history, physical examination, and EKG findings

  The role of echocardiography in this group of patients is to identify the presence of structural or organic heart disease, findings suggestive of an arrhythmic cause of syncope. The clinician may forego echocardiography in younger patients with no history of heart disease and an unremarkable physical examination. In these patients, the yield of echocardiography is quite low. In those >50 years of age, however, echocardiography should be considered even if the history, physical examination, and EKG findings are not consistent with heart disease.

- History, physical examination, and EKG findings support the presence of structural or organic heart disease

  If the initial assessment suggest the presence of structural or organic heart disease, the clinician should consider performing echocardiography. Echocardiography can not only confirm the presence of heart disease but can also provide information as to the severity and extent of the heart disease.

Exercise stress testing is recommended if either of the following hold true:

- Patient has syncope during or after exercise
- Clinical evaluation suggests presence of ischemic heart disease

In patients with exertional syncope, it is important to perform echocardiography before exercise stress testing to exclude hypertrophic obstructive cardiomyopathy.

If the echocardiography and/or exercise stress test confirm the presence of structural or organic heart disease, *Proceed to Step 9.*

If echocardiography or exercise stress testing do not reveal the presence of structural or organic heart disease, *Proceed to Step 12.*

STEP 9: *What are the Results of the Holtor Monitor?*

In patients with heart disease, the initial step in elucidating the etiology is prolonged EKG or Holtor monitoring. Prolonged EKG monitoring can detect an arrhythmic cause if the patient develops symptoms that correlate with the presence of an arrhythmia. Unfortunately, this correlation is identified in only 5% of patients. In 17% of patients, symptoms occur that do not correlate with an arrhythmia, thus excluding an arrhythmic cause of the syncope.

In the remaining 80% of patients, one of two outcomes is noted:

- No symptoms or rhythm disturbances documented
- Rhythm disturbances documented while patient is asymptomatic

These findings can be considered to be nondiagnostic. When there is a high pretest likelihood for arrhythmia, these nondiagnostic findings should not be considered reassuring. In these cases, the clinician should consult cardiology regarding the need for electrophysiology studies.

If the Holtor monitor reveals no rhythm disturbance during a time when the patient is symptomatic, then an arrhythmic cause has been excluded. *Proceed to Step 12.*

If the Holtor monitor reveals an arrhythmia during a time when the patient is symptomatic, then the evaluation and treatment should be directed at the arrhythmia identified.

If the Holtor monitor is nondiagnostic, *Proceed to Step 10.*

STEP 10: *Does the Patient Need Electrophysiologic Testing?*

Because of the infrequent nature of most arrhythmias that cause syncope, it is not unusual for prolonged EKG monitoring to be unrevealing. In those with heart disease, electrophysiologic testing should be considered to assess for arrhythmic causes of syncope. It is an invasive procedure that employs stimulation of the atria and ventricles to detect a clinically significant arrhythmia.

Simply inducing an arrhythmia during electrophysiologic testing does not establish that the arrhythmia is the cause of the syncope. Of particular value is the reproduction of symptoms (palpitations, near-syncope, syncope) when an arrhythmia is induced. Under these circumstances, the diagnosis is fairly certain. In other instances, however, an arrhythmia is induced but the patient remains asymptomatic. In these cases, the induced arrhythmia may not be the cause of the syncope. The clinician should also realize that not all arrhythmias are identified during electrophysiologic testing. In particular, bradyarrhythmias related to sinus or AV node dysfunction may not always be detected.

Tachyarrhythmias

The most common abnormality identified during electrophysiologic testing is sustained monomorphic ventricular tachycardia. When induced, this rhythm is the likely cause of the syncope. When electrophysiologic testing does not induce this rhythm, however, one cannot exclude ventricular tachycardia as the cause of the syncope. Predictors of ventricular tachycardia by electrophysiologic testing are listed in the following box.

Predictors of Ventricular Tachycardia by Electrophysiologic Testing	
Bundle branch block*	Organic heart disease
NSVT on Holtor monitoring	PVCs

*Up to 30% will have inducible ventricular tachycardia

The induction of nonsustained ventricular tachycardia or polymorphic ventricular tachycardia often represents a nonspecific response to aggressive stimulation of the ventricles. Therefore, the elicitation of the latter arrhythmias have little clinical significance. Very little clinical significance is also attached to the finding of ventricular fibrillation that occurs during electrophysiologic testing. When a supraventricular tachycardia is induced along with hypotension, the tachycardia may be presumed to be the cause of the syncope.

Bradyarrhythmias

After ventricular tachycardia, the two most common arrhythmic causes of syncope are sinus node dysfunction and AV block. Electrophysiologic testing may be used to detect these bradyarrhythmias. Predictors of bradyarrhythmia in those undergoing electrophysiologic testing are listed in the following box.

Predictors of Bradyarrhythmia	
Bundle branch block	Sinus bradycardia
First degree AV block	

Although electrophysiologic testing is often used to evaluate sinus node function, abnormal findings do not always indicate that sinus node dysfunction is the etiology of the syncope. A sinus node recovery time that exceeds 3 seconds is suggestive of sinus node dysfunction but it is preferable to demonstrate a clinical relationship between near-syncope and syncope and sinus node dysfunction. When no other cause for syncope can be found in the patient having a prolonged sinus node recovery time, many advocate the implantation of a pacemaker.

In the absence of documented high degree AV block by electrocardiography, it may be difficult to firmly link findings consistent with AV nodal dysfunction found on electrophysiologic testing to the syncope. An HV interval exceeding 100 msec or infranodal block induced by pacing are suggestive of a bradyarrhythmic cause of the syncope. However, block occurring within the AV node is not well detected by testing. The clinician should realize, however, that the underlying causes of AV nodal dysfunction also predispose patients to ventricular tachyarrhythmias. As a result, a thorough evaluation should be performed to exclude ventricular tachyarrhythmias in these patients. If no other cause of syncope can be identified, a prolonged HV interval can be considered to be the probable cause of the syncope.

If the electrophysiologic testing is positive, *Stop Here.*

If the electrophysiologic testing is negative, *Proceed to Step 11.*

STEP 11: *Should the Patient Have an Event Monitor?*

In patients who have had a negative electrophysiologic study, the incidence of sudden death is low. The study may, however, be falsely-negative in patients with sinus node dysfunction or AV block. To identify these patients, the clinician should consider long-term monitoring using an event monitor. The event monitor will have a greater yield in those who have recurrent syncope. With activation after a syncopal event, the monitor will capture the heart rhythm for some minutes before and after activation.

If the results of the event monitor reveal the cause of the syncope, *Stop Here.*

If the results of the event monitor do not reveal the cause of the syncope, *Proceed to Step 12.*

STEP 12: *What Should be Considered in the Patient With No Cause Identified?*

In many of these patients, the syncope will not recur. In others, further episodes may be rare. In those who have had a thorough evaluation (including extensive cardiac evaluation when indicated), the short-term prognosis is good.

However, the recurrence rate may be as high as 20% to 30%. Should repeat extensive evaluations be performed in this group of patients? In the majority of these patients, repeating an extensive evaluation is usually not helpful. Many of these patients may be suffering from neurally mediated (vasovagal) syncope or syncope related to psychiatric illness. These possibilities will be discussed in the remainder of this step.

Neurally-Mediated Syncope

Establishing a diagnosis of neurally-mediated syncope requires a tilt table test. Nearly 50% of patients with unexplained syncope have a positive tilt table test. The development of hypotension and/or bradycardia during upright tilt table testing is highly suggestive of spontaneous vasovagal syncope. Usually performed in the electrophysiology laboratory, this test is initially done as a passive test. If passive testing fails to establish the diagnosis, tilt testing may be performed using a pharmacologic agent such as isoproterenol. With the infusion of isoproterenol, the false-negativity rate of tilt table testing rises (30% vs 14%). Many authorities recommend stress testing prior to tilt table studies in men and women >45 and 55 years of age, respectively.

Not all patients with unexplained syncope require tilt table studies. Many experts do not perform tilt table studies in all patients with unexplained syncope. Often tilt table testing is reserved for those who have more than one episode of syncope.

Tilt table testing may also be helpful in the evaluation of carotid sinus hypersensitivity, another cause of recurrent unexplained syncope. In these patients, the diagnostic yield of carotid sinus massage during tilt table testing may be increased.

Carotid Sinus Syncope

Carotid sinus syncope is one type of neurally mediated syncope. The classic history of syncope precipitated by a tight collar, sudden turning, or shaving is often not present. Therefore, in elderly patients with recurrent syncope, carotid sinus syncope deserves consideration.

To confirm the diagnosis, carotid massage may be performed. Prior to the procedure, it is important to have a defibrillator readily available because, in rare instances, prolonged asystole or ventricular arrhythmias may be precipitated by massage. Other complications include transient or permanent neurological deficit or even sudden death. These complications, however, are very rare. Prior to performing carotid massage, the clinician should auscultate for bruits, suggestive of cerebrovascular disease.

The patient should be placed supine with the neck slightly extended. Bilateral massage should never be performed. Pressure should be applied for ten to fifteen seconds followed by a pause of 15 seconds prior to exerting more pressure either on the same side or the other side.

Massage may allow the diagnosis of one of the three forms of carotid sinus hypersensitivity. Cardioinhibitory carotid sinus hypersensitivity is present when cardiac asystole of 3 or more seconds is noted. The vasodepressor form is diagnosed when the systolic pressure falls more than 50 mm Hg. When features of both cardioinhibitory and vasodepressor forms are present, the patient is considered to have the mixed form of the disease. The diagnosis is established when one of these characteristic forms is identified in conjunction with symptoms. The lack of symptoms in a patient fulfilling the criteria for one of the above forms may also be considered to represent carotid sinus hypersensitivity, especially in patients with recurrent syncope who have had an otherwise negative evaluation.

Psychiatric Illness

Syncope has been well described in patients with psychiatric illness. Syncope has been reported in patients with generalized anxiety disorder, panic disorder, major depression, and somatization disorder. It is important to establish the diagnosis because this type of syncope tends to be recurrent. Screening tests are available to establish the presence of these various disorders. It deserves consideration particularly in younger patients with recurrent symptoms. Several studies have suggested that a hyperventilation maneuver be used in the identification of syncope associated with psychiatric illness. In these studies, investigators demonstrated that the development of near syncope or true syncope following open-mouthed hyperventilation was predictive of a psychiatric cause of syncope.

REFERENCES

Benditt DG, Lurie KG, and Fabian WH, "Clinical Approach to Diagnosis of Syncope. An Overview," *Cardiol Clin*, 1997, 15(2):165-76.

Forman DE and Lipsitz LA, "Syncope in the Elderly," *Cardiol Clin*, 1997, 15(2):295-311.

Grubb BP and Karas B, "Diagnosis and Management of Neurocardiogenic Syncope," *Curr Opin Cardiol*, 1997, 13(1):29-35.

Hayes OW, "Evaluation of Syncope in the Emergency Department," *Emerg Med Clin North Am*, 1998, 16(3):601-15.

Hurst's The Heart, Arteries and Veins, 9th ed, Alexander RW, Schlant RC, and Fuster V (eds), New York, NY: McGraw-Hill, 1998, 2473.

Kapoor WN, "Syncope," *N Eng J Med*, 2000, 343(25):1856-62 (review).

Kapoor WN, "Using a Tilt Table to Evaluate Syncope," *Am J Med Sci*, 1999, 317(2):110-6.

Linzer M, Yang EH, Estes NA, et al, "Diagnosing Syncope. Part 1: Value of History, Physical Examination, and Electrocardiography. Clinical Efficacy Assessment Project of the American College of Physicians," *Ann Intern Med*, 1997, 126(12):989-96 (review).

Linzer M, Yang EH, Estes NA, et al, "Diagnosing Syncope. Part 2: Unexplained Syncope. Clinical Efficacy Assessment Project of the American College of Physicians," *Ann Intern Med*, 1997, 127(1):76-86.

Meyer MD and Handler J, "Evaluation of the Patient With Syncope: An Evidence Based Approach," *Emerg Med Clin North Am*, 1999, 17(1):189-201.

Sutton R and Bloomfield DM, "Indications, Methodology, and Classification of Results of Tilt-Table Testing," *Am J Cardiol*, 1999, 84(8A):10Q-19Q.

Syncope: Mechanisms and Management, Grubb B and Olshansky B (eds), Armonk, NY: Futura Publishing Co, 1998, 43.

Wolff GS, "Unexplained Syncope: Clinical Management," *Pacing Clin Electrophysiol*, 1997, 20(8 Pt 2):2043-7.

SYNCOPE

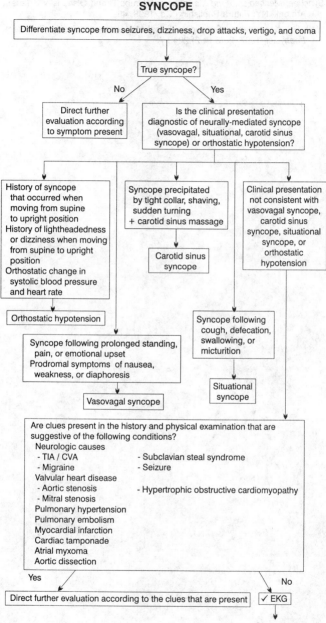

Differentiate syncope from seizures, dizziness, drop attacks, vertigo, and coma

True syncope?

No — Direct further evaluation according to symptom present

Yes — Is the clinical presentation diagnostic of neurally-mediated syncope (vasovagal, situational, carotid sinus syncope) or orthostatic hypotension?

History of syncope that occurred when moving from supine to upright position
History of lightheadedness or dizziness when moving from supine to upright position
Orthostatic change in systolic blood pressure and heart rate

Orthostatic hypotension

Syncope precipitated by tight collar, shaving, sudden turning + carotid sinus massage

Carotid sinus syncope

Clinical presentation not consistent with vasovagal syncope, carotid sinus syncope, situational syncope, or orthostatic hypotension

Syncope following prolonged standing, pain, or emotional upset
Prodromal symptoms of nausea, weakness, or diaphoresis

Vasovagal syncope

Syncope following cough, defecation, swallowing, or micturition

Situational syncope

Are clues present in the history and physical examination that are suggestive of the following conditions?
Neurologic causes
- TIA / CVA
- Migraine   - Subclavian steal syndrome
Valvular heart disease   - Seizure
- Aortic stenosis
- Mitral stenosis   - Hypertrophic obstructive cardiomyopathy
Pulmonary hypertension
Pulmonary embolism
Myocardial infarction
Cardiac tamponade
Atrial myxoma
Aortic dissection

Yes — Direct further evaluation according to the clues that are present

No — ✓ EKG

See next page

518

SYNCOPE
(continued)

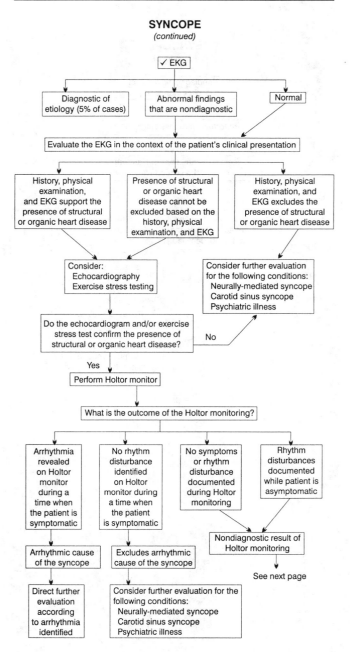

SYNCOPE
(continued)

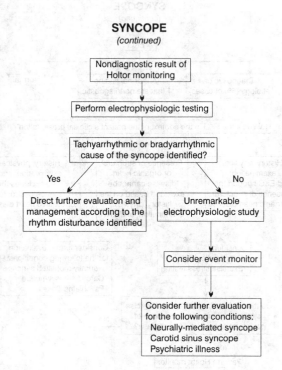

Nondiagnostic result of Holter monitoring

↓

Perform electrophysiologic testing

↓

Tachyarrhythmic or bradyarrhythmic cause of the syncope identified?

Yes ← → No

Direct further evaluation and management according to the rhythm disturbance identified

Unremarkable electrophysiologic study

↓

Consider event monitor

↓

Consider further evaluation for the following conditions:
Neurally-mediated syncope
Carotid sinus syncope
Psychiatric illness

VAGINAL DISCHARGE

STEP 1: *Does the Patient Have a Clinically-Significant Vaginal Discharge?*

Vaginal discharge is a commonly encountered problem in the outpatient setting, accounting for close to ten million office visits a year. It is the chief complaint in 30% of visits to sexually transmitted disease clinics. Prior to embarking on an evaluation, it is important to realize that vaginal discharge is not synonymous with vaginitis. Vaginitis is said to be present when the patient complains of an abnormal, pathologic discharge. To identify an abnormal vaginal discharge, the clinician must first recognize what constitutes a physiologic vaginal discharge.

The normal vaginal discharge is the result of substances secreted by various parts of the genital tract. The nature of the discharge in terms of amount and fluidity vary with the menstrual cycle. Around the time of ovulation, for example, cervical mucus becomes more fluid. Women commonly feel that this change in fluidity represents an abnormal discharge when, in fact, the change is physiologic. The amount of discharge often increases with stress, a fact that is not well appreciated by many women.

Although vaginal discharge alone may be the only manifestation of vaginitis, in many cases, other symptoms are present. These include irritation, odor, pruritus, frequency, or dysuria. The presence of any of these accompanying symptoms argues for a pathologic vaginal discharge. The clinician should consider these factors, then, in differentiating a physiologic from pathologic vaginal discharge.

If the vaginal discharge is physiologic, ***Stop Here.***

If the vaginal discharge is pathologic, ***Proceed to Step 2.***

STEP 2: *What are the Causes of a Pathologic Vaginal Discharge?*

Once the presence of a pathologic vaginal discharge has been established, the clinician should focus efforts on determining the etiology. Although there are infectious and noninfectious causes of vaginal discharge, most authorities maintain that up to 90% of cases are due to infectious organisms. In most of these cases, the vaginal discharge is accompanied by other symptoms such as frequency, dysuria, irritation, and pruritus.

When dysuria is present, the clinician should ascertain whether the dysuria is external or internal. External dysuria is present when pain and burning with urination only occur when the urine touches the vulva. External dysuria is not uncommon in patients with pathologic vaginal discharge. The presence of internal dysuria should prompt the clinician to consider cystitis rather than vaginitis.

The causes of a pathologic vaginal discharge are listed in the following box.

Causes of Vaginal Discharge	
Infectious Conditions	
Infectious vaginitis	Cervicitis
Bacterial vaginosis	*Chlamydia trachomatis*
Trichomoniasis	*Neisseria gonorrhoeae*
Vaginal candidiasis	Toxic shock syndrome
Noninfectious Conditions	
Allergy	Neoplasm
Atrophic vaginitis	Pemphigus syndromes
Behcet's disease	Retained products
Cervical ectropion	Postabortion
Cervical polyp	Postnatal
Chemical irritation	Tampons
Collagen vascular disease	Trauma (sexual aids, etc)
Erosive lichen planus	

Despite the numerous causes of vaginal discharge, nearly 90% are caused by infection. Of the infectious etiologies, the three major considerations are bacterial vaginosis, trichomoniasis, and vaginal candidiasis. Most of this chapter will focus on differentiating between these infectious causes of vaginitis.

Proceed to Step 3

STEP 3: *Are There Any Historical Clues That May Point to the Etiology of the Vaginal Discharge?*

Historical clues that may point to the etiology of the vaginal discharge are listed in the following table.

Historical Clue	Condition Suggested
Development of symptoms after recent change in sexual partner	Sexually transmitted disease
Multiple sexual contacts in the recent past	Sexually transmitted disease
Symptoms in partner	Sexually transmitted disease
Abrupt onset	Sexually transmitted disease
Oral contraceptive use	Vaginal candidiasis Physiologic discharge from oral contraceptive
Vaginal douche	Chemical vaginitis
Steroid use	Vaginal candidiasis
Current or recent antibiotic use	Vaginal candidiasis
Diabetes mellitus	Vaginal candidiasis
Premenstrual onset of symptoms	Vaginal candidiasis
Beginning during or immediately after menstrual period	Trichomoniasis
Abdominal pain*	Trichomoniasis (occasional)

*Abdominal pain is very uncommon in patients presenting with vaginal discharge. On occasion, it may be appreciated in trichomoniasis. If present, however, abdominal pain should prompt the clinician to consider urinary tract infection or pelvic inflammatory disease.

Unfortunately, historical features in the patient presenting with vaginal discharge are seldom helpful in establishing the etiology.

Proceed to Step 4

STEP 4: *Are There Any Clues in the Physical Examination That May Point to the Etiology of the Vaginal Discharge?*

Clues in the physical examination that may point to the etiology of the vaginal discharge are listed in the following table.

Physical Examination Clue	Condition Suggested
Diffuse perineal erythema	Trichomoniasis Vaginal candidiasis
Diffuse reddening with satellite lesions	Vaginal candidiasis
Severe perivaginal irritation	Argues against the diagnosis of bacterial vaginosis
Other genital lesions	Consider other sexually transmitted diseases

Like the history, the physical examination is seldom helpful in establishing the etiology.

Proceed to Step 5

STEP 5: *Does the Patient Have Cervicitis?*

Thirty-three percent of women who have gonococcal or chlamydial cervicitis report vaginal discharge. Because the diagnostic testing and treatment of cervicitis differs, it is absolutely essential that the clinician differentiate cervicitis from vaginitis. Cervicitis should be suspected if any of the following are present:

- Edema and erythema of cervix or cervical os
- Purulent or mucopurulent cervical discharge
- Ulcerative lesions of the cervix
- Cervical bleeding induced by swabbing the endocervical mucosa

If any of the above features of cervicitis are present, *Proceed to Step 6.*

If none of the above features of cervicitis are present, *Proceed to Step 7.*

STEP 6: *What is the Etiology of the Cervicitis?*

The three major causes of cervicitis include *Neisseria gonorrhoeae*, *Chlamydia trachomatis*, and herpes simplex virus. The symptoms of cervicitis do not allow the clinician to differentiate among these causes. Physical examination findings suggestive of cervicitis have been discussed in Step 5. In most cases, when signs of cervicitis are present, the manifestations do not allow the clinician to differentiate between the three major possibilities. Securing the diagnosis requires appropriate laboratory testing, which is described below.

Gonococcal Cervicitis

In all cases of cervicitis, a Gram's stain of the discharge should be performed. In up to 75% of gonococcal cervicitis, the Gram's stain will reveal the characteristic Gram-negative intracellular diplococci. Because the Gram's stain does not reveal the typical organisms in about 25% of cases, an unrevealing Gram's stain does not exclude the diagnosis of gonococcal cervicitis. As a result, a culture should always be obtained. The sensitivity of the endocervical culture is about 90%.

Chlamydial Cervicitis

In chlamydial cervicitis, a properly done Gram's stain of the cervical discharge will reveal increased numbers of polymorphonuclear cells. In the absence of significant numbers of vaginal epithelial cells, finding greater than 20 to 30 polymorphonuclear cells per 1000 X microscopic field is suggestive of cervicitis. The absence of Gram-negative organisms suggests chlamydial infection but the clinician should realize that the Gram's stain is unrevealing in 25% to 50% of gonococcal cervicitis. The definitive diagnosis requires specialized testing using immunofluorescence microscopy, DNA probes, enzyme immunoassays, PCR, or ligase chain reaction.

Herpetic Cervicitis

The visualization of multinucleated giant cells with characteristic intranuclear inclusions suggests the diagnosis of herpetic cervicitis. When cervical necrosis is present, however, the cytologic examination looking for multinucleated giant cells loses its reliability. Other techniques including culture, PCR, or DNA probes are available in establishing the diagnosis.

End of Section.

STEP 7: *What are the Clinical Presentations of the Major Causes of Infectious Vaginitis?*

Once cervicitis has been excluded as the cause of the vaginal discharge, the clinician can focus on elucidating the etiology of the vaginitis. As mentioned earlier, infectious causes represent about 90% of cases. Of the infectious etiologies, bacterial vaginosis, trichomoniasis, and vaginal candidiasis are the major considerations. The clinical presentation of these diseases are considered below.

Vaginal Candidiasis

Yeast, in small numbers, are a normal part of the vaginal flora. Under some circumstances, the yeast may gain a competitive advantage over the bacterial flora, resulting in signs and symptoms of vaginal candidiasis. Vaginal candidiasis is the second most common cause of infectious vaginitis. Although rarely occurring before menarche, by the age of 25, approximately 50% of women have had at least one episode of vaginal candidiasis. There are a number of factors that predispose women to the development of vaginal candidiasis. Chief among these are antibiotics. Other predisposing factors include pregnancy, oral contraceptives, diabetes mellitus, steroid use, obesity, and immunocompromise.

Infection with *Candida albicans* accounts for 80% to 90% of cases while *Candida glabarata* is responsible for 5% to 10%. Symptoms of vaginal candidiasis include pruritus and dysuria. The vaginal discharge is classically described as thick and curd-like ("cottage cheese"). In some cases, however, the discharge may be thin and loose. Vulvar erythema and edema are commonly appreciated on pelvic exam. Fissures and excoriations may be present. A clue to the diagnosis is the presence of satellite lesions, which are tiny papules or papulopustules. Inspection of the vaginal walls often reveals erythema with an adherent discharge.

Bacterial Vaginosis

Bacterial vaginosis is the most common cause of infectious vaginitis. The infection is characterized by an increase in the concentration of various organisms, many of which are listed in the following box.

Etiologic Organisms in Bacterial Vaginosis
Anaerobic Gram-negative rods
Bacteroides
Peptostreptococcus
Porphyromonas
Prevotella
Gardnerella vaginalis
Mobiluncus species
Mycoplasma hominis

In bacterial vaginosis, the vaginal discharge is often accompanied by an odor. Dysuria and dyspareunia are uncommonly appreciated. On occasion, mild abdominal discomfort may be noted.

Unlike vaginal candidiasis and trichomoniasis, inspection of the labia and vulva usually does not reveal erythema or edema. Vaginal erythema is uncommonly appreciated on speculum examination. The discharge is typically gray to white, thin, and homogenous. Not uncommonly, the discharge is adherent to the vaginal walls. During the examination, the clinician may notice a pungent, fishy odor.

Trichomoniasis

Vaginitis due to the parasite, *Trichomonas vaginalis*, is less common than vaginal candidiasis and bacterial vaginosis. Yet, it still accounts for about 25% of all cases. The organism is a unicellular, flagellated, protozoan parasite. Characteristic of this organism is the presence of 3-5 flagella, usually located on one end. Symptomatic trichomoniasis usually manifests with a malodorous discharge. The discharge is classically described as gray-green, copious, and frothy. Although uncommon, dysuria and dyspareunia may be present. Some patients complain of vaginal itching or irritation.

Physical examination may reveal vulvar erythema or edema. The classic "strawberry cervix" is fairly uncommon but its presence should certainly prompt consideration of trichomoniasis. The term refers to the presence of small, punctate cervical hemorrhages with ulcerations. Although uncommon (up to 5% of patients), this finding is very specific for trichomoniasis.

Proceed to Step 8

STEP 8: *What are the Results of Laboratory Testing?*

The clinical presentation, even when classic, seldom allows the clinician to determine the precise infectious etiology. As a result, the definitive diagnosis requires laboratory testing. Key to establishing the diagnosis is the performance of the following tests:

- Wet mount preparation
- KOH preparation and whiff test
- Litmus testing for pH

Each of these tests will be considered below.

Wet Mount Preparation

The clinician can develop the wet mount preparation by adding one or two drops of 0.9% NS to vaginal discharge that has been placed on a slide. Direct microscopy of the wet mount preparation allows the clinician to establish the diagnosis of trichomoniasis if the organism with its characteristic jerky mobility is seen. It is important to realize, however, that the sensitivity of the wet mount preparation is about 60%. The specificity of the test, however, is close to 99%.

Clue cells may also be appreciated on examination of the wet mount preparation. The presence of these cells are characteristic of bacterial vaginosis. These cells are said to be present when more than 20% of the epithelial cells have cell margins that are indistinct as a result of bacterial adherence. The following table summarizes the significance of various findings noted during direct microscopy of the wet mount preparation.

Wet Mount Preparation Finding	Condition Suggested
Motile organisms	Trichomoniasis
Clue cells	Bacterial vaginosis
Increased numbers of PMNs	Trichomoniasis Atrophic vaginitis
Fungal hyphae	Vaginal candidiasis
Round parabasal cells	Atrophic vaginitis

KOH Preparation and Whiff Test

A KOH preparation is obtained by adding 10% KOH to vaginal discharge placed on a slide. When the addition of KOH results in the elaboration of a "fishy" or amine odor (positive whiff test), the clinician should suspect bacterial vaginosis or trichomoniasis. The specimen should then be examined by direct microscopy for hyphae, mycelial tangles, and spores. The presence of any one or combination of these findings supports the diagnosis of vaginal candidiasis. The KOH preparation is positive in 50% to 70% of vaginal candidiasis cases. It is important to realize that the KOH preparation cannot be used to establish the diagnosis of trichomoniasis because the KOH destroys the trichomonad organisms.

Litmus Testing for pH

Litmus paper should be placed in the pooled vaginal secretions to determine the pH. The normal vaginal pH falls between 3.8 and 4.2. Both bacterial vaginosis and trichomoniasis are characterized by a pH >4.5. It is also important to realize that noninfectious causes of vaginitis, such as atrophic vaginitis, may also present with a similar pH.

The results of these four tests in combination with the patient's clinical presentation should allow the clinician to establish the infectious cause of the vaginitis. The clinician should realize that, not uncommonly, the patient with vaginal discharge may be infected with several different organisms. Herein lies the importance of performing all four of the above tests. The following table summarizes the findings that can be used to distinguish between the three infectious causes of vaginitis.

	Bacterial Vaginosis*	Vaginal Candidiasis	Trichomoniasis
Color of Discharge	Gray or white	White	Yellow-green
Consistency of Discharge	Homogenous (can be frothy)	Curdy ("cottage cheese")	Frothy (25%)
Dysuria	Uncommon	Common	Uncommon
Vulvar Irritation	May be present	Often present	Often present
Odor	Usually malodorous	Usually odorless	Usually malodorous
Labial Erythema	Usually absent	May be present	May be present
Satellite Lesions	Absent	May be present	Absent
Discharge Adherent to Vaginal Wall	Yes	Yes	No
Elevated pH (>4.5)	Yes	No	Yes
Wet Mount Preparation and KOH Preparation	Clue cells	Pseudohyphae Mycelial tangles Budding yeast cells	Motile organisms Many PMNs
Odor Appreciated on Whiff Test	Yes	No	Yes

*An accurate diagnosis of bacterial vaginosis is established in 90% of cases when three of the four following criteria are met: 1 - Thin, homogenous discharge; 2 - Positive "whiff" test; 3 - Vaginal pH >4.5; 4 - "Clue cells" present on microscopy

If one or more of the above causes of infectious vaginitis is identified, **Stop Here.**

If none of the above causes of infectious vaginitis is identified, **Proceed to Step 9.**

STEP 9: *Should a Culture be Performed?*

When the clinical presentation and standard laboratory testing described above does not reveal an infectious cause of the vaginitis, the clinician should perform cultures for vaginal candidiasis and trichomoniasis. In 30% to 50% of vaginal candidiasis cases, direct microscopy will fail to identify the yeast. In these patients, a positive culture supports the diagnosis with one caveat. Up to 25% of asymptomatic women are colonized with candidal organisms. Nonetheless, a positive culture in a woman with compatible signs and symptoms should prompt treatment for vaginal candidiasis.

Culture for *Trichomonas vaginalis* should also be performed when the wet mount preparation fails to reveal the motile organisms. This is not uncommon, occurring in 25% to 40% of cases. In these patients, a culture, which is the most sensitive test for trichomoniasis, should be obtained.

If the culture results are positive, **Stop Here.**

If the culture results are negative, **Proceed to Step 10.**

STEP 10: *Does the Patient Have Atrophic Vaginitis?*

After the three major causes of infectious vaginitis have been excluded, the clinician should consider atrophic vaginitis, the fourth most common cause of vaginitis. This should clearly be a consideration in postmenopausal women.

Most patients with atrophic vaginitis are asymptomatic. When symptomatic, patients complain of vaginal soreness, dyspareunia, and postcoital burning. Physical examination typically reveals diffuse redness and few or no vaginal folds. Vulvar atrophy may be noted in some patients. A serosanguineous or watery discharge is not uncommon in patients with atrophic vaginitis.

The pH of the vaginal discharge is usually above 4.5. Direct microscopy of the wet smear may reveal increased numbers of polymorphonuclear leukocytes along with rounded parabasal epithelial cells.

If the patient has atrophic vaginitis, *Stop Here.*

If the patient does not have atrophic vaginitis, *Proceed to Step 11.*

STEP 11: *What are Other Possibilities in the Patient Presenting With Vaginal Discharge?*

When infection and atrophic vaginitis are unlikely to be the cause of the vaginal discharge, the clinician should consider less common causes. In particular, a detailed history is warranted to elicit any substances that may have come into contact with the perineum. These substances may cause an allergic or chemically irritative vaginitis. Some of the offending agents include:

- deodorants
- soaps
- tampons or pads
- vaginal sprays
- colored or perfumed toilet tissue
- bubble bath
- laundry detergents
- fabric softeners
- swimming pools
- hot tubs
- vaginal contraceptives or condoms

If an allergic or chemically irritative vaginitis is not likely, the clinician should consider other causes of vaginitis. The other less common causes of vaginal discharge are listed in the box in Step 2.

End of Section.

REFERENCES

Carr PL, Felsenstein D, and Friedman RH, "Evaluation and Management of Vaginitis," *J Gen Intern Med*, 1998, 13(5):335-46 (review).

Coco AS and Vandenbosche M, "Infectious Vaginitis. An Accurate Diagnosis is Essential and Attainable," *Postgrad Med*, 2000, 107(4):63-6, 69-74 (review).

Egan ME and Lipsky MS, "Diagnosis of Vaginitis," *Am Fam Phys*, 2000, 62(5):1095-104 (review).

Haefner HK, "Current Evaluation and Management of Vulvovaginitis," *Clin Obstet Gynecol*, 1999, 42(2):184-95 (review).

Macsween KF and Ridgway GL, "The Laboratory Investigation of Vaginal Discharge," *J Clin Pathol*, 1998, 51(8):564-7 (review).

Sobel JD, "Bacterial Vaginosis," *Annu Rev Med*, 2000, 51:349-56 (review).

Sobel JD, "Vaginitis," *N Engl J Med*, 1997, 337(26):1896-903 (review).

Sobel JD, "Vulvovaginitis in Healthy Women," *Compr Ther*, 1999, 25(6-7):335-46 (review).

VAGINAL DISCHARGE

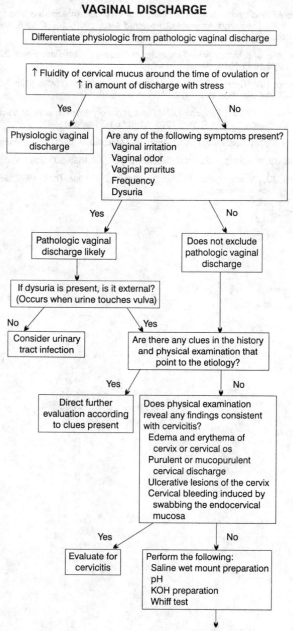

Differentiate physiologic from pathologic vaginal discharge

↓

↑ Fluidity of cervical mucus around the time of ovulation or
↑ in amount of discharge with stress

Yes → Physiologic vaginal discharge

No → Are any of the following symptoms present?
- Vaginal irritation
- Vaginal odor
- Vaginal pruritus
- Frequency
- Dysuria

Yes → Pathologic vaginal discharge likely

No → Does not exclude pathologic vaginal discharge

Pathologic vaginal discharge likely → If dysuria is present, is it external? (Occurs when urine touches vulva)

No → Consider urinary tract infection

Yes → Are there any clues in the history and physical examination that point to the etiology?

Yes → Direct further evaluation according to clues present

No → Does physical examination reveal any findings consistent with cervicitis?
- Edema and erythema of cervix or cervical os
- Purulent or mucopurulent cervical discharge
- Ulcerative lesions of the cervix
- Cervical bleeding induced by swabbing the endocervical mucosa

Yes → Evaluate for cervicitis

No → Perform the following:
- Saline wet mount preparation
- pH
- KOH preparation
- Whiff test

↓

See next page

VAGINAL DISCHARGE

(continued)

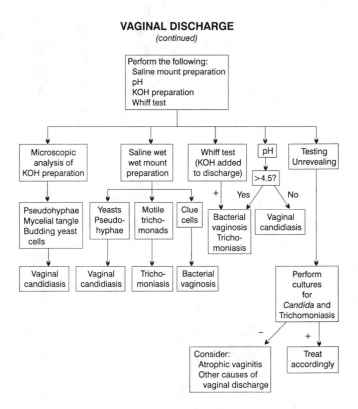

WEIGHT LOSS

STEP 1: *Does the Patient Have Weight Loss?*

Weight loss may be voluntary or involuntary. Involuntary weight loss is concerning for not only the patient but also the clinician. Of major concern is the possibility that the weight loss heralds the presence of a serious underlying physical or psychological disorder. This concern is understandable since about 25% of patients presenting with involuntary weight loss pass away in the year that follows their initial presentation.

Before embarking on an evaluation, which at times can be very extensive, it is important to verify that weight loss has truly occurred. Not all patients with weight loss report the complaint to the physician, particularly when the weight loss is unaccompanied by other symptoms. In fact, in many cases, it is the clinician who first detects the weight loss. Herein lies the importance of weighing patients at each visit.

Any complaint of weight loss should be confirmed by inspecting the patient's actual weight measurements. A 5% or greater reduction in weight over a period of six months establishes the presence of true weight loss.

If weight loss is not present, ***Stop Here.***

If weight loss is present, ***Proceed to Step 2.***

STEP 2: *What are the Causes of Weight Loss?*

The causes of weight loss are listed in the following box.

Causes of Weight Loss	
Chronic liver disease	Malignancy
Chronic obstructive pulmonary disease	Medications
Congestive heart failure	Neurologic causes
Connective tissue disease	CVA
Endocrine disorders	Dementia
Adrenal insufficiency	Parkinson's disease
Diabetes mellitus	Oral disorders
Hyperparathyroidism	Absence of teeth
Hyperthyroidism	Ill-fitting dentures
Hypothyroidism	Pain with eating
Pheochromocytoma	Psychiatric
Gastrointestinal disease	Alcoholism
Infection	Anxiety
Amebic abscess	Anorexia nervosa
Fungal disease	Bulimia
Subacute bacterial endocarditis	Depression
Tuberculosis	Uremia

Proceed to Step 3

STEP 3: *What are the Major Causes of Weight Loss?*

Several studies have been performed to elucidate the causes of weight loss. The findings of these studies are listed in the following table.

	Marton	Rabinovitz	Thompson
Cancer	19	36	16
GI Disorders	14	17	11
Cardiovascular	9	0	0
Alcohol	8	0	0
Pulmonary	6	0	0
Endocrine	4	4	9
Infectious	3	4	2
Inflammatory	2	1	0
Renal	0	4	0
Neurologic	0	0	7
Psychiatry	9	10	20
Unknown	26	23	24

Adapted from Wise GR and Craig D, "Evaluation of Involuntary Weight Loss. Where Do You Start?," *Postgrad Med*, 1994, 95(4):143-6, 149-50 (review); also adapted from Yamada T, *Textbook of Gastroenterology*, Baltimore, MD: Lippincott Williams & Wilkins, 1999, 762.

The conditions associated with weight loss will be discussed in more detail below.

Malignancy

Malignancy should be a major consideration in the patient presenting with weight loss because of the seriousness of this diagnosis. Malignancy occurring in any organ can result in weight loss. In many patients, there are signs and symptoms suggestive of malignancy. In others, however, weight loss may be the initial presentation of an occult malignancy. In fact, malignancy is the major consideration when weight loss is unaccompanied by other signs and symptoms. Although any malignancy can present with weight loss alone, the clinician should be wary of gastrointestinal malignancy, especially pancreatic cancer. Other malignancies that commonly present with weight loss include hepatoma, lymphoma, leukemia, prostate cancer, and ovarian cancer.

The etiology of weight loss in patients with malignancy is thought to be multifactorial. Anorexia is a common complaint in patients with malignancy. Some cancers interfere with the digestion and absorption of food while others increase metabolism. Cancer patients are often depressed, another factor predisposing to weight loss.

Gastrointestinal Disorders

Various gastrointestinal disorders may be associated with weight loss. Some of the causes include the following:

- Peptic ulcer disease
- Gastrointestinal obstruction
- Motility disorders
- Pancreaticobiliary disorders
- Chronic hepatitis / cirrhosis
- Malabsorption
- Chronic mesenteric ischemia

The mechanism of the weight loss varies depending on the condition, often being multifactorial. Anorexia, vomiting, inflammation, fear of eating, and malabsorption are some possible mechanisms in the conditions described above.

Cardiac Disease

Although many patients with congestive heart failure have weight gain, there is a subset of patients, particularly those with severe chronic congestive heart failure (functional class III or IV) who may have weight loss. Causes of weight loss in these patients include anorexia, dietary restriction, increased metabolic demands, and abdominal angina.

Alcoholism

Weight loss is not uncommon in alcoholic patients, who often consume large amounts of empty calories. In addition to poor nutrition, another cause of weight loss in this population is diarrhea which may be due to alcohol-induced alteration in small bowel function. Alternatively, diarrhea may be the result of exocrine pancreatic insufficiency. Alcoholics who have developed chronic liver disease or cirrhosis often have accompanying weight loss. Alcoholics are certainly predisposed to malignancy, which is the second leading cause of death in this population after cardiovascular disease. These patients are at increased risk of developing cancers of the head and neck, esophagus, liver, and pancreas. Depression often coexists with alcoholism, a further impetus for weight loss.

Pulmonary Disease

Weight loss is not uncommon in patients with chronic obstructive pulmonary disease, particularly when the underlying disease is advanced. In these patients, shortness of breath may develop during eating, thereby limiting their food consumption. In others, accessory muscle use may play a large role in caloric consumption.

Medications

Although any medication could be a potential cause of weight loss, common offenders include those that are listed in the following box.

Medications Commonly Causing Weight Loss	
Antibiotics	Clofibrate
Anticholinergics	Cytotoxins (cancer chemotherapeutic)
Antihistamines	Griseofulvin
Antipsychotics	Hypoglycemic agents
Cardiovascular agents	L-dopa
ACE-inhibitors	NSAIDs
Antiarrhythmics	Opiates
Clonidine	Serotonin reuptake inhibitors
Digoxin	Sucralfate
Diuretics	Theophylline
Reserpine	Tricyclic antidepressants

Endocrine Disorders

Common manifestations of hyperthyroidism include nervousness, insomnia, tremors, emotional lability, excessive sweating, and heat intolerance. Although weight loss often accompanies these classic manifestations, on occasion, isolated weight loss may be the initial presentation of hyperthyroidism.

Weight loss is also commonly found in patients with diabetes mellitus. Its presence suggests poorly controlled diabetes mellitus and, as such, is usually accompanied by polyuria, polydipsia, and polyphagia. On occasion, however, isolated weight loss may be the only clue to the presence of diabetes mellitus. Both diabetes mellitus and hyperthyroidism may be associated with an increased appetite.

Other less common endocrine disorders that are also associated with weight loss include adrenal insufficiency, panhypopituitarism, hypothyroidism, and hyperparathyroidism.

Infection

Weight loss is more typical of chronic infection. Unexplained weight loss should prompt consideration of tuberculosis, subacute bacterial endocarditis, osteomyelitis, and abscess. HIV infection is also a consideration.

Renal Disease

Anorexia commonly accompanies uremia, oftentimes leading to weight loss.

Connective Tissue Disease

Anorexia, malaise, and nausea are frequently found in patients with systemic lupus erythematosus, rheumatoid arthritis, polyarteritis nodosa, polymyositis, ankylosing spondylitis, scleroderma, polymyalgia rheumatica, and temporal arteritis. Scleroderma is also associated with esophageal dysmotility and altered gastrointestinal motility, two other factors that predispose to weight loss.

Oral Disorders

Nearly 50% of individuals have lost most of their teeth by the age of 65. Even in patients who have dentures, there are problems with chewing that may be the result of ill-fitting dentures. Ulcerations of the tongue and oral mucosa may also interfere with eating.

Neurologic Disease

The prevalence of dementia increases with age. Early in the course of dementia, patients may have difficulty with memory loss or judgment. These cognitive losses may prevent the patient from buying food or preparing meals. With advancing disease, many may not recognize the need to eat. Others have difficulty feeding themselves, often relying on caregivers. Many patients with dementia are depressed, yet another factor that predisposes to weight loss.

Many neurologic conditions are associated with swallowing difficulty. Examples include Parkinson's disease, CVA, ALS, and poliomyelitis. Depression may also be a factor in these patients as well.

Psychiatric Conditions

Psychiatric illnesses associated with weight loss include depression, anxiety, bereavement over an extended period of time, and eating disorders. When a medical or physical cause of weight loss is not identified, the clinician should consider psychiatric etiologies.

Proceed to Step 4

> **STEP 4: *Are There Any Clues in the History That Point to the Etiology of the Weight Loss?***

Clues in the patient's history that point to the etiology of the weight loss are listed in the following table.

Historical Clue	Condition Suggested
Onset before the age of 25 in female patient	Anorexia nervosa
Onset after the age of 25 in female patient	Argues against diagnosis of anorexia nervosa
Increase in appetite	Hyperthyroidism Diabetes mellitus Malabsorption Painful oral disorders
Episodes of binge eating	Anorexia nervosa Bulimia
Fear of becoming obese	Anorexia nervosa Bulimia
Feeling "fat"	Anorexia nervosa
Ill-fitting dentures	Oral disorder
Chronic diarrhea	Malabsorption Inflammatory bowel disease
Blood in stools	Gastrointestinal carcinoma
Increased thirst (polydipsia)	Diabetes mellitus
Increased volume of urine (polyuria)	Diabetes mellitus
Feelings of guilt or depression after eating	Bulimia
Fever	Chronic infection
Palpitations	Hyperthyroidism

Abdominal pain after eating	Gastrointestinal illness
	   Chronic pancreatitis
	   Chronic mesenteric ischemia
	   Partial gastric outlet obstruction
	   Gastric or pancreatic carcinoma

Difficulty swallowing	Oropharyngeal or esophageal disorder
Dyspnea on exertion Orthopnea PND	Congestive heart failure
Smoking history	Malignancy COPD
Hematuria	Malignancy (urologic)
Homosexual Sexual promiscuity Intravenous drug abuse	HIV / AIDS
Alcohol abuse	Alcoholism
Heat intolerance	Hyperthyroidism
Fluctuation in weight	Bulimia
Absence of teeth	Oral disorder
Alteration in bowel habits	Gastrointestinal cancer

Proceed to Step 5

> **STEP 5:** *Are There Any Clues in the Patient's Physical Examination That may Point to the Etiology of the Weight Loss?*

Clues in the patient's physical examination that point to the etiology of the weight loss are listed in the following table.

Physical Examination Finding	Condition Suggested
Fever	Chronic infection
Tremor	Hyperthyroidism
Warm, moist skin	Hyperthyroidism
Tachycardia	Hyperthyroidism
Lymphadenopathy	Malignancy
Abdominal mass	Malignancy
Dupuytren's's contracture Gynecomastia Palmar erythema Spider angioma Testicular atrophy	Chronic liver disease or cirrhosis
Dental erosions	Bulimia
Hyperpigmentation	Adrenal insufficiency
Murmur	Subacute bacterial endocarditis
Breast mass	Malignancy
Rectal mass	Malignancy
Prostate nodule or induration	Malignancy
Edema Elevated jugular venous pressure S3	Congestive heart failure
Mass in oral cavity	Impairment of adequate oral intake
Ulcerations of tongue and oral mucosa	Impairment of adequate oral intake
Poor dentition	Impairment of adequate oral intake

If there are clues in the patient's history and physical examination that point to the etiology of the weight loss, the evaluation should be directed accordingly.

If there are no clues in the patient's history and physical examination that point to the etiology of the weight loss, *Proceed to Step 6.*

> **STEP 6:** *What are the Results of the Laboratory Tests?*

In most cases, a thorough history and physical examination reveals clues that may point the clinician in a certain direction. In the study by Morton, approximately 50% of the patients had a chief complaint that directed the ensuing evaluation. This study and others have found that physical or medical causes of weight loss are present in 60% to 70% of patients.

In the absence of clues pointing to the etiology of the weight loss, laboratory tests and other studies that should be obtained are included in the following list.

- CBC
- Serum BUN / creatinine
- Serum electrolytes
- Fasting glucose
- Liver function tests (AST, ALT, alkaline phosphatase)
- Albumin
- Calcium
- Urinalysis
- TSH
- CXR
- HIV
- ESR

An abnormal result of any of the above tests warrants an investigation to determine the cause of the abnormality. Further laboratory testing is not warranted in the patient with normal results of the above tests.

If abnormal laboratory tests are identified, the evaluation should be directed at elucidating the etiology of the abnormal lab tests. *Stop Here.*

If laboratory tests are normal, *Proceed to Step 7.*

STEP 7: *What are the Results of Cancer Screening?*

A very real concern for both patients and clinicians is the possibility of occult malignancy in the patient who has an unremarkable history, physical examination, and laboratory testing. But in the absence of any findings, an exhaustive evaluation searching for a malignancy is not indicated. Many clinicians decide to perform abdominal and chest CT scans in the hopes of detecting an occult malignancy. The yield of abdominal and chest CT scan in the absence of symptoms, signs, and abnormal laboratory data is very low. As a result, CT scanning is not recommended in these cases.

Rather the clinician should perform age-appropriate screening for cancer as recommended by the American Cancer Society. This includes the following:

- Fecal occult blood testing (age ≥40)
- Pap smear in women
- Mammography (age >40)
- PSA (age ≥50)
- Flexible sigmoidoscopy (if fecal occult blood test is negative and patient is ≥50 years)

If the results of these age-appropriate cancer screening studies are abnormal, the clinician should tailor the evaluation accordingly.

If the results of these age-appropriate cancer screening studies are normal, *Proceed to Step 8.*

STEP 8: *Is the Weight Loss Secondary to a Social, Functional, or Economic Cause?*

When an organic cause of the weight loss is unlikely, the clinician should consider social, functional, and economic causes of weight loss. These factors are listed in the following box.

Social, Functional, and Economic Causes of Weight Loss
Social isolation
No transportation
Inadequate cooking facilities
Inadequate facilities to store food
Dependence on caregivers or institution for food
Reduced mobility
Arthritis
Neurologic deficit

If one or more of the above factors are present and the weight improves with correction of the above factors, **Stop Here.**

If one or more of the above factors are present but the weight does not improve with correction of the above factors, **Proceed to Step 9.**

If none of the above factors are present, **Proceed to Step 9.**

STEP 9: Is the Weight Loss Due to a Psychiatric Condition?

Depression is thought to affect close to 20 million people in the United States alone, many of which do not realize that they suffer from depression. Not uncommonly, depression presents with weight loss and anorexia. Oftentimes, these patients do not realize that this is the result of an emotional problem. Weight loss is a common presentation of depression, particularly in the elderly. Because it can be difficult for clinicians to recognize depression, every patient with unexplained weight loss should be screened for depression using a standardized screening tool. Anxiety and bereavement over an extended period of time are other psychiatric causes of weight loss.

Anorexia nervosa and bulimia also deserve consideration, particularly when weight loss occurs in young, previously healthy women. These are eating disorders that have a predilection for middle class white women. Central to both of these disorders is the pursuit of thinness. Food intake is curtailed in anorexia nervosa. In bulimia, there are episodes of binge eating followed by vomiting and excessive use of laxatives. Criteria from the *Diagnostic and Statistical Manual of Mental Disorders* (DSM-IV) are used to establish the diagnosis of these two disorders. These criteria are listed in the following boxes.

Diagnostic Criteria for Anorexia Nervosa
1. Refusal to maintain body weight at or above a minimally normal weight for age and height (eg, weight loss leading to maintenance of body weight less than 85% of that expected; or failure to make expected weight gain during period of growth, leading to body weight less than 85% of that expected).
2. Intense fear of gaining weight or becoming fat, even though underweight.
3. Disturbance in the way in which one's body weight or shape is experienced, undue influence of body weight or shape on self-evaluation, or denial of the seriousness of the current low body weight.
4. In postmenarchal females, amenorrhea (ie, the absence of at least three consecutive menstrual cycles). (A woman is considered to have amenorrhea if her periods occur only following hormone, eg, estrogen administration).

Diagnostic Criteria for Bulimia
1. Recurrent episodes of binge eating. An episode of binge eating is characterized by both the following: a. Eating, in a discrete period of time (eg, within any two-hour period), an amount of food that is definitely larger than most people would eat during a similar period of time and under similar circumstances.   b. A sense of lack of control over eating during the episode (eg, a feeling that one cannot stop eating or control what or how much one is eating).
2. Recurrent inappropriate compensatory behavior in order to prevent weight gain, such as self-induced vomiting, misuse of laxatives, diuretics, or other medications; fasting; or excessive exercise.
3. The binge eating and inappropriate compensatory behaviors both occur, on average, at least twice a week for three months.
4. Self-evaluation is unduly influenced by body shape and weight.
5. The disturbance does not occur exclusively during episodes of anorexia nervosa.

Adapted from *Diagnostic and Statistical Manual of Mental Disorders*, 4th ed, (DSM-IV), Washington, DC: American Psychiatric Association, 1994.

If the patient's weight loss is due to a psychiatric condition, ***Stop Here.***

If the patient's weight loss is not due to a psychiatric condition, ***Proceed to Step 10.***

STEP 10: *What is the Approach to the Patient With Weight Loss Who Has No Etiology Identified?*

When the history, physical examination, and laboratory data do not reveal the etiology of the weight loss, a careful follow-up is recommended. Because organic disease is rarely found in patients having a normal history, physical examination, laboratory tests, and screening studies, a period of watchful waiting is unlikely to result in a poor outcome.

There is no evidence to suggest that further testing is necessary unless the patient develops signs and symptoms suggestive of a particular illness. In the latter setting, a directed evaluation is warranted.

REFERENCES

Gazewood JD and Mehr DR, "Diagnosis and Management of Weight Loss in the Elderly," *J Fam Pract*, 1998, 47(1):19-25 (review).

Reife CM, "Involuntary Weight Loss," *Med Clin North Am*, 1995, 79(2):299-313 (review).

Robbins LJ, "Evaluation of Weight Loss in the Elderly," *Geriatrics*, 1989, 44(4):31-4, 37 (review).

Williams B, Waters D, and Parker K, "Evaluation and Treatment of Weight Loss in Adults With HIV Disease," *Am Fam Phys*, 1999, 60(3):843-54, 857-60 (review).

Wise GR and Craig D, "Evaluation of Involuntary Weight Loss. Where Do You Start?" *Postgrad Med*, 1994, 95(4):143-6, 149-50 (review).

WEIGHT LOSS

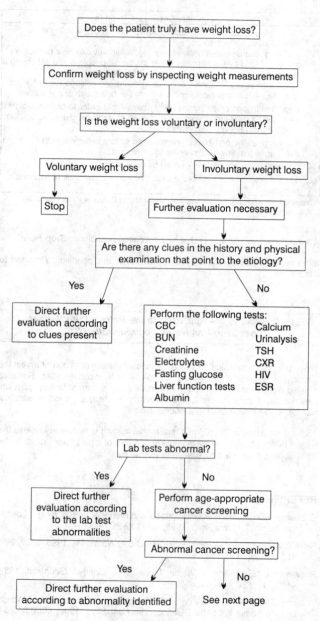

Does the patient truly have weight loss?

Confirm weight loss by inspecting weight measurements

Is the weight loss voluntary or involuntary?

Voluntary weight loss

Involuntary weight loss

Stop

Further evaluation necessary

Are there any clues in the history and physical examination that point to the etiology?

Yes

No

Direct further evaluation according to clues present

Perform the following tests:
CBC	Calcium
BUN	Urinalysis
Creatinine	TSH
Electrolytes	CXR
Fasting glucose	HIV
Liver function tests	ESR
Albumin	

Lab tests abnormal?

Yes

No

Direct further evaluation according to the lab test abnormalities

Perform age-appropriate cancer screening

Abnormal cancer screening?

Yes

No

Direct further evaluation according to abnormality identified

See next page

WEIGHT LOSS
(continued)

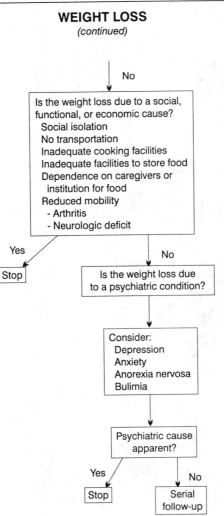

TOPIC INDEX

F

R

NOTES

Other titles offered by

DRUG INFORMATION HANDBOOK (International edition available)
by Charles Lacy, RPh, PharmD, FCSHP; Lora L. Armstrong, RPh, PharmD, BCPS; Morton P. Goldman, PharmD, BCPS; and Leonard L. Lance, RPh, BSPharm

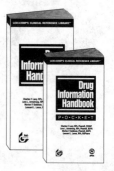

Specifically compiled and designed for the healthcare professional requiring quick access to concisely-stated comprehensive data concerning clinical use of medications.

The Drug Information Handbook is an ideal portable drug information resource, providing the reader with up to 29 key points of data concerning clinical use and dosing of the medication. Material provided in the Appendix section is recognized by many users to be, by itself, well worth the purchase of the handbook.

All medications found in the *Drug Information Handbook*, are included in the abridged *Pocket* edition (select fields were extracted to maintain portability).

PEDIATRIC DOSAGE HANDBOOK (International edition available)
by Carol K. Taketomo, PharmD; Jane Hurlburt Hodding, PharmD; and Donna M. Kraus, PharmD

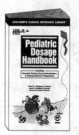

Special considerations must frequently be taken into account when dosing medications for the pediatric patient. This highly regarded quick reference handbook is a compilation of recommended pediatric doses based on current literature, as well as the practical experience of the authors and their many colleagues who work every day in the pediatric clinical setting.

Includes neonatal dosing, drug administration, and (in select monographs) extemporaneous preparations for medications used in pediatric medicine.

GERIATRIC DOSAGE HANDBOOK
by Todd P. Semla, PharmD, BCPS, FCCP; Judith L. Beizer, PharmD, FASCP; and Martin D. Higbee, PharmD, CGP

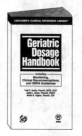

Many physiologic changes occur with aging, some of which affect the pharmacokinetics or pharmacodynamics of medications. Strong consideration should also be given to the effect of decreased renal or hepatic functions in the elderly, as well as the probability of the geriatric patient being on multiple drug regimens.

Healthcare professionals working with nursing homes and assisted living facilities will find the drug information contained in this handbook to be an invaluable source of helpful information.

An International Brand Name Index with names from 22 different countries is also included.

To order call toll free anywhere in the U.S.: 1-800-837-LEXI (5394)
Outside of the U.S. call: 330-650-6506 or online at www.lexi.com

Other titles offered by

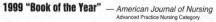
LEXI-COMP, INC

DRUG INFORMATION HANDBOOK *for* ADVANCED PRACTICE NURSING by Beatrice B. Turkoski, RN, PhD; Brenda R. Lance, RN, MSN; and Mark F. Bonfiglio, PharmD   Foreword by: Margaret A. Fitzgerald, MS, RN, CS-FNP

1999 "Book of the Year" — *American Journal of Nursing*
Advanced Practice Nursing Category

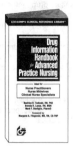

Designed specifically to meet the needs of nurse practitioners, clinical nurse specialists, nurse midwives, and graduate nursing students. The handbook is a unique resource for detailed, accurate information, which is vital to support the advanced practice nurse's role in patient drug therapy management. Over 4750 U.S., Canadian, and Mexican medications are covered in the 1000 monographs. Drug data is presented in an easy-to-use, alphabetically organized format covering up to 46 key points of information (including dosing for pediatrics, adults, and geriatrics). Cross-referenced to Appendix of over 230 pages of valuable comparison tables and additional information. Also included are two indexes, Pharmacologic Category and Controlled Substance, which facilitate comparison between agents.

DRUG INFORMATION HANDBOOK *for* NURSING
by Beatrice B. Turkoski, RN, PhD; Brenda R. Lance, RN, MSN; and Mark F. Bonfiglio, PharmD

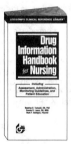

Registered Professional Nurses and upper-division nursing students involved with drug therapy will find this handbook provides quick access to drug data in a concise easy-to-use format.

Over 4000 U.S., Canadian, and Mexican medications are covered with up to 43 key points of information in each monograph. The handbook contains basic pharmacology concepts and nursing issues such as patient factors that influence drug therapy (ie, pregnancy, age, weight, etc) and general nursing issues (ie, assessment, administration, monitoring, and patient education). The Appendix contains over 230 pages of valuable information.

DRUG INFORMATION HANDBOOK *for* PHYSICIAN ASSISTANTS
by Michael J. Rudzinski, RPA-C, RPh and J. Fred Bennes, RPA, RPh

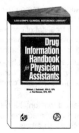

This comprehensive and easy-to-use handbook covers over 4100 drugs and also includes monographs on commonly used herbal products. There are up to 26 key fields of information per monograph, such as Pediatric and Adult Dosing With Adjustments for Renal/Hepatic Impairment, Labeled and Unlabeled Uses, Drug & Alcohol interactions, and Education & Monitoring Issues. Brand (U.S. and Canadian) and generic names are listed alphabetically for rapid access. It is fully cross-referenced by page number and includes alphabetical and pharmacologic indexes.

To order call toll free anywhere in the U.S.: 1-800-837-LEXI (5394)
Outside of the U.S. call: 330-650-6506 or online at www.lexi.com

Other titles offered by

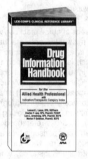 LEXI-COMP, INC

DRUG INFORMATION HANDBOOK FOR THE ALLIED HEALTH
PROFESSIONAL by Leonard L. Lance, RPh, BSPharm; Charles Lacy, RPh, PharmD, FCSHP; Lora L. Armstrong, RPh, PharmD, BCPS; and Morton P. Goldman, PharmD, BCPS

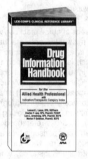

Working with clinical pharmacists, hospital pharmacy and therapeutics committees, and hospital drug information centers, the authors have assisted hundreds of hospitals in developing institution-specific formulary reference documentation.

The most current basic drug and medication data from those clinical settings have been reviewed, coalesced, and cross-referenced to create this unique handbook. The handbook offers quick access to abbreviated monographs for generic drugs.

This is a great tool for physician assistants, medical records personnel, medical transcriptionists and secretaries, pharmacy technicians, and other allied health professionals.

DRUG-INDUCED NUTRIENT DEPLETION HANDBOOK
by Ross Pelton, RPh, PhD, CCN; James B. LaValle, RPh, DHM, NMD, CCN; Ernest B. Hawkins, RPh, MS; Daniel L. Krinsky, RPh, MS

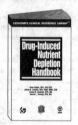

A complete and up-to-date listing of all drugs known to deplete the body of nutritional compounds.

This book is alphabetically organized and provides extensive cross-referencing to related information in the various sections of the book. Drug monographs identify the nutrients depleted and provide cross-references to the nutrient monographs for more detailed information on Effects of Depletion Symptoms, of Deficiencies, RDA, Dosage Range, and Dietary Sources. This book also contains a Studies & Abstracts section, a valuable Appendix, and Alphabetical & Pharmacological Indexes.

NATURAL THERAPEUTICS POCKET GUIDE
by James B. LaValle, RPh, DHM, NMD, CCN; Daniel L. Krinsky, RPh, MS; Ernest B. Hawkins, RPh, MS; Ross Pelton, RPh, PhD, CCN; Nancy Ashbrook Willis, BA, JD

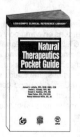

Provides condition-specific information on common uses of natural therapies. Each condition discussed includes the following: review of condition, decision tree, list of commonly recommended herbals, nutritional supplements, homeopathic remedies, lifestyle modifications, and special considerations.

Provides herbal/nutritional/nutraceutical monographs with over 10 fields including references, reported uses, dosage, pharmacology, toxicity, warnings & interactions, and cautions & contraindications.

The Appendix includes: drug-nutrient depletion, herb-drug interactions, drug-nutrient interaction, herbal medicine use in pediatrics, unsafe herbs, and reference of top herbals.

To order call toll free anywhere in the U.S.: 1-800-837-LEXI (5394)
Outside of the U.S. call: 330-650-6506 or online at www.lexi.com

Other titles offered by

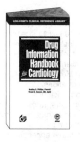
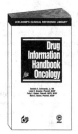
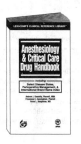

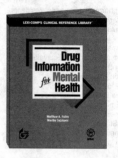
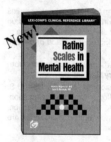
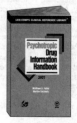

Other titles offered by

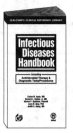
LEXI-COMP, INC

INFECTIOUS DISEASES HANDBOOK by Carlos M. Isada, MD; Bernard L. Kasten Jr., MD; Morton P. Goldman, PharmD; Larry D. Gray, PhD; and Judith A. Aberg, MD

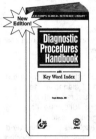

This four-in-one quick reference is concerned with the identification and treatment of infectious diseases. Each of the four sections of the book (disease syndromes, organisms, laboratory tests, and antimicrobials) contain related information and cross-referencing to one or more of the other three sections. The disease syndrome section provides the clinical presentation, differential diagnosis, diagnostic tests, and drug therapy recommended for treatment of more common infectious diseases. The organism section presents the microbiology, epidemiology, diagnosis, and treatment of each organism. The laboratory diagnosis section describes performance of specific tests and procedures. The antimicrobial therapy section presents important facts and considerations regarding each drug recommended for specific diseases of organisms. Also includes an International Brand Name Index with names from 22 different countries.

DIAGNOSTIC PROCEDURE HANDBOOK by Frank Michota, MD

A comprehensive, yet concise, quick reference source for physicians, nurses, students, medical records personnel, or anyone needing quick access to diagnostic procedure information. This handbook is an excellent source of information in the following areas: allergy, rheumatology, and infectious disease; cardiology; computed tomography; diagnostic radiology; gastroenterology; invasive radiology; magnetic resonance imaging; nephrology, urology, and hematology; neurology; nuclear medicine; pulmonary function; pulmonary medicine and critical care; ultrasound; and women's health.

LABORATORY TEST HANDBOOK & CONCISE version
by David S. Jacobs MD, FACP; Wayne R. DeMott, MD, FACP; Harold J. Grady, PhD; Rebecca T. Horvat, PhD; Douglas W. Huestis, MD; and Bernard L. Kasten Jr., MD, FACP

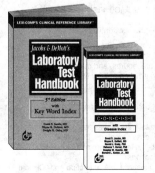

Contains over 900 clinical laboratory tests and is an excellent source of laboratory information for physicians of all specialties, nurses, laboratory professionals, students, medical personnel, or anyone who needs quick access to most routine and many of the more specialized testing procedures available in today's clinical laboratory. Including updated AMA CPT coding, each monograph contains test name, synonyms, patient care, specimen requirements, reference ranges, and interpretive information with footnotes and references. The *Laboratory Test Handbook Concise* is a portable, abridged (800 tests) version and is an ideal, quick reference for anyone requiring information concerning patient preparation, specimen collection and handling, and test result interpretation.

To order call toll free anywhere in the U.S.: 1-800-837-LEXI (5394)
Outside of the U.S. call: 330-650-6506 or online at <u>www.lexi.com</u>

Other titles offered by

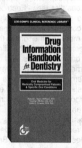
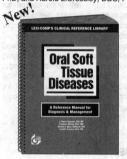
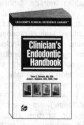

Other titles offered by

LEXI-COMP, INC

DENTAL OFFICE MEDICAL EMERGENCIES
by Timothy F. Meiller, DDS, PhD; Richard L. Wynn, BSPharm, PhD; Ann Marie McMullin, MD; Cynthia Biron, RDH, EMT, MA; and Harold L. Crossley, DDS, PhD

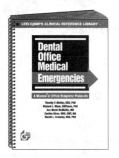

Designed specifically for general dentists during times of emergency. A tabbed paging system allows for quick access to specific crisis events. Created with urgency in mind, it is spiral bound and drilled with a hole for hanging purposes.

- Basic Action Plan for Stabilization
- Allergic / Drug Reactions
- Loss of Consciousness / Respiratory Distress / Chest Pain
- Altered Sensation / Changes in Affect
- Management of Acute Bleeding
- Office Preparedness / Procedures and Protocols
- Automated External Defibrillator (AED)
- Oxygen Delivery

POISONING & TOXICOLOGY COMPENDIUM
by Jerrold B. Leikin, MD and Frank P. Paloucek, PharmD

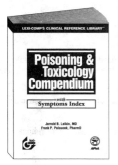

A six-in-one reference wherein each major entry contains information relative to one or more of the other sections. This compendium offers comprehensive, concisely-stated monographs covering 645 medicinal agents, 256 nonmedicinal agents, 273 biological agents, 49 herbal agents, 254 laboratory tests, 79 antidotes, and 222 pages of exceptionally useful appendix material.

A truly unique reference that presents signs and symptoms of acute overdose along with considerations for overdose treatment. Ideal reference for emergency situations.

POISONING & TOXICOLOGY HANDBOOK
by Jerrold B. Leikin, MD and Frank P. Paloucek, PharmD

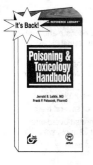

It's back by popular demand! The small size of our Poisoning & Toxicology Handbook is once again available. Better than ever, this comprehensive, portable reference contains 80 antidotes and drugs used in toxicology with 694 medicinal agents, 287 nonmedicinal agents, 291 biological agents, 57 herbal agents, and more than 200 laboratory tests. Monographs are extensively referenced and contain valuable information on overdose symptomatology and treatment considerations, as well as, admission criteria and impairment potential of select agents.

Designed for quick reference with monographs arranged alphabetically, plus a cross-referencing index. The authors have expanded current information on drugs of abuse and use of antidotes, while providing concise tables, graphics, and other pertinent toxicology text.

To order call toll free anywhere in the U.S.: 1-800-837-LEXI (5394)
Outside of the U.S. call: 330-650-6506 or online at www.lexi.com

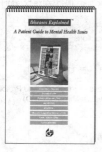
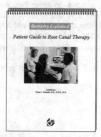
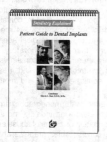

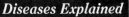
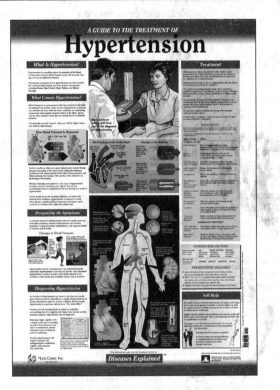

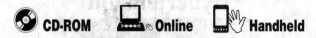